PSYCHOSOMATIC SYNDROMES
AND
SOMATIC SYMPTOMS

PSYCHOSOMATIC SYNDROMES
AND
SOMATIC SYMPTOMS

by

Robert Kellner, M.D., Ph.D.

Professor and Vice Chairman
Department of Psychiatry
The University of New Mexico
Albuquerque, New Mexico

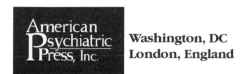

American Psychiatric Press, Inc.

Washington, DC
London, England

Copyright © 1991 American Psychiatric Press, Inc.
ALL RIGHTS RESERVED
Manufactured in the United States of America on acid-free paper.
94 93 92 91   4 3 2 1
First Edition

American Psychiatric Press, Inc.
1400 K Street, N.W., Washington, DC 20005

Library of Congress Cataloging-in-Publication Data
Kellner, Robert.
    Psychosomatic syndromes and somatic symptoms / Robert Kellner.
        p. cm.
    Includes index.
    ISBN 0-88048-110-2
    1. Somatoform disorders. 2. Somatoform disorders—Treatment. I. Title.
    [DNLM: 1. Hypochondriasis. 2. Somatoform Disorders. 3. Somatoform
    Disorders—case studies. WM 178 K295p]
    RC552.S66K45 1992
    616'.0019—dc20
    DNLM/DLC   91-4867
    for Library of Congress   CIP

British Library Cataloguing in Publication Data
A CIP record is available from the British Library.

Contents

Acknowledgments

This book was made possible in its present form only with the generous help of many people. Several colleagues read various chapters and recommended numerous changes; nonpsychiatric physicians, all experts in their field, expressed their opinion on the summarized research and on my conclusions. Dr. Denis McCarthy reviewed the chapters on dysphagia and esophageal motility disorders, non-ulcer dyspepsia, and the irritable bowel syndrome (Chapters 4, 5, and 6, respectively). Dr. Frederick Koster reviewed the chapter on chronic fatigue (Chapter 2), and Drs. Wolfgang Schmidt-Nowara and David Benahum reviewed sleep studies and rheumatological studies, respectively, in the chapter on fibromyalgia and fibrositis (Chapter 1). Dr. John Slocumb discussed with me several times research on pelvic pain, and my conclusions (see Chapter 9) stem in part from articles we published together. Drs. Laura Lane and Tina Walch reviewed the remaining chapters and pointed out errors and inconsistencies. I am, of course, entirely responsible for the views I have expressed.

Ms. Elynn Cowden's help was invaluable; she edited the manuscript and tolerated innumerable changes and revisions; Ms. Betty Bierner and Ms. Heidilisa Hunt did secretarial and library work and carried out many other tasks. In spite of my daily requests and impositions, these three crucial collaborators have remained delightful friends. Dr. Walter Winslow allowed me to take a half-time sabbatical during which most of the work on this volume was done. Finally, Dr. Diana Kellner managed to find time in her busy career to act as a sounding board and critic apart from being a supporting wife. To all these persons the book is gratefully dedicated.

An abridged version of Chapter 10 has been previously published as "Somatization: Theories and Research" in the *Journal of Nervous and Mental Disease* (178:150–160, 1990) and is reproduced with the publisher's permission.

Lest I create the unwarranted impression of scholarship in the history of medicine, I should like to acknowledge various authors from whom I have copied the following historical quotations: those by J. M. Charcot (E. D. Acheson), William James (M. Schuster), J. Hope (W. Katon), John Howship (M. Ruoff), D. H. Tuke (I. Veith), J. C. Williams (P. W. Skerrit), and Robert Whytt (H. Merskey).

Preface

This volume deals with psychobiological and psychiatric aspects of bodily symptoms. It is an extension of an earlier book that addressed predominantly hypochondriasis (Kellner 1986). The present volume explores some psychosomatic syndromes—meaning syndromes in which psychological factors may play a substantial role—and the relationship of these syndromes to somatization in general. The aim is to review the empirical literature on the nature and treatments of these disorders.

The volume is intended for general psychiatrists and psychologists who encounter many of these syndromes and for physicians who treat somatizing patients as a large part of their daily practice. For psychiatrists who work in consultation-liaison and for mental health professionals who work in behavioral medicine, I hope it will serve as a partial survey of the psychological and psychiatric research on these topics.

The topic of psychosomatics is vast; I have had to choose artificial boundaries because I could not find them in nature. I have placed emphasis on syndromes that are common, or that may be distressing—those that are only briefly discussed in the psychiatric literature that add to the understanding of somatization. Psychiatric somatoform disorders that are traditionally described in textbooks of psychiatry (e.g., conversion disorder and hypochondriasis) are discussed only to the extent that they throw light on the nature of somatization or because of recent pertinent research. I have summarized, briefly, biological research and, more extensively, studies on the role of psychological and psychiatric factors.

This volume, however, does not address the psychological aspects of physical disease in which emotions may influence the course of illness (e.g., hypertension, coronary heart disease, bronchial asthma, peptic ulcer, ulcerative colitis). These topics have been extensively discussed by others in many volumes of behavioral medicine.

The relationship between physical and mental diseases is almost as much a philosophical issue as it is a biological one. (For example, see Merskey 1986 for a learned discourse on this topic.) Whenever possible, I have tried to classify symptoms of ill health by the use of the traditional dichotomy: those caused by tissue pathology and those that belong to the realm of physiology and psychology. Many syndromes and symptoms—for example, gastric discomfort associated with hyperemia and hyperactivity of the gastric musculature (Stenbäck 1960a, 1960b)—cannot be confidently placed into one or the other of these categories, and in many other disorders, such as chronic fatigue syndrome, there is a complex interaction of psychological and physical causes. Yet, often it is important for this distinction to be made. Some psychosomatic diseases, unlike functional somatic symptoms, can be life threatening, and their etiology as well as their treatment tends to be different (Kellner 1975).

In Part I of this volume, various psychosomatic syndromes are described. In Part II an overview of processes that lead to the voicing of bodily complaints is provided. This includes a review of theories and research on somatization, and a brief description of the traditional psychiatric somatoform syndromes and their relationship to the other syndromes discussed in previous chapters. The reader who is not acquainted with current views on these topics might prefer to read Part II before turning to the individual syndromes.

In many of the syndromes I have described, pathological or physiological factors are important causes; in several, controversy persists among experts on their etiology. I have summarized the research and have tried to reach conclusions on the nature of these syndromes and the implications for treatment. In view of the complexity of the syndromes and ongoing research, many of the interpretations of the findings need to be regarded as tentative.

Throughout the text I have summarized several patient histories. Case histories are a biased source of information because of the liability of distortions by the patient and by the clinician. Even with the best intentions, one can mislead with such uncontrolled information. However, I have included them because they often portray effectively a clinical event, draw attention to an unusual case, and tend to be less dull than the information contained in tables. I have also selected mostly successful cases. Failures of treatment are common and usually less interesting; moreover, improvement or recovery indicates, perhaps, that the treatment was appropriate and contributed to the improvement, and that such treatment may be considered by the reader for future studies. In all cases, I have disguised the identity of the patients.

I have tried to give credit to the original author when quoting opinions; when several authors concurred, I have not quoted them all because this would have involved a large number of references. There may have been occasions when I expressed opinion without quoting the source, believing that it was my own conclusion; over the years I may have forgotten who first expressed a particular view and since then may have adopted it as my own. I find such an adoption of views difficult to avoid, and it has been unintentional. If my colleagues recognize an opinion that they published many years ago and do not find that I have given them credit, I beg them to regard this as a compliment and not an attempt to deprive them of the authorship.

Definitions of Terms

The terms in the psychosomatic literature resemble each other and tend to be confusing, in part because there is incomplete agreement among authors on definitions. While the disorders, nomenclature, and theories concerning somatization are discussed elsewhere, a summary of the definitions of terms as used in this volume is presented here.

Somatoform disorders— These comprise a group of disorders listed in DSM-III-R. The "essential features" of these disorders are physical symptoms in the absence of physical disease (American Psychiatric Association 1987, p. 255).

Somatization disorder— This is one of the somatoform disorders of DSM-III-R. Patients classified with somatization disorder have multiple somatic complaints (at least 13) beginning usually before the age of 30. The disorder has a chronic, fluctuating course.

Somatization— This is a term that has been used to describe a subconscious process by which a patient translates emotional distress into bodily complaints. A more recent usage—which has been adopted for this volume—is the presentation of somatic symptoms in the absence of disease or tissue damage, regardless of the diagnostic category. For other commonly used definitions and a discussion of the concept of somatization, see Chapter 10.

Functional somatic symptoms— These are the symptoms of somatizing patients as defined in the previous paragraphs. This term has been used by several authors who are quoted in this volume. The term as used herein does not imply that the symptoms serve a function for the patient.

Physiological symptoms— These are symptoms that reflect physiological changes; for example, symptoms that coincide with contractions of the smooth muscle of the intestine.

Psychophysiological processes— These are processes in which physiological changes are secondary to psychological factors. Examples include sweating or racing of the heart at times of fear or anxiety.

Psychosomatic or psychobiological— The term *psychosomatic* indicates a mind-body relationship. It comprises psychophysiological processes as well as physical diseases that may be influenced by psychological factors (e.g., bronchial asthma or peptic ulcer). Psychosomatic syndromes, or psychosomatic disorders, are physical disorders in which emotional processes play a role in some patients.

Neurosis (neurotic disorders)— Neurotic disorders are mental disorders without any demonstrable organic basis into which the patient may have considerable insight and has unimpaired reality testing in that he or she does not usually confuse his or her morbid subjective experiences and fantasies with external reality. (This definition is adopted from the International Classification of Diseases and Causes of Death, Ninth Edition [ICD-9] [World Health Organization 1977].)

Hypochondriacal concerns— These are either inordinate fears of disease or false beliefs of having a disease.

Conversion— A conversion is an alteration or loss of physical functioning without evidence of damage to tissues. Conversions usually mimic symptoms of neurological disease such as paralysis, anesthesia, or disturbance of coordination. Some authors believe that patients invariably gain by conversion.

Hysteria— This term describes several syndromes and includes conversion disorder. The various meanings of the term are discussed in Chapter 11.

Diagnostic Classification

I have used the diagnostic classifications of the Diagnostic and Statistical Manual of Mental Disorders, Third Edition, Revised (DSM-III-R) (American Psychiatric Association 1987), and the draft of the 10th Edition of the International Classification of Diseases and Causes of Death (ICD-10) (World Health Organization 1988). When two codes are listed, the first refers to the DSM-III-R and the second to the draft of the ICD-10. I did not know which should be the correct order of these two codes; I solved the conflict in the way I did because of the alphabetical order of the two titles and because of the provisional nature of the current ICD-10 classification.

References

American Psychiatric Association: Diagnostic and Statistical Manual of Mental Disorders, 3rd Edition, Revised (DSM-III-R). Washington, DC, American Psychiatric Association, 1987

Kellner R: Psychotherapy in psychosomatic disorders: a survey of controlled studies. Arch Gen Psychiatry 32:1021–1030, 1975

Kellner R: Somatization and Hypochondriasis. New York, Praeger-Greenwood, 1986

Merskey H: A variable meaning for the concept of disease. J Med Philos 11:215–232, 1986

Stenbäck A: Gastric neurosis, pre-ulcer conflict, and personality in duodenal ulcer. J Psychosom Res 4:282–296, 1960a

Stenbäck A: Hypochondria in duodenal ulcer. Adv Psychosom Med 1:307–312, 1960b

World Health Organization: Manual of the International Classification of Diseases, Injuries, and Causes of Death, 9th Revision (ICD-9). Geneva, World Health Organization, 1977

World Health Organization: Draft of the 10th Revision of the International Classification of Diseases. Geneva, World Health Organization, 1988

PART I

PSYCHOSOMATIC SYNDROMES

No man, I am satisfied, can ever be a sound Pathologist, or a judicious Practitioner, who devotes his attention to any of these systems [the mental and the organic] in preference to or [to] the exclusion of the other; through life they are perpetually acting and inseparably linked together.

J. C. Williams
*Practical Observations
on Nervous and Sympathetic
Palpitations of the Heart, as
Well on Palpitation, the
Result of Organic Disease
(1836)*

Chapter 1

Fibromyalgia, Fibrositis, and Myofascial Pain Syndrome

Disease does not change. It is we who change, learn more about disease, and perceive it differently.

J. M. Charcot *Leçons du mardi à la Salpetrière (1886)*

Muscular aches and pains are the main features of *fibromyalgia,* or *fibrositis.* A substantial proportion of patients attending rheumatology clinics suffer from this syndrome.

History of the Concept

The history of the concept of fibromyalgia has been summarized by several authors, including Ruhmann (1940), Moldofsky (1976), Goldenberg (1987), and Hadler (1986). The most comprehensive review was written by Reynolds (1983), who also surveyed the earliest history of the concept of *rheumatism,* starting in the 16th century. Rheumatism was introduced into medicine as a musculoskeletal disorder, not merely a disease of joints, by Bailloun in 1592 (Ruhmann 1940). According to Goldenberg (1987), Balfour (1824a, 1824b) described *tender points* in rheumatism. In 1841 Valleix described referred pains from various tender points that could be elicited only by pressure.

Sir William Gowers (1904) coined the term *fibrositis* and expressed the opinion that it was muscular rheumatism, or muscular fibrosis, a type of inflammation. Stockman (1904), a contemporary of Gowers, described palpable indurations and tenderness and reported inflammatory changes at these sites. Subsequently, the infection theory was abandoned because no specific histological abnormalities were found in the muscles of the patients examined.

Travell and Rinzler (1952) introduced the term *myofascial pain syndrome* and used this diagnosis to include the radiating pain occurring upon pressure to soft tissues in various locations. Smythe (1972, 1986) described a set of diagnostic criteria for fibromyalgia-fibrositis; these criteria have been only slightly modified by later authors. The term fibromyalgia is currently preferred because there is no evidence of histological changes consistent with inflammation (Yunus 1989). In this chapter, however, the terms are used synonymously, because the authors' original terms have been retained as their studies are summarized.

Symptoms and Signs

Most of the patients presenting to physicians have chronic complaints. Conventionally, the diagnosis of fibromyalgia is not made unless the condition has lasted for 3 months or longer.

The main complaints are generalized aches, pains, stiffness, and tender points at various anatomical sites. There is no evidence of other illness causing these symptoms except in cases of secondary fibromyalgia. Other commonly reported symptoms are disturbed sleep, complaints of swelling and numbness, and pain in the neck and shoulders. A characteristic sign is tenderness at specific "tender points." A recent multicentered research study used as its research diagnostic criteria point tenderness at 11 or more out of 18 specified sites in the body (Wolfe 1989). Most rheumatologists require a minimum of 8 tender points to make the diagnosis (Schumacher 1988).

Fibromyalgia can occur in various degrees of severity, and patients differ in the number and kind of associated symptoms experienced (Goldenberg 1987; Smythe 1985; Wolfe et al. 1985; Yunus et al. 1981). The prevalence of various symptoms in patients with fibromyalgia who attended a rheumatology clinic are listed in Table 1-1.

Several authors distinguish between fibromyalgia on the one hand and myofascial pain syndrome on the other (Bennett 1987; Simons 1988; Skootsky et al. 1989). In fibromyalgia, the characteristic features are multiple and widespread tender points with a sleep disorder, fatigue in the morning, and morning stiffness. In the myofascial pain syndrome, the characteristic features are trigger points; the pain is localized, and most of the systemic features of fibromyalgia are absent (Wolfe 1988).

Prevalence

The prevalence of fibromyalgia varies with the method and the site of the study. This disorder belongs among the three most commonly diagnosed disorders in the practice of rheumatology. Its prevalence in rheumatology clinics is 15% to 20%, and in a general medical clinic, 6% to 11% (Skootsky et al. 1989; Wolfe 1986, 1989). Masi and Yunus (1986) have suggested that the prevalence depends on the inclusion criteria because the disorders form a spectrum. On one end there are patients with a few tender points without symptoms of pain; with mild pain without tender points; or with mild pain and a few tender points. These patients usually do not attend clinics, nor do they seek help from physi-

Table 1-1. **Percent frequency of selected manifestations in 50 primary fibromyalgia patients and matched healthy control subjects**

Manifestations	Patients	Controls
Symptoms		
Generalized aches and pains	98	†
Tiredness	92	10**
Stiffness	84	†
Anxiety	70	18**
Sleep problem	56	12**
Bothersome headaches	44	16*
Irritable bowel symptoms	34	8*
Subjective swelling[a]	32	6*
Numbness	26	4*
Tender points		
One or more found	100	48**
Mean number	12	1.1**
Range	4–38	0–4**

†Individuals with significant aches, pains, or stiffness were excluded from the control group.
[a]Periarticular, or diffusely in the fingers.
*$P<.01$; **$P<.001$.
Source. From Yunus et al. 1981. Reprinted with permission of the author and editor, and W.B. Saunders. Copyright 1981, W.B. Saunders.

cians. On the other end is a disorder with multiple tender points and generalized fibromyalgia; this form is often associated with other psychosomatic disorders such as chronic fatigue. Patients with this disorder frequently attend rheumatology clinics. Between these two extremes there are patients with symptoms that vary in kind, severity, and course.

Etiology and Pathology

Fibromyalgia is more common in women and occurs usually between the ages of 25 and 40 (Yunus et al. 1981). The female-to-male ratio is about 5 to 1 (Wolfe 1986).

Sedimentation rate, muscle enzyme levels, rheumatoid factors, antinuclear antibody, and other laboratory results are typically normal. In addition, there is no evidence of pathology on sacroiliac radiographs. When fibromyalgia coexists with a connective tissue disorder such as rheumatoid arthritis, the disorder has been termed *secondary fibromyalgia* (Wolfe and Cathey 1983, 1984).

Dinerman et al. (1986) carried out a controlled study of 118 patients with fibromyalgia and examined the patients and healthy employee control subjects for evidence of immune disorders. They found that 30% of the fibromyalgia patients and 6% of the control subjects described a classic Raynaud's phenome-non. In about one half of the patients the Raynaud's phenomenon preceded onset of fibromyalgia, and in the others it either appeared concurrently or oc-curred after the onset of fibromyalgia. In addition, 18% of the patients had sicca symptoms (dry eyes and mouth and positive Schirmer test), and one third also had evidence of keratitis sicca. In a subsample, 11% were found to have im-munoglobulin IgG deposits in the dermal-epidermal junction. Fourteen percent had at least one positive antinuclear antibody test, and 7% of the patients had at least one lower-third component of serum complement (C3). The patients with Raynaud's phenomenon had significantly higher prevalence of sicca symptoms, positive antinuclear antibody test, or a lower-third component of serum com-plement (C3) when compared with the patients who did not have Raynaud's phenomenon. The authors concluded that a subset of patients with fibro-myal-gia may have features suggestive of a systemic connective tissue disorder. On follow-up that lasted between 1 and 3 years, none of the patients developed another physical disease such as systemic lupus erythematosus, rheumatoid ar-thritis, or scleroderma. Caro (1984) found in three quarters of patients with pri-mary fibromyalgia, deposits of immunoglobulin (IgG) at the dermal-epidermal junction on skin biopsy.

Among the findings that suggest a metabolic basis of the fibromyalgia syn-drome are low levels of free tryptophan (a precursor of serotonin [5-hydroxytryptamine]) in patients with severe fibromyalgia (Moldofsky and Warsh 1978). A low concentration of serotonin has been associated with hyper-algesia and low pain-threshold disturbance of non-REM sleep (Harvey and Lints 1965; Tenen 1967).

Moldofsky and Scarisbrick (1976) found that patients with the fibromyalgia syndrome took longer to fall asleep and slept, on the average, for a shorter time than did a nonfibromyalgia control group. Several authors have found sleep disturbance of various kinds in patients with the syndrome compared with con-trol subjects. Moldofsky and Scarisbrick (1976) demonstrated in six healthy males that increased muscle tenderness could be induced by deprivation of non-REM sleep, but not by deprivation of REM sleep. Moldofsky and Lue (1980) found during a drug trial that alpha intrusion during REM and non-REM sleep correlated with overnight increase in pain and hostility and decrease in energy, whereas the presence of delta waves during non-REM sleep was related to over-night decrease in pain, anxiety, hostility, and increased energy. The authors proposed that nonrestorative sleep is an etiological factor in this syndrome. Moldofsky and Warsh (1978) examined total tryptophan, plasma free trypto-phan, self-rated pain severity, pain threshold at tender points, and self-rated mood in eight patients with fibromyalgia. Plasma free tryptophan was nega-tively correlated to the severity of self-rated pain but was not related to the patients' self-rated mood. A small study suggests that patients with fibromyalgia may also have more sleep apnea than do control subjects (Molony et al. 1986).

Kraft et al. (1968) and Moldofsky et al. (1975) did *not* find increased muscle tension in patients with these complaints.

Moldofsky et al. (1988) studied patients with fibromyalgia that started with a febrile illness of unknown cause. They compared these patients with those patients having fibromyalgia who did not attribute the onset of symptoms to a febrile illness. Ten asymptomatic volunteers served as control subjects. The authors found that both patient groups showed an alpha electroencephalographic non-REM anomaly and had similar tender points and self-ratings of musculoskeletal pain. The authors concluded that patients with postfebrile fibromyalgia have a nonrestorative sleep disorder that is characteristic of patients with fibromyalgia syndrome, and that these patients share similar symptoms with patients who have chronic fatigue syndrome.

Gupta and Moldofsky (1986) compared sleep electroencephalographic studies of six patients with fibromyalgia and the same number of patients with dysthymic disorder. There were several significant differences between the two groups. All dysthymic subjects showed episodic (theta) bursts of high amplitude, whereas the fibromyalgia patients had more alpha activity in non-REM sleep.

Generalized fatigue occurs in a large proportion of patients with fibro-myalgia and has been regarded as one of the minor diagnostic criteria. Several authors have suggested that, at least in some patients, the etiology of the fibromyalgia syndrome is similar to that of chronic fatigue syndrome. Yunus and Masi (1986) compared female patients with primary fibromyalgia syndrome ($n = 52$) to patients with rheumatoid arthritis and healthy control subjects. The authors examined in these three groups the prevalence of other stress-related syndromes: irritable bowel syndrome, tension headaches, primary dysmenorrhea, and premenstrual tension syndrome. Irritable bowel syndrome, tension headaches, and primary dysmenorrhea were significantly more common in patients with the diagnosis of fibromyalgia than in the other two groups.

Various other pathological changes and metabolic abnormalities, including altered muscle physiology and cold reactivity, have been reported (Bennett 1989b; Caro 1989; Caro and Quismorio 1986; Moldofsky 1989; Russell et al. 1986; Sheon 1986; Yunus 1988; Yunus and Kalyan-Raman 1989; Yunus et al. 1986).

Other studies have shown increased experimental muscular fatigue (Bengtsson et al. 1986a), reduced high-energy phosphate levels in biopsy samples of trigger points (Bengtsson et al. 1986b), decreased oxygen tension in muscle near trigger points (Lund et al. 1986), and reversal of the effects of injection of a local anesthetic into trigger points by naloxone (thus suggesting a fault in the endogenous opioid system) (Fine et al. 1988). One study showed a 10-fold increase in muscle myoglobin after massage of areas of pain (Danneskiold-Samsoe et al. 1982). An eye motility derangement was found in a substantial proportion of patients, which suggests brain dysfunction (Rosenhall et al. 1987).

One study showed a positive correlation of induced flares and number of tender points in patients with fibromyalgia and dermatographia (Littlejohn et al. 1987). Another study found muscle fibers connected by a network of reticular or elastic fibers that are absent in normal muscle (Bartels and Danneskiold-Samsoe 1986).

The description of the above studies lies beyond the scope of this chapter. For a comprehensive review of the studies in fibromyalgia, the reader is referred to the proceedings of a symposium on this subject (Bennett 1986a, 1986b; Goldenberg 1986; McCain and Scudds 1988; Miller and Seifert 1987; Moldofsky 1989; Simons 1986; Wolfe 1988; Yunus 1988).[1]

Psychological and Psychiatric Studies

Several studies have compared patients having fibromyalgia with other patients using either psychological inventories or observer ratings. Ahles et al. (1984) administered the Holmes-Rahe Life Events Inventory to patients with fibromyalgia and to healthy control subjects as well as to patients with rheumatoid arthritis. Stressful life events were reported more frequently in the fibromyalgia group. Kellner and Sheffield (1973) administered a symptom questionnaire to psychiatric patients and to random employees; psychiatric patients reported more muscular aches and pains than did the control subjects (see Table 1-1).

Payne et al. (1982) administered the Minnesota Multiphasic Personality Inventory (MMPI) to patients with fibromyalgia (n = 30) and two control groups: one with rheumatoid arthritis (n = 41) and the other with arthritis from other causes (n = 30). The patients were hospitalized and admitted for diagnosis and treatment of rheumatic disease. The scales of hypochondriasis (Hs), hysteria (Hy), psychopathic deviancy (Pd), paranoia (Pa), schizophrenia (Sc), and mania (Ma) were all significantly higher in the fibromyalgia group than in the rheumatoid arthritis group. The authors concluded that the population consisted of patients having different psychological disturbances, with stiffness and musculoskleletal pain as their principal and common symptoms. Ahles et al. (1984), in the study summarized above, also administered the MMPI and the Assertiveness-Aggressiveness Inventory. The fibromyalgia group scored significantly higher than did the rheumatoid arthritis group on the Hs, Hy, Sc, and Pt (psychasthenia) scales. Compared with the healthy control subjects, the fibromyalgia patients scored higher on eight of the MMPI scales. When subgrouped according to MMPI profiles, 31 were judged to be psychologically dis-

---

[1]
  After this chapter was completed, the proceedings of a symposium on fibromyalgia were published (Bennett 1989a). Numerous articles on recent studies were presented at this symposium.

turbed, 33 had a typical chronic pain profile, and 36 were within the normal range.

Wolfe et al. (1984) compared 46 patients with primary fibromyalgia (F) whose mean duration of illness was over 10 years and who had been exposed to various treatments; 32 patients with fibromyalgia occurring in association with rheumatoid arthritis (FRA); and two groups of a total of 76 patients with rheumatoid arthritis (RA). The authors administered several psychological inventories. The MMPI scores were classified by the number of elevated neurotic scales based on comparison with previous results from chronic pain patients. The protocols were also blindly classified by two psychologists into the categories of normal, somatically concerned, and psychologically disturbed. The other scales were a self-report scale of family stress, the Family Inventory of Life Events (FILE); self-ratings of anxiety and depression from the Arthritis Impact Measurement Scales (AIMS); the Multidimensional Health Locus of Control; and a self-rated self-motivation scale. The FRA patients scored significantly higher on most MMPI scales, as well as on anxiety and depression, than did the RA patients. The FRA patients scored significantly higher than matched RA control subjects on the Hs and Si (social introversion) scales. The other MMPI classifications showed that F and FRA patients resembled each other, but differed significantly from RA patients. Clinical profiles were judged to be normal in 28% of the F patients, 25% of the FRA patients, and 51% and 60% of the patients from the two RA groups. Those patients judged as psychologically disturbed composed 37% of the F group, 31% of the FRA group, and 11% and 16% of the RA groups. There were no significant differences among the groups on the other scales.

Clark et al. (1985a) administered the Beck Depression Inventory (BDI), the Spielberger State-Trait Anxiety Inventory, and the Johns Hopkins Symptom Checklist-90–Revised (SCL-90-R) to 22 patients with fibromyalgia and 22 general medical outpatients. The fibromyalgia patients were selected from a survey: about 600 patients attending general medicine and medical subspecialty clinics completed a brief questionnaire concerning musculoskeletal symptoms and sleep disturbance. Of those who were believed to have possible fibromyalgia, 22 fulfilled the criteria for the diagnosis. None of the psychological tests revealed differences between the fibromyalgia patients and the other medical patients. The authors commented that most patients with fibromyalgia have a self-limited disease; that is, they learn to live with their pain and have not sought rheumatological care. The patients who are referred to rheumatologists probably have more severe or chronic disease, or have not responded to therapy and might be expected to have a higher incidence of psychological abnormality.

Ahles et al. (1987) administered the Zung Depression Scale to patients with fibromyalgia and to patients with rheumatoid arthritis. In both groups a substantial proportion of patients had depressive symptoms (29% and 31% of the patients, respectively, in the fibromyalgia and rheumatoid arthritis groups); there was no significant difference between the two study groups.

Hudson et al. (1985) and Goldenberg (1986) evaluated 31 fibromyalgia patients, 14 patients with rheumatoid arthritis, 24 female outpatients with depression, and 41 first-degree relatives of schizophrenic patients as control subjects. The authors administered the Diagnostic Interview Schedule (DIS). Of the fibromyalgia group, 71% had either current or past depression and 26% had anxiety disorders. Current depression was present in 26% of the fibromyalgia patients, and in over one half of these patients depression had preceded the onset of fibromyalgia. Subsequently, the authors administered the DIS to an additional 51 patients, and the results were similar. Primary affective disorders were significantly more common among relatives with fibromyalgia than among relatives with rheumatoid arthritis. Scores from the Hamilton Rating Scale for Depression were 13.1 in the fibromyalgia group and 7.3 in the rheumatoid arthritis group, showing that the fibromyalgia group rated as significantly more depressed. There was no evidence of personality disorder among the fibromyalgia patients. The authors concluded that fibromyalgia is not associated with a character disorder, that the use of the MMPI and similar psychological inventories is unsuitable to make such a judgment, and that these inventories are unsuitable to interpret pain conditions.

Kirmayer et al. (1988) compared 20 patients having fibromyalgia with 23 patients having rheumatoid arthritis who attended the clinic of a rheumatologist in Montreal. A trained lay interviewer using the DIS rated the patients, and the authors administered the Center for Epidemiologic Studies Depression Scale (CES-D) and a modified version of the SCL-90 somatization scale. There were no significant differences between the groups in rating or self-rating of depression, and there was a nonsignificant trend for a history of depression to be more common in the fibromyalgia patients. There were several significant differences between the groups, including the following: the fibromyalgia patients 1) had significantly more somatic symptoms without medical explanation in systems other than the musculoskeletal, including more pain and more headaches; 2) were more likely to view themselves as sickly; and 3) were more likely to miss time from work for medically unexplained illness.

Leichner-Hennig and Vetter (1986) administered several psychological inventories (i.e., Freiburger Personality Inventory, Giessen Test, Revised Multidimensional Pain Scale) to patients with fibromyalgia and to those with rheumatoid arthritis (N = 20). There were no differences in scores between the two groups, but the group with fibromyalgia "tended to characterize themselves as being psychosomatically disturbed" (p. 139). The measure of significant correlation between the pain scales and the personality scales was larger in the fibromyalgia group; the authors interpreted this finding as being caused by alexithymia in the fibromyalgia group.

Quimby et al. (1988) compared 43 patients with primary fibromyalgia, 23 patients with a diagnosis of "nonarticular rheumatism excluding fibromyalgia," 30 patients with rheumatoid arthritis, and 29 patients with osteoarthritis. They examined pain tolerance on tender points as well as generalized pain tolerance on control sites. The authors administered the following self-rating scales: the BDI, the State-Trait Anxiety Inventory, the Eysenck Personality Inventory (EPI), forms C and D of Cattell's 16 Personality Factor Questionnaire, and the Pennebaker Index of Limbic Languidness (PILL). The symptoms that differentiated between articular and nonarticular rheumatism were moderate to severe diffuse musculoskeletal pain, stiffness, and aching; feeling tired upon awakening; headaches (all kinds); symptoms of irritable bowel syndrome; numbness; and anxiety. Patients with nonarticular rheumatism scored higher on physicians' ratings of emotional disturbance and on the PILL scale, the State-Trait Anxiety Inventory, Cattell's emotional stability scale, and the neuroticism scale of the EPI. There were no differences on psychological scales between patients with fibromyalgia and those with other "nonarticular rheumatism." Unlike the findings by Campbell et al. (1983), there was *no* significant difference in pain tolerance at tender points and control sites.

The authors concluded that patients with fibromyalgia do not differ from other patients with generalized nonarticular rheumatism except for the presence of tender points. The presence of tender points is merely a reflection of the patient's general pressure-pain sensitivity and is not indicative of any special localized pathological phenomenon. The authors concluded that patients with nonarticular rheumatism show a high frequency of manifold disagreeable symptoms, that these patients have a general low tolerance for discomfort, that characteristic tender points do not exist, and that the causes of generalized nonarticular rheumatism are unknown.

Crook et al. (1987) compared tenderness of trigger points and control points in patients with fibromyalgia and in normal control subjects. The greatest tenderness difference between the fibromyalgia patients and the control subjects was not in the tender points but in the control points.

Comment

In the studies by Kirmayer et al. (1988) and Hudson et al. (1985), the authors rated depression in patients with fibromyalgia and rheumatoid arthritis. Fibromyalgia patients were significantly more depressed in the Hudson et al. study than in the Kirmayer et al. study. Kirmayer et al. point out that in their study a lay interviewer used the DIS, whereas in the Hudson study an experienced research psychiatrist did so, but that the comparison of the results of the two studies suggests that this was not a reason for the differences between the findings. They believe that one of the reasons for the differences may have been that their study was carried out in Canada; the patients have universal health insurance and therefore no financial disincentive to seek medical care, and patients who have fibromyalgia and no concurrent depression may seek medical treatment more readily than their United States counterparts. The fibromyalgia patients, however, had significantly more unexplained somatic symptoms and were more often diagnosed with somatization disorder. Kirmayer et al. further point out that their results "are consistent with those of other . . . studies . . . that have used the MMPI depression scale or the Zung Self-Rating Depression Scale" and "do not support the view of fibromyalgia as a form of masked or somatized depression . . ." (p. 953). The authors conclude that "fibromyalgia patients exhibit a pattern of reporting more somatic symptoms, multiple surgical procedures, and help seeking that may reflect a process of somatization rather than a discrete psychiatric disorder" (p. 950).

The studies on depression in fibromyalgia are conflicting; some studies, but not others, show substantially more depression in patients with fibromyalgia than in those with rheumatoid arthritis. The studies all show, however, that patients with fibromyalgia have decidedly more other psychopathology, as measured by various inventories, than do patients with rheumatoid arthritis or random control subjects.

There is one exception among these studies. Clark et al. (1985a) found no more psychopathology in fibromyalgic patients than in other medical patients. They studied patients with fibromyalgia who had *not* been referred to a rheumatology clinic but had attended a general medical clinic for complaints other than fibromyalgia. Clark et al. concluded that patients who attend rheumatology clinics differ from those who do not seek medical care for fibromyalgia in that they have less psychopathology. The various possible explanations for these differences are as follows: either the patients who attend rheumatology clinics have more severe pain, or the patients who are neurotic or depressed as well as having fibromyalgia are self selected, or will be selectively referred to rheumatology clinics. Patients with neuroses as well as fibromyalgia may be less capable of tolerating the symptoms of their disorder, or are more concerned about them, or both, and therefore seek treatment for fibromyalgia. There may be a third group in which fibromyalgia is caused by a stressor, meaning that it is a biological consequence of stress, a condition that was termed in the past as *psychogenic rheumatism.* This would be consistent with the view expressed by Moldofsky et al. (1988). All three relationships probably play a role to an extent that varies among patients.

Goldenberg (1989a, 1989b) has argued that most psychological and psychiatric studies with fibromyalgia have used inventories such as the MMPI that do not control for pain, and these results may be misleading. He advocates studies with fibromyalgia patients with varying levels of severity of symptoms and utilization of health care.

Leichner-Hennig and Vetter (1986) concluded that the lower number of significant correlations between personality scales and pain scales in fibromyalgia than in rheumatoid arthritis suggests evidence of alexithymia in the former.

However, this may not be an adequate explanation. First, patients with fibromyalgia complain of pain as well as of psychological distress, which does not suggest alexithymia (see Chapter 10, pp. 205–207); second, the reason for the difference may be that in patients with rheumatoid arthritis, psychopathology is proportionate to the degree of pain, as in other patients in whom physical disease causes pain (see Chapter 9, pp. 168–169). Patients with fibromyalgia (at least those who attend rheumatology clinics) tend to have more psychopathology; they may seek help in part because of psychological distress, not merely because of pain, which would result in a lower correlation between these two sets of measures.

Moldofsky et al. (1988) have suggested that the altered sleep physiology is a biological correlate to the subjective experience of light or restless, unrefreshing sleep; chronic fatigue; widespread musculoskeletal pain; and localized tenderness at specific anatomic sites. The alpha intrusion during sleep is a physiological indicator of an arousal disorder during sleep coincident with these symptoms. This sleep disorder and subsequent fibromyalgia symptoms may be induced by emotional stress or other disturbances of sleep such as involuntary leg movements or sleep apnea, and by nocturnal pain caused by inflamed joints during an acute flare of rheumatoid arthritis.

Yunus et al. (1989) concluded that primary fibromyalgia belongs to a spectrum of well-recognized stress-related syndromes. They found that other stress disorders such as tension headaches and the irritable bowel syndrome occur more often in patients with fibromyalgia than in other patients.

Diagnosis

The history is suggestive; the patient complains of musculoskeletal aching and stiffness with tender points, impaired sleep, and other associated symptoms that have been described above. Connective tissue disorders that can cause secondary fibromyalgia need to be excluded.

Wolfe et al. (1985) compared symptoms of patients having fibromyalgia with those of patients having other rheumatic diseases and healthy control subjects. Tender-point count separated patients with fibromyalgia from other patients better than historical data.

Yunus and Masi (1986) carried out a multivariate statistical analysis of patients with fibromyalgia and three control groups. They identified six historical features and seven pairs of tender points that yielded a sensitivity of 89%. The authors believe that these data will provide effective criteria for primary fibromyalgia. If emotional factors play a substantial role, the DSM-III-R classification of *psychological factors affecting physical conditions* (316.00) and the corresponding classification of the draft of ICD-10 (F54) are appropriate.

Treatments

Drug Treatments

Numerous drugs have been used in the treatment of fibromyalgia (see Miller and Seifert 1987). The most common drugs and analgesics have been aspirin and nonsteroidal anti-inflammatory drugs. Cathey et al. (1986) questioned patients with fibromyalgia and reported their treatments as follows: many patients had nonnarcotic analgesics, corticosteroids, and hypnotics; 33% had been treated with estrogen, 22% with diuretics, 18% with various medications that act on the gastrointestinal tract; 22% had vitamins and 22% had minerals; and 13% were using narcotic analgesics. Only 2.5% of the patients were without drugs.

In one study, systemic prednisone was no more effective than placebo (Clark et al. 1985b). Corticosteroids have also been used as injections into trigger areas, but there are to date no controlled studies of this treatment. Other drugs that have been used are topical application of salicylates and various analgesics such as propoxyphene, and various muscle relaxants.

Wysenbeck et al. (1985), in an uncontrolled study, judged imipramine to be largely ineffective. In a controlled study, Moldofsky and Lue (1980) found 100 mg chlorpromazine at night more effective than 5 g L-tryptophan for ameliorating pain and mood symptoms. Carette et al. (1986) compared the effects of amitriptyline, 50 mg, and placebo in a double-blind study. Twenty-seven patients completed the trial with amitriptyline and 32 with placebo. The authors used analogue scales to measure pain and sleep quality, and the tenderness was tested with a dolorimeter. Patients who were treated with amitriptyline improved significantly in morning stiffness, pain, sleep, and physician's global assessment compared with baseline scores; no such changes occurred in the placebo group. Tenderness did not improve in either group.

Goldenberg et al. (1986) compared the effects of 25 mg of amitriptyline at night, 500 mg of naproxen twice daily, a combination of amitriptyline and naproxen, and placebo in a 6-week double-blind trial. There were 19 patients in each group initially and only a few dropouts. The patients were evaluated on several visual analogue scales. The amitriptyline groups improved significantly on all outcome measures, including patient's and physician's global assessment, pain, sleep difficulties, fatigue on awakening, and rating of tender points. The combination of naproxen-amitriptyline was not significantly better than amitriptyline alone, suggesting that amitriptyline was the effective ingredient of the combination.

Bennett et al. (1988) compared cyclobenzaprine to placebo in a controlled trial of 120 patients with fibromyalgia. (In pharmacological studies cyclobenzaprine has effects similar to those of the structurally related tricyclic antidepressants, including peripheral and central anticholinergic effects and sedation.) One half of the placebo patients and only 16% of those taking the drug dropped out. Patients taking cyclobenzaprine experienced a decrease in severity of pain and a nonsignificant trend for improvement in fatigue. Morning stiffness remained unchanged. Tender point and muscle tightness also decreased significantly.

Injection of Local Anesthetics

Several studies suggest short-term efficacy of injections of local anesthetics into tender points (see Fine et al. 1988). Jaeger and Skootsky (1987) compared the effects of injection of procaine, saline, and dry needling (insertion of needle without injection) into tender points. Injection of a solution, whether saline or procaine, was significantly better in reducing referred symptoms than was dry needling. Dry needling was poor in reducing the intensity of referred symptoms, but was as effective as injection of saline and procaine in reducing local trigger-point tenderness. Reduction in local trigger-point tenderness appeared to depend only on penetration of the trigger point with a needle. The reduction in the referred symptoms was greater with injection of a solution, but there was no significant difference between procaine and saline.

Fisher et al. (1989) compared a homeopathic medicine, *Rhus toxicodendron* 6c, with placebo in a double-blind crossover trial of 30 patients. The assessment comprised the number of tender spots, a visual analogue scale of pain and sleep, and overall assessment. The comparisons were made between values at the end of active and placebo treatment. The medicine was found to be significantly more effective than placebo.

Psychotherapy, Rehabilitation, and Physical Exercise

Draspa (1959) published a controlled study of psychotherapy of patients with muscular pain. These were all patients who had attended various clinics and for whose pain no obvious physical cause had been found. The proportion that would have been classified by today's standards as suffering from fibromyalgia is not known.

Patients who had muscular pain for which no organic cause was found (n = 112) were matched with the same number of patients having the same complaint. Both groups had physical treatments, but the experimental group also had psychological treatments. Psychotherapy consisted of 1) teaching the patients first passive, then active, relaxation; 2) reassuring them that the pain was only muscular and posed no immediate danger; and 3) "giving insight into the causes of excessive muscular contraction and so promoting self-adjustment to changed internal or external environmental situations" (p. 110). In both the experimental and control groups, assessment of the degree of recovery was made by the same physician or surgeon who had made the initial diagnosis. Almost twice as many patients in the experimental as in the control group became free from pain. The mean number of attendances for the experimental group was only half that of the control group, and recovery took twice as long in the control group.

Biofeedback

Ferraccioli et al. (1987), in an uncontrolled study, treated patients who had fibromyalgia with electromyographic biofeedback. In over half of the patients a substantial improvement occurred. The improvement was largely limited to those patients who had no overt psychopathological features. In a subsequent controlled study, 6 patients were treated with true electromyographic biofeedback and 6 with false feedback in a blind study of 15 sessions twice weekly each. The patients in the control group were not instructed to learn to relax and received no signal that indicated the degree of relaxation of their muscle tension. The treated group was instructed to continue the same relaxation procedure at home twice weekly for the 6-month follow-up. The treated group showed significant improvement in tender points, clinical questionnaire, and individual analogue scales in pain and morning stiffness. In the control group only the tender points decreased significantly.

Physical Exercise

McCain (1986) and colleagues (see McCain et al. 1988) evaluated the effect of cardiovascular fitness training in patients with fibromyalgia. They decided to test the effects of exercise because of one of Moldofsky and Scarisbrick's (1976) observations: these authors had found in an experimental induction of fibromyalgia by non-REM sleep deprivation that fibromyalgic tender points could not be induced in a marathon runner. The authors hypothesized that the patient's unusual fitness prevented him from acquiring the experimental fibromyalgia syndrome.

Thirty-four patients with fibromyalgia were randomly assigned either to cardiovascular fitness training or to a program that consisted only of flexibility exercises. The patients met in supervised groups three times weekly for a 20-week observation period. The fitness group underwent gradual heart rate–elevated training using a bicycle ergometer. The patients in the cardiovascular fitness groups had significant improvements in pain as measured by a visual analogue scale, by total scores on pain threshhold on fibrositic tender points, by percentage of total body area affected as measured by self-administered pain diagrams, and by global assessment scores from both patients and physicians. Ratings on several of the scales of the SCL-90-R also improved in the cardiovascular fitness group compared with those in the control subjects.

Graff-Radford et al. (1987) described the outcome of a rehabilitation program with 25 chronic myofascial head- and neck-pain patients. The average number of previous consultations was 4.7. The program emphasized planning of self-management skills, and combined physical treatments and cognitive-behavioral therapy. There was a substantial decrease in pain and analgesics consumption, and none of the patients had sought additional treatment for the pain on a 1-year follow-up.

Several other methods of rehabilitation have been proposed by various authors, and uncontrolled studies suggest that patients benefit from these treatments. However, there are no published controlled studies on the effects of these treatments (Buckelew 1989).

Comment

Draspa's study that pioneered work in the psychotherapy of bodily complaints has some flaws and was less well designed than subsequent studies in therapeutics. Without information to the contrary, we must assume that the physician who assessed outcome knew which patient was in the experimental group and which in the control group; the methods of rating improvement were not described, nor was the duration of follow-up. This is, however, the largest study of its kind to date, and was superior in design to most other studies of psychotherapy conducted at the time. The uniformity of the results, with the findings that the duration to recovery was shorter and the number of attendances needed were fewer in the experimental group, suggests that the psychotherapeutic techniques accelerated recovery.

The controlled study with electromyographic biofeedback combined with regular relaxation suggests that the patients benefited from those treatments. The number of patients was small and would merit replication. The effects of rehabilitation programs appear promising. McCain's study suggests that aerobic exercise is an important ingredient of these programs.

Numerous other physical treatments have been used. These include massage, diathermy, ultrasound, transcutaneous electrical nerve stimulation (TENS), heat, cold, ethylchloride spray, postisometric relaxation (Lewit and Simons 1984), and acupuncture. Success has been claimed for all these treatments in uncontrolled studies. These treatments have been reviewed by McCain (1989) and Miller and Seifert (1987).

Recommended Treatments

The recommendation for treatment was summarized by Yunus (1989, p. 475) as follows:

> The management includes firm diagnosis and assurance regarding its benign nature, explanation of the probable mechanisms of pain, gradually increasing physical activity, use of simple analgesics, prescribing tricyclic agents in small doses, and occasional injections of a limited number of tender points with a local anaesthetic and a corticosteroid preparation. Successful management is facilitated by a caring and understanding doctor who gently but firmly guides the patient to assume responsibility for her own well being.

Much can be achieved by doctors who recognise the fibromyalgia syndrome as a characteristic clinical entity and treat their patients with understanding.

The author is an internationally recognized expert, and it is with reluctance that I alter his recommendations. The injection of local anesthetics and corticosteroids has had inadequate support from controlled studies to date. These treatments should be tried only after other methods have failed.

Cardiovascular fitness training should be included in a rehabilitation program. It is conceivable that psychotherapy has a greater role to play than is currently believed—at least Draspa's study would suggest so. No recommendations can be made about the kind of psychotherapeutic strategies until more is known. The methods used by Draspa should be used if formal psychotherapy is attempted. If other treatments fail, electromyographic biofeedback combined with relaxation training merits a trial.

Little is known about the effects of larger doses of tricyclic antidepressants that have been used in controlled studies in patients who have not responded to the conventional doses. It is conceivable that bolder treatment with psychotropic drugs could improve the outcome in more patients.

Exercise, psychotropic drugs, and psychotherapy each may benefit some patients with this syndrome. There are no adequate data to guide the choice of treatment for any individual. The safest and simplest treatments should be tried first.

Case History

The patient G.A. was a 33-year-old female who had been referred with incapacitating pain in her forearms. She is a professional artist who had not been painting lately because she was too busy with her household and children. Her husband is a successful architect.

The referring internist wrote as follows:

She has extreme muscle pain with movements of her arms, but no myalgia in her legs. The pain is not localized to her joints. She can attain relief if she puts her arm in a sling. She has seen two orthopedic doctors and has had multiple X-rays that were all normal, and negative bone scans. The laboratory tests done by these physicians indicate a normal ESR [erythrocyte sedimentation rate] and a normal rheumatoid factor. It is difficult to evaluate the strength of these muscles because of the pain. There is no pain with passive movement of the arms. No vesiculation nor muscle atrophy was observed. I ordered numerous tests. Dr. B. [a neurologist] found no neurologic disease. The patient's entire chemistry profile was within normal limits, and her antinuclear antibody (ANA) was negative, suggesting that an autoimmune process was not present. The EMG studies were normal. I would at least have expected her CPK [creatine phosphokinase] to be elevated if she had an endogenous muscle disease. I hope you can help this lady with her fibromyositis.

The patient revealed that the onset of pain 2 years previously was sudden but was initially mild and had become progressively worse. It "came and went," but now it was continuous, including at night. The pain was so bad that she said she could not do even the simplest chores; the arms were often painful even when she was resting.

Her mother had osteoarthritis; she had died 2 years and 3 months previously. There was no other family history of significance. G.A. was dissatisfied with her marriage because her husband had no time for the family. She resented her husband's neglect of her and her children and retaliated by refusing sex, which caused frequent quarrels.

Her mother's death caused her grief; it preceded the onset of pain by 3 months. The husband's former wife had always been in the picture and the patient described her as "a real pain." The former wife called frequently at the slightest pretense, was sarcastic and insulting, and had brought numerous legal suits against her husband asking for more child support or for other reasons. The patient believed that the former wife deliberately coached her husband's teenage children who lived with their mother to be rude and insulting. (Subsequently, in the course of psychotherapy, I told the patient that I had known teenagers who managed to be like that even without coaching.)

G.A. described the various treatments that she had received. Analgesics had not relieved the pain. One orthopedist said she had tendinitis and injected her with cortisone on five occasions. This helped, according to the patient, "a little bit." Her internist prescribed triazolam because the patient slept very little. At one time G.A. resolved she would have no more treatment. She tried to resume dancing classes and volleyball, but this made the pain worse. Before her physician prescribed triazolam, she had difficulty in falling asleep, and some nights she hardly slept at all.

On the Brief Problems List she checked as "extremely distressing" the following items: difficulties with children, loneliness, death of a family member, feeling blue, crying easily, temper outbursts that you could not control, soreness of muscles, heavy feelings in arms and legs, feeling angry, and feeling of hate.

The patient was conspicuously depressed. She said she did not enjoy any of her activities and had lost interest in sex. The forearms were somewhat more tender than other muscles, but there were no definite tender points.

I prescribed imipramine, 10 mg at night, to be gradually increased depending on her tolerance. I saw the patient a week later; she had increased the dose of imipramine to 40 mg at night and the pain in her arms was somewhat better. The patient returned after another week and said that the pain in the arms had gone. She had a few days when she felt "great." Subsequently, the pain returned intermittently, and the dose of imipramine was increased to 60 mg at night. The blood level of imipramine and desipramine combined was 67 mg.

Three months later the patient said that she was feeling "very well," had returned to dancing, was playing volleyball, and had no pain. She continued in psychotherapy for 2 years for various problems unrelated to her pain. Although she had recurrences of mild to moderate depression when there was tension and disharmony in the family, there was no recurrence of the muscle pain.

In the course of 3 years, she was weaned several times from all medications, but resumed taking tricyclic drugs or doxepin intermittently at times when she could not sleep. She had no recurrence of discomfort in her arms.

Comment

After 1 1/2 years of continuous severe pain, the patient remitted while being treated with a small dose of tricyclic antidepressants. Although the blood level of tricyclic drugs was below the usual therapeutic range, she responded rapidly. It is unlikely that this was a placebo effect, because the patient had numerous treatments from other physicians previously, including steroid injections, without remission of the incapacitating pain. It is of interest that after the patient stopped the tricyclic drugs 9 months later, the muscular pain did not return, although she had subsequent episodes of minor depression.

This patient could not be classified as having classical fibromyalgia because she did not meet the necessary criteria. The case is described here because of muscular pain in which emotional distress played apparently a substantial role; the incapaciting pain appeared to be an unusual symptom of a depression. The patient's symptoms did not appear to be a grief-related facsimile of the illness of her mother, who had died before the onset of the patient's pain (Zisook and DeVaul 1976–1977), because her mother had various joint pains, whereas the patient had muscular pains limited to the forearms. There was no evidence of reinforcement; on the contrary, the pain stopped her from dancing and playing volleyball, the two activities she enjoyed most. There appeared to be no adequate explanation for the cause and site of the pain in this patient; the old term for this syndrome was *psychogenic rheumatism*.

Prognosis

The socioeconomic impact of fibromyalgia was studied by Cathey et al. (1986), in whose studies 6.3% of fibromyalgia patients described themselves as disabled. The number of physicians visited was lower than that for rheumatoid arthritis but was no different from that of patients with osteoarthritis. The rate of hospitalization for fibromyalgia patients was higher than in patients with other musculoskeletal disorders, including osteoarthritis, rheumatoid arthritis, and lower back pain. The disability was the same as in back pain, but lower than in rheumatoid arthritis and osteoarthritis, and the number of days away from work because of illness was similar to that of lower back pain and almost double that of osteoarthritis.

Felson and Goldenberg (1986) followed up 39 treated patients with fibromyalgia; the illness had lasted on the average 1.3 years before inclusion in the study. Throughout the follow-up, more than 60% of the patients had moderate to severe continuing symptoms, and almost all took medication regularly to control symptoms. Younger patients with less severe symptoms at the initial survey and those with Raynaud's phenomenon were more likely to have improved 2 years later, although the remission was usually transitory.

According to Masi and Yunus (1986), the prognosis of fibromyalgia depends on the nature, duration, and severity of the disorder. These authors differentiate between patients who remit after one attack, those who have an intermittent course with freedom from pain between painful episodes, those with a fluctuating course but some pain between attacks, and those with a nonremitting course. Thus, any study of prognosis needs to take into account the duration of the disorder, the course so far, and the initial severity. Patients who are detected in a community survey are likely to have a better prognosis than patients attending rheumatology clinics or those with nonremitting symptoms.

Discussion

Patients who attend rheumatology clinics with fibromyalgia tend to be more emotionally distressed than patients with rheumatoid arthritis and healthy control subjects. In medical outpatients who have fibromyalgia but attend clinics for illnesses other than fibromyalgia (probably mild cases), anxiety, depression, and other neurotic symptoms are no different from those of other medical patients. Medical patients, however, have more psychopathology than do subjects in the community who are not patients (Fava et al. 1982). To my knowledge, there have been no psychological studies of fibromyalgia of individuals in the community who choose not to seek treatment.

Several of the studies in the literature suggest a physiological disturbance or anomaly in patients with fibromyalgia. The relationship of these abnormalities to the symptoms and signs, including tender points, is controversial and will require a great deal more research. One of the difficulties in evaluating the majority of the studies that showed physiological abnormalities—including most of the studies that found a non-REM sleep anomaly and studies such as those on ocular motility dysfunction and dermatographia—was that the control groups were made up of healthy control subjects. These patients' sleep architecture differs from that of patients who have dysthymic disorder, but it is not yet known how it would compare with that of patients who are anxious or depressed, or who have multiple somatic symptoms but no fibromyalgia. The study that showed that deprivation of non-REM sleep induced muscle pain requires replications. It is conceivable that the sleep anomaly is a consequence of pain rather than a cause.

It seems likely that multiple etiological factors contribute to fibromyalgia, and the etiology differs probably from one patient to another. A study by Pellegrino et al. (1989) suggests a genetic component. This study, however, requires replication using a larger sample with control groups.

The extent to which psychological factors play a part is not known with certainty. There is some evidence to suggest that psychological treatment is helpful for a substantial proportion of patients, but this does not preclude an organic etiology, because there are several examples of organic diseases (e.g., peptic ulcer) in which psychotherapy alters outcome (Chappell and Stevenson 1936; Sjödin et al. 1986).

Amitriptyline has been found to relieve symptoms of fibromyalgia, but this is not necessarily evidence for psychological causation, because the drug could have specific effects, either peripherally or indirectly, by improving the quality of non-REM sleep. Moreover, there is evidence that tricyclic antidepressants raise the pain threshold; for example, patients with rheumatoid arthritis also benefit from tricyclic antidepressants even though the etiology of this condition seems to be substantially different from that of the fibromyalgia syndrome.

Based on the research summarized in this chapter and on the views of the authors of this research, a simplified and tentative scheme can be presented as follows: various stressors can cause a stage-4 sleep anomaly and aroused and nonrestorative sleep; these stressors include some of the physical diseases, emotional trauma, depression, other psychopathology, and pain. These stressors are associated with low serotonin concentrations that in turn may decrease pain threshold and induce the formation of tender points in susceptible individuals. Other unknown endocrine biochemical or immune mechanisms may be involved. Secondary fibromyalgia may share some of the pathology of the primary disorder (see Figure 1-1).

Summary and Main Conclusions

Fibromyalgia is a complex and controversial topic. Fibromyalgia is the term currently preferred over fibrositis because there is no evidence of inflammation. The symptoms are predominantly muscular aches, pains, and stiffness, and there are tender points at various anatomical sites. In one study, there was a significant difference in pain threshold between the characteristic tender points and control points. Another study, however, failed to replicate this result; it found a generally low muscle pain threshold. In addition, there is no evidence of increased muscle tension. Some authors distinguish between fibromyalgia and the myofascial pain syndrome, both of which have somewhat different manifestations.

Fibromyalgia can be secondary to other diseases; for example, Raynaud's phenomenon is more common in patients with fibromyalgia than in control subjects, and a subgroup of patients shows evidence of a connective tissue disorder. By definition, the results of routine laboratory investigations in primary fibromyalgia are within the normal ranges, yet there are numerous findings from studies in which special techniques were used that suggest pathology, at least in some patients (e.g., a larger prevalence of immunoglobulin [Ig] at the dermal-epidermal junction).

About 6% of patients in a medical clinic and 15% to 20% of patients in a rheumatology clinic present with fibromyalgia. The prevalence depends to a large extent on the diagnostic criteria; muscle pains are less severe, and incomplete syndromes are more common.

About 6% of the patients with fibromyalgia describe themselves as disabled. The rate of hospitalization is higher than that for rheumatoid arthritis. The number of days lost from work is similar to that for lower back pain and double that of osteoarthritis.

A study of a small number of families of patients with fibromyalgia suggests a genetic component, possibly with dominant autosomal inheritance. Several studies have shown impaired sleep associated with fibromyalgia. In a study

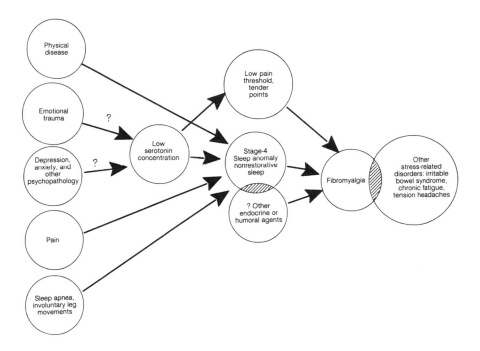

Figure 1-1. A tentative schematic presentation of current views on the pathology and psychological factors in fibromyalgia. The diagram is based on the conclusions and diagrams of authors of the studies summarized in this chapter: after Bennett 1986a, 1986b; Masi and Yunus 1986; Moldofsky and Scarisbrick 1976; Moldofsky and Warsh 1978; Moldofsky et al. 1988; Yunus 1989.

with healthy volunteers, increased muscle tenderness was induced by deprivation of non-REM sleep but not of REM sleep. The sleep architecture of patients
with fibromyalgia is similar to that of patients with chronic fatigue syndrome,
but differs from that of patients with dysthymic disorder. The findings suggest
that nonrestorative sleep may be one of the causes of fibromyalgia.

There are several psychological studies in which patients with fibromyalgia
were compared with other patients, including patients with rheumatoid arthritis
and healthy control subjects. Studies in which psychological inventories were
used and those in which psychiatric disorders were diagnosed by interviews
show that patients with fibromyalgia who attend rheumatology clinics have
more psychopathology than do other patients and control subjects. An exception is a study in which patients with fibromyalgia were compared with other
medical patients, and there was no difference in distress or psychopathology
between the two. These were patients who had symptoms of fibromyalgia but
who attended a general medical clinic and had not sought treatment for
fibromyalgia; either they may have suffered from a less severe disorder, or because of less psychopathology they may have chosen not to seek treatment for
fibromyalgia.

The findings on depression have not been uniform. Some studies show substantially more depression in patients with fibromyalgia than in other medical
patients. One study showed a higher prevalence of primary affective disorder in
relatives of patients with fibromyalgia than in relatives of patients with rheumatoid arthritis.

Although there is evidence that some patients with fibromyalgia have physiological abnormalities or tissue pathology, the extent to which this occurs is
unknown. The pathology and psychobiology of fibromyalgia are not fully understood. The current findings suggest a process as follows: various factors, including physical disease, psychopathology, and low serotonin concentration,
can cause a stage-4 sleep anomaly. This in turn decreases pain threshold and
induces the characteristic features of fibromyalgia. Other unknown biochemical
or immune mechanisms may be involved. In the more severe cases, other stress
syndromes (e.g., chronic fatigue, the irritable bowel syndrome, and headaches)
occur in conjunction with fibromyalgia, perhaps because of shared stressors or
shared psychopathology. The characteristics of many of the patients are similar
to those of somatizing patients, and similar psychological processes may be involved. The role of various etiological factors differs probably from one individual to the next.

In one study of medically unexplained muscular pains, psychotherapy combined with physiotherapy was substantially more effective than physiotherapy
alone. In a small controlled study, electromyographic biofeedback was more
effective than placebo treatment. In a further study, cardiovascular fitness training was more effective than a control treatment.

Patients with fibromyalgia have been exposed to numerous drug treatments.

Controlled drug studies to date have shown results as follows: amitriptyline in small doses was significantly more effective than both placebo and naproxen. Cyclobenzaprine was more effective than placebo. *Rhus toxicodendron,* a homeopathic remedy, was also more effective than placebo. The effects of systemic steroids did not differ from those of placebo. There are no controlled studies of corticosteroid injections into trigger points. Injections of local anesthetics are frequently being used, and there is some evidence for short-term relief, but their efficacy on follow-up has not been tested in controlled studies.

In one follow-up study, 60% of the patients still had substantial symptoms and continued to take medication. Prognosis of fibromyalgia appears to depend on the duration and severity of the disorder.

References

Ahles TA, Yunus MB, Riley SD, et al: Psychological factors associated with primary fibromyalgia syndrome. Arthritis Rheum 27:1101–1106, 1984

Ahles TA, Yunus MB, Masi AT: Is chronic pain a variant of depressive disease? The case of primary fibromyalgia syndrome. Pain 29:105–111, 1987

Balfour W: Illustrations of the efficacy of compression and percussion in the cure of rheumatism and sprains, scrofulous affections of the joints and spine, chronic pains arising from a scrofulous taint in the constitution, lameness, and loss of power in the hands from gout, paralytic debility of the extremities, general derangement of the nervous system; and in promoting digestion, with all the secretions and excretions, Part I. London Medical and Physician's Journal 51:446–462, 1824a

Balfour W: Illustrations of the efficacy of compression and percussion in the cure of rheumatism and sprains,…, Part II. London Medical and Physician's Journal 52:104–115, 200–208, 284–291, 1824b

Bartels EM, Danneskiold-Samsoe B: Histological abnormalities in muscle from patients with certain types of fibrositis. Lancet 1:755–757, 1986

Bengtsson A, Henriksson K-G, Jorfeldt L, et al: Primary fibromyalgia: a clinical and laboratory study of 55 patients. Scand J Rheumatol 15:340–347, 1986a

Bengtsson A, Henriksson K-G, Larsson J: Reduced high-energy phosphate levels in painful muscle in patients with primary fibromyalgia. Arthritis Rheum 29:817–821, 1986b

Bennett RM: Current issues concerning management of the fibrositis/fibromyalgia syndrome. Am J Med 81 (suppl 3A):15–18, 1986a

Bennett RM (ed): The Fibrositis/Fibromyalgia Syndrome: Proceedings of a Symposium (special supplement). Am J Med Vol 81, Suppl 3A, 1986b

Bennett RM: Fibromyalgia (editorial). JAMA 257:2802–2803, 1987

Bennett RM (ed): The Palm Springs Fibromyalgia Symposium. Palm Springs, CA, Annenberg Center for Health Sciences, 1989a

Bennett RM: Physical fitness and muscle metabolism in the fibromyalgia syndrome: an overview. J Rheumatol 16 (suppl 19):28–29, 1989b

Bennett RM, Gatter RA, Campbell SM, et al: A comparison of cyclobenzaprine and placebo in the management of fibrositis. Arthritis Rheum 31:1535–1542, 1988

Buckelew SP: Fibromyalgia—a rehabilitation approach: a review. Am J Phys Med Rehabil 68:37–42, 1989

Campbell SM, Clark S, Tindall EA, et al: Clinical characteristics of fibrositis, I: a "blinded," controlled study of symptoms and tender points. Arthritis Rheum 26:817–824, 1983

Carette S, McCain GA, Bell DA, et al: Evaluation of amitriptyline in primary fibrositis: a double-blind, placebo-controlled study. Arthritis Rheum 29:655–659, 1986

Caro XJ: Immunofluorescent detection of IgG at the dermal-epidermal junction in patients with primary fibrositis syndrome. Arthritis Rheum 27:1174–1179, 1984

Caro XJ: Is there an immunologic component to the fibrositis syndrome? Rheum Dis Clin North Am 15:169–186, 1989

Caro XJ, Quismorio FP: IgG subclass distribution of deposits at the dermal-epidermal junction of skin in primary fibrositis syndrome (abstract). Arthritis Rheum 29:588, 1986

Cathey MA, Wolfe F, Kleinheksel SM, et al: Socioeconomic impact of fibrositis: study of 81 patients with primary fibrositis. Am J Med 81 (suppl 3A):78–84, 1986

Chappell MN, Stevenson TI: Group psychological training in some organic conditions. Mental Hygiene 20:588–597, 1936

Charcot JM: Leçons du mardi a la Salpetrière, 2 vols (1872–1893), in Oeuvres Completes, Vol 7. Paris, 1886–1890

Clark S, Campbell SM, Forehand ME, et al: Clinical characteristics of fibrositis, II: a "blinded," controlled study using standard psychological tests. Arthritis Rheum 28:132–137, 1985a

Clark S, Tindall E, Bennett RM: A double-blind cross-over trial of prednisone versus placebo in the treatment of fibrositis. J Rheumatol 12:980–983, 1985b

Crook DJ, Tunks E, Normal G, et al: A comparative study of tenderness thresholds in trigger points and non-trigger points in normal and fibromyalgia patients. Pain, Suppl 4 (Abstr no 589, S307), 1987

Danneskiold-Samsoe B, Christiansen E, Lund B, et al: Regional muscle tension and pain ("fibrositis"): effect of massage on myoglobin in plasma. Scand J Rehabil Med 15:17–20, 1982

Dinerman H, Goldenberg DL, Felson DT: A prospective evaluation of 118 patients with the fibromyalgia syndrome: prevalence of Raynaud's phenomenon, sicca symptoms, ANA, low complement, and Ig deposition at the dermal-epidermal junction. J Rheumatol 13:368–373, 1986

Draspa LJ: Psychological factors in muscular pain. Br J Med Psychol 32:106–116, 1959

Fava GA, Pilowsky I, Pierfederici A, et al: Depressive symptoms and abnormal illness behavior in general hospital patients. Gen Hosp Psychiatry 4:171–178, 1982

Felson DT, Goldenberg DL: The natural history of fibromyalgia. Arthritis Rheum 29:1522–1526, 1986

Ferraccioli G, Ghirelli L, Scita F, et al: EMG-biofeedback training in fibromyalgia syndrome. J Rheumatol 14:820–825, 1987

Fine PG, Milano R, Hard BD: The effects of myofascial trigger point injections are naloxone reversible. Pain 32:15–20, 1988

Fisher P, Greenwood A, Huskisson EC, et al: Effect of homoeopathic treatment on fibrositis (primary fibromyalgia). Br Med J 299:365–366, 1989

Goldenberg DL: Psychologic studies in fibrositis. Am J Med 81 (suppl 3A):67–70, 1986

Goldenberg DL: Fibromyalgia syndrome: an emerging but controversial condition. JAMA 257:2782–2787, 1987

Goldenberg DL: An overview of psychologic studies in fibromyalgia. J Rheumatol 16 (suppl 19):12–14, 1989a

Goldenberg DL: Psychiatric and psychologic aspects of fibromyalgia syndrome. Rheum Dis Clin North Am 15:105–114, 1989b

Goldenberg DL, Felson DT, Dinerman H: A randomized, controlled trial of amitriptyline and naproxen in the treatment of patients with fibromyalgia. Arthritis Rheum 29:1371–1377, 1986

Gowers WR: Lumbago: its lessons and analogues. Br Med J 114:117–121, 1904

Graff-Radford SB, Reeves JL, Jaeger B: Management of head and neck pain: the effectiveness of altering perpetuating factors in myofascial pain. Headache 27:186–190, 1987

Gupta MA, Moldofsky H: Dysthymic disorder and rheumatic pain modulation disorder (fibrositis syndrome): a comparison of symptoms and sleep physiology. Can J Psychiatry 31:608–616, 1986

Hadler NM: A critical reappraisal of the fibrositis concept. Am J Med 81 (suppl 3A):26–30, 1986

Harvey JA, Lints CE: Lesions in the medial forebrain bundle: delayed effects on sensitivity to electric shock. Science 148:250–252, 1965

Hudson JI, Hudson MS, Pliner LF, et al: Fibromyalgia and major affective disorders: a controlled phenomenology and family history study. Am J Psychiatry 142:441–446, 1985

Jaeger B, Skootsky SAP: Double-blind controlled study of different myofascial trigger point injection techniques. Abstract from the International Association for the Study of Pain, Hamburg, FRG, August 1987

Kellner R, Sheffield BF: A self-rating scale of distress. Psychol Med 3:88–100, 1973

Kirmayer JL, Robbins JM, Kapusta MA: Somatization and depression in fibromyalgia syndrome. Am J Psychiatry 145:950–954, 1988

Kraft GH, Johnson EW, LaBan MM: The fibrositis syndrome. Arch Phys Med Rehabil 49:155–162, 1968

Leichner-Hennig R, Vetter GW: Relation between pain experience and psychological markers in patients with fibrositis syndrome and patients with rheumatoid arthritis. Z Rheumatol 45:139–145, 1986

Lewit K, Simons DG: Myofascial pain: relief by post-isometric relaxation. Arch Phys Med Rehabil 65:452–456, 1984

Littlejohn GO, Weinstein C, Helme RD: Increased neurogenic inflammation in fibrositis syndrome. J Rheumatol 14:1022–1025, 1987

Lund N, Bengtsson A, Thorborg P: Muscle tissue oxygen pressure in primary fibromyalgia. Scand J Rheumatol 15:165–173, 1986

Masi AT, Yunus MB: Concepts of illness in populations as applied to fibromyalgia syndromes. Am J Med 81 (suppl 3A):19–25, 1986

McCain GA: Role of physical fitness training in the fibrositis/fibromyalgia syndrome. Am J Med 81 (suppl 3A):73–77, 1986

McCain GA: Nonmedicinal treatments in primary fibromyalgia. Rheum Dis Clin North Am 15:73–90, 1989

McCain GA, Scudds RA: The concept of primary fibromyalgia (fibrositis): clinical value, relation, and significance to other chronic musculoskeletal pain syndromes. Pain 33:273–287, 1988

McCain GA, Bell DA, Francois MM, et al: A controlled study of the effects of a supervised cardiovascular fitness training program on the manifestations of primary fibromyalgia. Arthritis Rheum 31:1135–1141, 1988

Miller DR, Seifert RD: Management of fibromyalgia, a distinct rheumatologic syndrome. Clin Pharm 6:778–786, 1987

Moldofsky H: Fibrositis syndrome or psychogenic rheumatism, in Modern Trends in Psychosomatic Mcdicine, Vol 3. Edited by Hill O. London, Butterworth, 1976, pp 187–195

Moldofsky H: Sleep and fibrositis syndrome. Rheum Dis Clin North Am 15:91–103, 1989

Moldofsky H, Lue FA: The relationship of alpha and delta EEG frequencies to pain and mood in "fibrositis" patients treated with chlorpromazine and L-tryptophan. Electroencephalogr Clin Neurophysiol 50:71–80, 1980

Moldofsky H, Scarisbrick P: Induction of neurasthenic musculoskeletal pain syndrome by selective sleep state deprivation. Psychosom Med 38:35–44, 1976

Moldofsky H, Warsh JJ: Plasma tryptophan and musculoskeletal pain in non-articular rheumatism ("fibrositis syndrome"). Pain 5:65–71, 1978

Moldofsky H, Scarisbrick P, England R, et al: Musculoskeletal symptoms and non-REM sleep disturbance in patients with fibrositis syndrome and healthy subjects. Psychosom Med 37:341–351, 1975

Moldofsky H, Saskin P, Lue FA: Sleep and symptoms in fibrositis syndrome after a febrile illness. J Rheumatol 15:1701–1704, 1988

Molony RR, MacPeek DM, Schiffman PL: Sleep, sleep apnea, and the fibromyalgia syndrome. J Rheumatol 13:797–800, 1986

Payne TC, Leavitt F, Garron DC, et al: Fibrositis and psychologic disturbance. Arthritis Rheum 25:213–217, 1982

Pellegrino MJ, Waylonis GW, Sommer A: Familial occurrence of primary fibromyalgia. Arch Phys Med Rehabil 70:61–63, 1989

Quimby LG, Block SR, Gratwick GM: Fibromyalgia: generalized pain intolerance and manifold symptom reporting. J Rheumatol 15:1264–1270, 1988

Reynolds MD: The development of the concept of fibrositis. J Hist Med Allied Sci 38:5–35, 1983

Rosenhall U, Johansson G, Orndahl G: Eye motility dysfunction in chronic primary fibromyalgia with dysesthesia. Scand J Rehabil Med 19:139–145, 1987

Ruhmann W: The earliest book on rheumatism. Br J Rheumatol 2:140–162, 1940

Russell IJ, Vipraio GA, Morgan WW, et al: Is there a metabolic basis for the fibrositis syndrome? Am J Med 81 (suppl 3a):50–54, 1986

Schumacher HR Jr (ed): Fibrositis-fibromyalgia syndrome, in Primer on the Rheumatic Diseases, 9th Edition. Edited by Schumacher HR Jr. Atlanta, GA, Arthritis Foundation, 1988, pp 227–230

Sheon RP: Regional myofascial pain and the fibrositis syndrome (fibromyalgia). Compr Ther 12:42–52, 1986

Simons DG: Fibrositis/fibromyalgia: a form of myofascial trigger points? Am J Med 81 (suppl 3A):93–98, 1986

Simons DG: Myofascial pain syndromes: Where are we? Where are we going? Arch Phys Med Rehabil 69:207–212, 1988

Sjödin I, Svedlund J, Ottosson JO, et al: Controlled study of psychotherapy in chronic peptic ulcer disease. Psychosomatics 27:187–200, 1986

Skootsky SA, Jaeger B, Oye RD: Prevalence of myofascial pain in general internal medicine practice. West J Med 151:157–160, 1989

Smythe HA: Nonarticular rheumatism and the fibrositis syndrome, in Arthritis and Allied Conditions, 8th Edition. Edited by Hollander JL, McCarty DJ. Philadelphia, PA, Lea & Febiger, 1972, pp 874–884

Smythe HA: Nonarticular rheumatism and psychogenic musculoskeletal syndromes, in

Arthritis and Allied Conditions, 10th Edition. Edited by McCarty DJ. Philadelphia, PA, Lea & Febiger, 1985, pp 1083–1093

Smythe HA: Tender points: evolution of concepts of the fibrositis/fibromyalgia syndrome. Am J Med 81 (suppl 3A):2–6, 1986

Stockman R: The causes, pathology, and treatment of chronic rheumatism. Edinburgh Med J 15:107–116, 1904

Tenen SS: The effects of *p*-chlorophenylalanine, a serotonin depletor, on avoidance acquisition, pain sensitivity, and related behavior in the rat. Psychopharmacology (Berlin) 10:204–219, 1967

Travell J, Rinzler SH: The myofascial genesis of pain. Postgrad Med 11:425–434, 1952

Valleix F: Traité des Néuralgies au Affections Douloureuses des Nerfs. Paris, JB Baillière, 1841, pp 654–671

Wolfe F: The clinical syndrome of fibrositis. Am J Med 81 (suppl 3A):7–14, 1986

Wolfe F: Fibrositis, fibromyalgia, and musculoskeletal disease: the current status of the fibrositis syndrome. Arch Phys Med Rehabil 69:527–531, 1988

Wolfe F: Fibromyalgia: the clinical syndrome. Rheum Dis Clin North Am 15:1–18, 1989

Wolfe F, Cathey M: Prevalence of primary and secondary fibrositis. J Rheumatol 10:965–968, 1983

Wolfe F, Cathey M: Fibrositis (fibromyalgia) in rheumatoid arthritis. J Rheumatol 11:814–818, 1984

Wolfe F, Cathcy MA, Klcinhcnksel SM, et al: Psychological status in primary fibrositis and fibrositis associated with rheumatoid arthritis. J Rheumatol 11:500–506, 1984

Wolfe F, Hawley DJ, Cathey MA, et al: Fibrositis: symptom frequency and criteria for diagnosis. J Rheumatol 12:1159–1163, 1985

Wysenbeck AJ, Mor F, Lurie Y, et al: Imipramine for the treatment of fibrositis: a therapeutic trial. Ann Rheum Dis 44:752–753, 1985

Yunus MB: Diagnosis, etiology, and management of fibromyalgia syndrome: an update. Compr Ther 14:8–20, 1988

Yunus MB: Fibromyalgia syndrome: new research on an old malady. Br Med J 298:474–475, 1989

Yunus MB, Kalyan-Raman UP: Muscle biopsy findings in primary fibromyalgia and other forms of nonarticular rheumatism. Rheum Dis Clin North Am 15:115–134, 1989

Yunus MB, Masi AT: Association of primary fibromyalgia syndrome (PFS) with stress-related syndromes (abstracts S88, D34). 50th annual meeting of the American Rheumatism Association, Louisiana, June 3–7, 1986

Yunus MB, Masi AT, Calabro JJ, et al: Primary fibromyalgia (fibrositis): clinical study of 50 patients with matched normal controls. Semin Arthritis Rheum 11:151–171, 1981

Yunus MB, Denko CW, Masi AL: Serum ß-endorphin in primary fibromyalgia syndrome: a controlled study. J Rheumatol 13:183–186, 1986

Yunus MB, Masi AT, Aldag JC: A controlled study of primary fibromyalgia syndrome: clinical features and association with other functional syndromes. J Rheumatol 16 (suppl 19):62–71, 1989

Zisook S, DeVaul RA: Grief-related facsimile illness. Int J Psychiatry Med 7:329–336, 1976–1977

Chapter 2

Chronic Fatigue and Chronic Fatigue Syndrome

Chronic fatigue is a common symptom, the main feature of which is a pervasive feeling of being tired, and there may be several associated physical and psychiatric symptoms. Chronic fatigue *as a symptom* needs to be distinguished from the chronic fatigue *syndrome* that is described in the next paragraph.

Symptoms and Signs

Holmes et al. (1988), a working group of several experts on infectious diseases, defined a syndrome for research purposes as characterized primarily by chronic or recurrent debilitating fatigue, aggravated after exertion, that has lasted for at least 6 months. Other symptoms include sore throat, lymph node pain and tenderness, headache, myalgia, arthralgia, weakness, fever (reported by the patient), decreased memory, confusion, depression, decreased ability to concentrate on tasks, and various other complaints in the absence of abnormal signs and abnormal laboratory values. They recommended that this syndrome should be renamed the *chronic fatigue syndrome* because there was no definite evidence that the syndrome was caused by the Epstein-Barr virus (EBV). The disorder comprising these symptoms characterizes only a subgroup of patients; most patients with chronic fatigue have only some of these symptoms.

Etiology

The nature of the chronic fatigue syndrome is not known with certainty. Several authors, including Valdini (1985), Straus (1987), Holmes et al. (1988), Kennedy (1988), Komaroff et al. (1989), and White (1989), have recently reviewed research on its etiology. The relationship between chronic fatigue and myalgic encephalomyelitis has been reviewed by Byrne (1988).

Many studies have been published on the topic, and these have been listed in the above reviews. A few that illustrate the nature of the problem and are pertinent to the topic of this volume are summarized below.

31

Physiology

The relationship of tiredness and exhaustion as a consequence of physical exertion is summarized in textbooks of physiology. There also is an established relationship between sustained mental activity on the one hand and a temporary decrease in attention, concentration, and performance on the other. There are, however, substantial differences among individuals before the point of physical exhaustion is reached or before mental performance becomes impaired. For example, inactive persons and smokers report more fatigue on a treadmill test than do other persons (Hughes et al. 1984). Some of the major experiments on the physiology and psychology of fatigue are surveyed by Kennedy (1988).

In the chronic fatigue syndrome the resting cardiac function is normal, but there is a slower acceleration of the heart rate. Fatigue of the exercised muscles occurs long before peak heart rate is achieved (Montague et al. 1989). Maximum isometric strength does not differ from that of healthy control subjects, but there is some impairment in the rate of recovery (Lloyd et al. 1988). Stokes et al. (1988) tested patients who complained of excessive fatigue on a cycle ergometer for fatigability and maximal isometric contraction. The authors concluded that during the experiment the patients were neither weaker nor more fatigable than were control subjects; they further concluded that increased perception of effort is caused by a central, rather than a peripheral, mechanism.

Physical Disease

There are numerous physical diseases that cause lack of energy or fatigue, and these symptoms are also side effects of many drugs. Holmes et al. (1988) compiled a list of physical diseases that need to be excluded in patients with chronic fatigue; these include malignancy, autoimmune disease, localized infection, chronic or subacute bacterial disease (such as endocarditis or tuberculosis), fungal disease, parasitic disease, disease related to human immunodeficiency virus (HIV), chronic use of drugs, chronic inflammatory disease (such as sarcoidosis), neuromuscular disease (such as multiple sclerosis or myasthenia gravis), endocrine disease, drug dependency or abuse, side effects of a chronic medication, and other chronic pulmonary, cardiac, gastrointestinal, hepatic, renal, and hematological diseases. Apart from the specific methods used to exclude these diseases, the authors recommend serial weight measurements, serial morning and afternoon temperature measurements, and complete blood count. If any of the results from these tests are abnormal, the physician should search for other conditions that may cause such a result; only if no such conditions are detected on a reasonable evaluation are the criteria for exclusion satisfied.

The role of infections in the chronic fatigue syndrome is the most controversial and the most difficult one to evaluate. Tobi et al. (1982) reported elevated titers that they believed were evidence of an EBV infection in a group of patients with chronic fatigue, and this finding was subsequently confirmed by several other authors (Jones et al. 1985; Straus et al. 1985). Later investigators cast doubt on the value of positive EBV serologic results (Buchwald et al. 1987; Hellinger et al. 1988; Holmes et al. 1987). Elevated titers are only a part of polyclonic activation of antibody responses to various antigens, including measles and cytomegalovirus (CMV). In a group of patients with high EBV viral capsid antigen titers and chronic fatigue, Gold et al. (1990) found no evidence of active viral infection.

It lies beyond the scope of this chapter to discuss in detail the virology of chronic fatigue. There are several review papers that have dealt with the consequences of persistent viral infections and the postinfectious disease syndrome (see Bannister 1988; Southern and Oldstone 1986). Other review papers have dealt with epidemic myalgic encephalomyelitis, Iceland disease, Royal Free disease, or epidemic neuromyasthenia (Acheson 1959; Byrne 1988; Dawson 1987). Only some of the studies on the virology of chronic fatigue syndrome are discussed in this chapter.

Hellinger et al. (1988) compared 30 patients with chronic fatigue who had highly elevated titers of antibody to early antigen (a sensitive test of EBV infection) with 30 matched fatigue control subjects who were negative for this test. There was no clinical difference between these two groups. On follow-up there was no difference in outcome between the patients and the control subjects. The authors concluded that, in view of the large proportion of healthy symptom-free individuals who have measurable antibody and the lack of prognostic value, the test is not helpful in the clinical evaluation of patients with chronic fatigue. (See, also, footnote 3 on p. 45.)

Kroenke et al. (1988) evaluated patients with fatigue in two family clinics. Routine laboratory testing did not reveal unsuspected physical disease and did not help in determining the cause of the fatigue. The impairment caused by fatigue was of the same order as that of patients with major medical illness.

Other authors have found evidence for infections other than the EBV. Behan et al. (1985) found evidence that Coxsackie viruses play an important role in the postviral fatigue syndrome, and these authors believe that other viruses may cause a similar disease. They expressed the opinion that the disease is caused by a metabolic disorder that, in turn, is caused by a persistent virus infection and is associated with defective immune regulation. Jamal and Hansen (1985) studied single-fiber electromyography (SFEMG) in 40 of these patients. About 75% had abnormal results, suggesting an abnormality in the peripheral part of the motor unit, probably the muscle fiber. Other virus infections that have been found to be associated with chronic fatigue are herpes simplex viruses 1 and 2, measles virus, and human herpesvirus 6 (HHV-6) (Holmes et al. 1988), but the results are inconclusive. Archard et al. (1988) compared skeletal muscle biopsy specimen from 96 patients with postviral fatigue syndrome who had myalgic encephalomyelitis up to 20 years previously with those of healthy control subjects. The authors used enterovirus-specific probes for Coxsackie B virus (CBV) to detect virus-specific RNA. The probes were positive in 20 of the 96 patients, and the remainder were indistinguishable from the control subjects. The authors concluded that enterovirus RNA is present in skeletal muscles of some patients with postviral fatigue syndrome up to 20 years after the onset of the disease. They further suggested that a persistent virus infection has an etiological role in chronic fatigue.

Bell et al. (1988) studied CBV titers in newly admitted psychiatric patients. It was found that 12.5% of the psychiatric patients had significantly raised CBV titers, compared with 4% to 5% of the control subjects. The authors did not specify whether fatigue was a symptom in the patients with raised CBV titers.

In patients with the postviral syndrome, 50% were found to have evidence of chronic enterovirus infection and 20%, evidence of active infection with EBV (Hotchin et al. 1989). Yousef et al. (1988) investigated 76 patients with the fatigue syndrome and 30 control subjects. Postviral-positive cultures of enteroviruses were obtained from 22% of the patients and 7% of the control subjects. An enterovirus-group–specific monoclonal antibody was found in 51% of another group of patients with chronic fatigue. One year later, in the patients from the first group, the same virus was isolated again from 29%; 53% were positive for antigen in the serum. The authors concluded that chronic infection is present in many patients with the chronic fatigue syndrome. This method of detection of enterovirus antigen in the serum, however, has not been independently validated.

Numerous other abnormalities have been reported in the chronic fatigue syndrome, including functional deficiency in natural killer (NK) cells (Caligiuri et al. 1987). The "low natural killer cell syndrome" and chronic fatigue immune deficiency syndrome (CFIDS) (Aoki et al. 1987; Caligiuri et al. 1987) are characterized by fatigue, remittent fever, and lowered NK cell activity. It has not been established, however, that a deficiency of NK cells has clinical implications.[1]

In a study of patients with chronic fatigue, morning cortisone levels were lower than those in control subjects (Poteliakhoff 1981).

Central nervous system involvement may occur in a substantial proportion of patients. Bastien (1989) found several neuropsychological deficits in patients with chronic fatigue syndrome, including the following: 1) more severe impairment was evident on the performance section of the Wechsler Adult Intelligence Scale—Revised (WAIS-R) than on the verbal section; and 2) verbal mem-

---

[1] Since this chapter was written, DeFreitas et al. (1990) presented a report of immunological studies of patients with the chronic fatigue syndrome. A substantially larger proportion of patients with this syndrome showed evidence of retrovirus infection than did control subjects.

ory was 68% below the mean T score; and visual sequencing and nonverbal problem-solving ability were also substantially impaired.[2]

Seventy-one percent of the patients with CFS were found to have temporal lobe hypoperfusion on single-photon emission computed tomography (SPECT) scanning; interlobar differences were found in 25% of the patients as opposed to 4% in healthy control subjects (Mena and Villanueva-Meyer 1990).

Straus et al. (1988) reviewed the literature on chronic fatigue and allergy. The authors concluded that atopy coexists with chronic fatigue in greater than 50% of the patients. The significance of this observation has not been adequately explored.

Fatigue and Psychiatric Disorders

Beard (1880), in what was an influential book at the time, described neurasthenia as a disorder that was characterized by a large number of symptoms, and these included exhaustion, aches, excessive sweating, trembling attacks, and palpitations that had a variable and fleeting character. Since then, studies have shown a consistent association between fatigue or lack of energy and psychiatric disorders. For example, Chen (1986) found that self-reported depression, anxiety, and emotional stress were highly associated with fatigue. Students who reported uncommon tiredness in a questionnaire study rated themselves as significantly more depressed and anxious than did other students, and described themselves as more time-pressured by problems and as more competitive (Montgomery 1983). Between 78% and 86% of neurotic psychiatric patients affirmed the symptom "feeling tired and lacking in energy" in two studies; this proportion was significantly higher than that found in random employees (Kellner and Sheffield 1973).

There are numerous reports on the coexistence of fatigue and depression. Fatigue can range from a lack of zest to severe psychomotor retardation or even depressive stupor. Conversely, in the hypomanic and manic phase of a bipolar disorder, the previously lethargic patients may have episodes of sustained mental activity and striking physical energy that persist in spite of excessive exertion. These observations show that a mood disorder can cause a feeling of fatigue and lassitude on the one hand and energy and mental and physical stamina on the other.

There are also numerous studies in the literature on *neurasthenic neurosis,* a disorder in which fatigue is the prominent symptom. Most of the studies with this syndrome, however, were carried out before the current specific tests for

---

2
  A recent study failed to confirm cognitive impairment in chronic fatigue. On the contrary, on all tests but one, subjects' performances were rated significantly higher than those in the normative data (Altay et al. 1990).

viral infections were available, so some of the patients may have suffered from the consequences of viral infections.

Some textbooks and diagnostic classifications describe the category of neurasthenic neurosis, or neurasthenic reactions (Slater and Roth 1969). The draft of the ICD-10 (World Health Organization 1988) has retained the concept of neurasthenia (chronic fatigue); it describes fatigue, weakness, and exhaustion after minimal effort with accompanying symptoms of reduced interest, irritability, insomnia, hypersomnia, poor concentration, and various physical symptoms. Chatel and Peele (1970) and White (1989) have reviewed the concept and studies of neurasthenia.

Verhaest and Pierloot (1980) carried out a hierarchical cluster analysis from the responses to a questionnaire from 183 psychiatric outpatients. The study revealed a cluster of somatic complaints that was, in part, distinct from anxiety and depressed mood and included fatigue as one of the symptoms. The cluster was similar to the neurasthenic syndrome of various other authors.

Manu et al. (1988) examined psychiatric diagnoses in 100 patients who complained of chronic fatigue. In five patients a physical disease was subsequently diagnosed, which probably accounted at least in part for the fatigue. Sixty-six percent of the patients had psychiatric diagnoses that were judged to be a major cause of their chronic fatigue; of these, over one third had major depression, 15% had a somatization disorder, and the remaining patients had various other psychiatric disorders, including anxiety disorders. In a subsequent study, Manu et al. (1989) found that 15% of the patients with chronic fatigue had somatization disorder. Gold et al. (1990) found that in patients with chronic fatigue syndrome, 50% had a history of one or more episodes of depression before the onset of chronic fatigue. Kruesi et al. (1989) also reported a high prevalence of psychiatric illness in patients with the chronic fatigue syndrome, and, in several patients, psychiatric disorders appeared to precede fatigue rather than follow it. Most patients believed that the cause of their symptom was medical and cited viral infections or hormonal imbalance as the reasons for their symptoms; one quarter believed that their symptoms were of psychological origin (Manu et al. 1989).

There are several studies that suggest that stress, particularly loneliness, can have effects on decreased immune competency (Glaser et al. 1985; Kiecolt-Glaser et al. 1984a, 1984b; Locke et al. 1981). In most studies, the effects of feeling lonely on the one hand and lack of social integration on the other have not been separately evaluated (Kellner, in press). Some of the findings of decreased immune competency in the chronic fatigue syndrome could be explained, at least in part, by psychosocial stress; incapacitating fatigue is a stressor in itself that could contribute to a vicious cycle of stress, decreased immune competency, and chronic fatigue.

Diagnosis

Because in most cases the exact etiology is often unknown, psychiatric classification of the chronic fatigue syndrome is not feasible. For the DSM-III-R classification (American Psychiatric Association 1987), fatigue is one of the symptom complexes characteristic of an *undifferentiated somatoform disorder* (300.70) provided that "appropriate evaluation uncovers no organic pathology" (p. 267). The failure to uncover organic pathology by routine laboratory investigation does not guarantee, of course, that the syndrome is not caused by the complications of a viral infection. This is one of the situations in which accurate communication is more important than choosing the appropriate code. If the syndrome is clearly secondary to a viral infection and the patient also has psychiatric symptoms, the classification on Axis I is "psychological factors affecting condition" (316.00 in DSM-III-R; F54 in ICD-10), and the physical disease is listed on Axis III. In the remaining, and probably the majority, of cases, the diagnosis should be chronic fatigue syndrome (316.00 or 300.70 in DSM-III-R); on Axis III the description should be "exact cause uncertain." The corresponding ICD-10 diagnosis is neurasthenia (chronic fatigue, F48.0) with a similar qualifying statement.

For clinical work, the type of investigations and their limits depend in part on the physician's belief of the nature of the disorder and his or her temperament and philosophy. For research purposes, the history, clinical examination, and laboratory investigations suggested by Holmes and his fellow experts (1988), as summarized above (see pp. 31–32), should be carried out.

Treatment

Treatment should depend, of course, on the cause; however, in many cases the cause is unknown. Even if one of the etiological factors, such as an immune response to a viral infection, has been identified, the extent to which other factors contribute to the symptoms is usually unknown.

There are no controlled studies to date that demonstrate the efficacy of antiviral drugs. Such treatment is controversial at present. Straus et al. (1988) evaluated the effects of acyclovir in a placebo-controlled study. There were no significant differences between the effects of acyclovir and placebo on fatigue. Neither acyclovir nor clinical improvement correlated with alterations of laboratory findings such as antibody to EBV or levels of circulating immune complexes. Self-ratings of anxiety, depression, and confusion as measured by the Profile of Mood States (POMS) were less on placebo. Fatigue was negatively correlated with improved mood.

In an uncontrolled study, Wessely et al. (in press) treated patients with severe and chronic fatigue (average duration 4 1/2 years) with a combination of treatments. Because this study describes the largest group of patients with the chronic fatigue syndrome treated by psychiatric and psychological methods to date, and because it contains a detailed description of treatment of this syndrome and the promising outcome, we summarize its findings as follows.

The authors discuss their model of the chronic fatigue syndrome. They view it as a combination of infective physical, behavioral, and psychological factors. In many patients there is an infective trigger with associated fatigue, myalgia, and inactivity that begins a cycle in which attributive and cognitive factors induce avoidant behavior, which itself sustains symptoms. The authors place these interactions within a psychosocial framework and address each component during treatment.

The first phase is a detailed assessment that includes a search for a coexistent depression to learn exactly what the patient thinks about the problem, the extent of the impairment, and the reasons for the restricted life. The second phase is the engagement and offer of treatment. According to the authors, "No treatment can proceed until this hurdle is overcome," because many patients are hostile to a psychological approach. The third phase is the treatment of coexisting depression, if necessary, with antidepressant drugs. Cognitive therapy consists of encouraging the patient to see the full range of etiological factors, not merely the physical ones, and the therapist avoids the body-mind dichotomy. Therapy involves more explanation and education than during conventional cognitive therapy. The patient is encouraged to increase gradually the amount of physical activity with realistic goals. Once increased activity has been accomplished, the patient gains a perception of control over symptoms. The authors adopt the approach to exercise that has been found beneficial in the treatment of fibromyalgia (see Chapter 1, this volume).

Of the 32 patients who agreed to participate in the treatment, 6 did not walk and were either confined to bed or in wheelchairs. These patients were treated for 2 months as inpatients, and the remainder were treated as outpatients.

Five patients dropped out of treatment; of these, one reported that he felt better. Of the remaining 27 patients, 16 rated themselves as "very much better," 6 as "better," 4 as the "same," and 1 as "much worse." At the time of publication, the patients had been followed up for 3 months; one of the patients who had improved at the end of the treatment had relapsed.

Comment

The magnitude of the specific effects of treatment, if any, cannot be asssessed without comparison with changes in an untreated control group or a group treated by other methods. Spontaneous recovery cannot be ruled out in an uncontrolled study. This seems an unlikely explanation for the improvement in this study because of the severity and chronicity of the disorder and because improvement coincided with psychiatric treatment. However, the follow-up was short, and the long-term outcome will be of interest.

Recommended Treatments

There are no agreed upon treatments for the chronic fatigue syndrome and no controlled studies that demonstrate the efficacy of antiviral drugs or of any other treatments. The choice of treatments, including the recommendations that follow, depend on the author's bias, so the recommendations herein should be regarded only as guidelines. The same treatment is apparently not equally suited for all patients, because there are large differences in outcome among patients with the same treatment.

The decision of whether to use antiviral drugs is not one the psychiatrist or psychologist is called upon to make. If the presence of treatable physical disease has been excluded, physical rehabilitation and the treatment of emotional, cognitive, and behavioral components of the disorder are all that can be done for the patient.

Because there are no controlled studies of psychotherapy in chronic fatigue, the methods described here are based on psychotherapeutic strategies of somatization in general, which, in turn, are based on controlled studies with somatizing patients, on Wessely et al.'s study (see above), and on my experience of individual psychotherapy with fatigued patients.

The patient may have to be persuaded to choose such a course rather than to continue to pursue endless laboratory investigations and to attend for more physical treatments. Numerous patients will cancel the initial appointment with the psychiatrist, some will drop out early in treatment, and others will persist in asking for additional laboratory investigations. They are usually knowledgeable about the syndrome and have read reports of patients with chronic fatigue who were successfully treated after the organic disease causing the syndrome was discovered and appropriate treatment instituted. The patient should not be told that the cause is psychological; the therapist ought to be frank about the doubts and the existing controversies. He or she should emphasize that the likelihood of a dangerous or even treatable physical disease is small after the thorough investigations the patient has completed. The therapist should further explain that the aim of treatment is rehabilitation and treatment of several of the concomitants of the syndrome. This approach merits a trial regardless of the cause. An analogy may be presented of a fit sportsman whose muscle has become weak after prolonged immobilization necessitated by a severe injury. After the patient understands the aims of the treatment, coexisting psychiatric disorders such as depression or anxiety should be energetically treated by appropriate methods.

Psychotherapy consists of support, guidance about ways to cope with the disability, and guidance about changing a life-style that is often devoid of pleasure. Psychotherapy should include treatment of depression and neurotic attitudes that perpetuate distress.

The value of exercise in the chronic fatigue syndrome has not been tested in a controlled study. The study by Wessely et al. included gradual increase in physical activity, and the treatment seemed to be successful. There is evidence for antidepressant effects of exercise in depression (Kellner 1988; Lobstein et al. 1983) as well as other nonpsychotic mental disorders (Martinsen 1989). Physical exercise is apparently of value in the treatment of neurocirculatory asthenia (Shoenfeld et al. 1978) and fibromyalgia (see Chapter 1, this volume), and symptoms of somatic anxiety are fewer in subjects who exercise regularly (Schwartz et al. 1978). Because fatigue is more common in people who are physically inactive (Chen 1986; Farmer et al. 1988; Hughes et al. 1984), it is worthwhile to try to persuade the patient to gradually increase the amount of physical activity with definite realistic targets and monitoring of progress. Apart from the various physical benefits that aerobic exercise entails (Phelps 1987), it may help to relieve depression, increase physical fitness, and perhaps reduce the sensation of fatigue.

If the patient is convinced that his or her illness has a serious physical cause in spite of thorough investigations, is demanding more tests, and is seeking the opinion of more experts in infectious diseases, the therapist may need to wait until the patient completes one more round of investigations. Then methods of persuasion need to be tried similar to those described in Chapter 10 (p. 216). The management of disease conviction in the presence of physical disease, or when doubts exist in the therapist's mind, often poses special problems. The physician must combine truthfulness, reasonable precautions, and education with reassurance, yet must avoid denying the possibility of a physical component in the syndrome (Kellner 1986, pp. 256–257). The patient will need to be convinced that it is possible to feel extremely exhausted even while being physically healthy.

Some patients no longer feel tired after treatment of the psychiatric disorder with psychotropic drugs. In depressed patients, tricyclic antidepressants, which can be extremely sedating in some patients, will diminish fatigue and tiredness when the depression is successfully treated. Even drugs that are central nervous system depressants, such as diazepam, can increase self-rated vigor when anxiety and the associated depression are effectively treated (Uhlenhuth et al. 1977).

Case Histories

In the two case histories that follow, the symptoms were similar, but apparently the etiology and course were different. In the first patient, it seems that a viral infection coincided with the onset of severe fatigue.

Case History 1

J.B., a 27-year-old sales manager for a large and prestigious corporation, was unusually successful. He won sales prizes and was awarded unusually large bonuses because of his achievements, until 2 years before his first attendance, when he began to feel exhausted. The patient was a biology graduate who was highly intelligent and had acquired an expert knowledge on research on chronic fatigue. His fatigue had begun after a febrile episode associated with liver tenderness. The fatigue was incapacitating; he slept up to 15 hours a day and felt exhausted for the remainder. He also had a feeling of weakness, dizziness, disorientation, blurred vision, a feeling of pressure in his head, an impairment of memory, mild headaches, and nausea.

There was a disagreement among two expert virologists on the presence of antibody HHV-6. One immunologist interpreted his laboratory studies as abnormal, showing evidence of infection, but another did not agree with this interpretation. The T4/T8 ratio was 0.9, with T4 helper cell deficiency. The patient had low immunoglobulin (IgG) subclass 3 and 4 and low B cell numbers. He was treated with intravenous acyclovir, and, after treatment, the T4/T8 ratio rose to 1.9. There was disagreement by two radiologists on the interpretation of magnetic resonance imaging, which, according to one report, showed small demyelinated foci.

Neuropsychological testing showed a verbal IQ of 129 (superior) and a performance IQ of 91 (average), suggesting a deterioration from a premorbid IQ. Several of the performance tests were in the mildly impaired range, and memory tests indicated mildly impaired, delayed verbal memory.

The patient was conspicuously depressed and attributed his depression to the way he felt physically. He said that on days when he felt physically well, he was in a good mood.

J.B. agreed to try treatment of his depression with drugs. He had been previously treated with doxepin, 50 mg daily, which did not relieve his depression; when the dose was increased to 100 mg daily it made him even more tired. I tried slowly increasing doses of several tricyclic antidepressants. All were tried until a dose failed to relieve his symptoms, yet caused unpleasant side effects. While taking tricyclic antidepressants he slept fewer hours, but the agents had no appreciable effect on mood, nor on the feeling of fatigue. The effects of fluoxetine were similar, and lithium was ineffective. The patient did not want to try monoamine oxidase inhibitors.

I treated the patient in part with insight-oriented and cognitive therapy, but he did not appear to benefit. He said he could not increase the amount of physical activity even in small increments, an approach that I had recommended.

There appeared to be some improvement after treatment with acyclovir and gamma globulin, but the symptoms were still incapacitating. After several months of treatment the patient returned to work part-time, but he found it an ordeal because of the overwhelming tiredness.

After 3 years he recovered; for the past 6 months he has had no symptoms of fatigue and has regained his previous ability to work long hours. He is now able to concentrate and is optimistic about the future.

Case History 2

R.S. was a 30-year-old law student. He was older than his fellow students because he had served as an officer in the military and had had a successful sales
job for 4 years before he resumed his studies. He was referred because of unexplained severe fatigue. The family physician was psychologically minded and
believed that the patient was physically healthy. By today's standards the patient had had only minimal and inadequate investigations to exclude a physical
disease. The patient's only complaint was exhaustion. He was tired when he got
up in the morning, and the tiredness became worse during the day. He said he
was so tired that it was an effort to climb even a few stairs. He attempted to study
until midnight every evening and about 12 to 14 hours on weekends. After
opening his books to study he usually felt overwhelmed by exhaustion and
often fell asleep with his head on the table, only to wake up several hours later.
The patient was convinced that there was a physical cause for his tiredness that
his physician had missed, and he was reluctant to accept a psychological explanation. During the first two sessions the patient talked only about his bodily
complaints, but with encouragement he began to discuss other problems during the next three sessions.

He revealed that his life had changed substantially. His war service was ardu-
ous but exciting. After leaving the army, he got a job as a salesman for a firm that
manufactured expensive road-building machinery, and he was paid on com-
mission. He traveled a great deal; it was a time when this equipment was selling
well and he was prosperous. He enjoyed his life, spent freely, and had several
girlfriends in various cities. He decided eventually to apply for law school because it had been an early ambition and he said that he did not want to sell
machines for the rest of his days.

Starting in law school was a formidable change. The other students were
substantially younger than he was, and he found them immature, so he had not
made any friends. He found studying difficult, took very little time off, and studied excessive hours to compensate for what he believed was a poor memory
and poor concentration. His savings were adequate for living expenses only.
Instead of eating in expensive restaurants as he had been used to, he made
himself sandwiches for lunch and cooked frugal suppers. When he was
wealthy, he had had no difficulty in befriending attractive women he had met in
expensive bars, whereas now "none [of the beautiful young women] were interested in a broke law student who was getting on in years." He had parted some
time ago with a woman friend, which he now regretted.

Initially, I believed that the patient had a physical illness and that the referral
to a psychiatrist had been premature, but after I learned the history, I suspected
that these changes in his life, the excessive hours he worked, and the lack of
leisure and pleasurable activities had caused a depression. At this stage I asked
him to enumerate in detail his daily activities during the past week. He de-

scribed his difficulties again, but he also described a Saturday that was unusual. He chose to play rugby with his friends, which he had not done for a long time. He said that his muscles were so sore for 3 days afterward that he believed that he had polio, which was still a common and dreadful disease at that time. After the game the team went for a meal and for drinks in a pub and then went to a party. At the party he danced most of the time, spoke to several girls, made a date, and finally went to bed after 3:00 A.M. When I asked him about tiredness, he replied that at no time during that day did he feel tired. The next day his exhaustion returned and was undiminished. At this point I told him that his endurance on that Saturday made it most unlikely that his tiredness was caused by a physical disease; it was far more likely to be caused by a depression that temporarily lifted when his life became pleasant and exciting. I also told him that excessive hours of work and lack of pleasure were adequate to explain his feeling of exhaustion.

During that session the patient talked more about his feelings. He felt so lonely that he was often near tears; he missed his girlfriend, and he accused himself of having made a "stupid mistake" of having parted with her. She had left town and found another man friend, and when he tried to renew their affair, she wrote to him that she did not love him anymore.

At times he regretted that he had left his well-paying job and joyful life for what he called "endless drudgery." He had doubts whether he would enjoy working as a lawyer.

After this session, the patient had become more open and talked freely about his frustrations. After 7 weeks he had made several changes. He spoke to his former boss, who offered him a summer job as a salesman during his vacation. This relieved his worry about money because he had spent too much of his savings. He had a date with the girl he had met recently, and they agreed to meet more frequently. He decided that he would study less and would set aside certain times of the week for pleasurable activities other than studying. He had previously told me that he disliked studying. His practice had been of setting himself goals of a large number of pages each day, which would eventually allow time for several revisions, but these goals proved to be overambitious and impossible to achieve. I advised him that instead of his current practice, he should set aside a certain time for studying without a set plan unless he was reviewing a large amount of material just prior to an examination. He should read the parts that interested him most at the time rather than trying to memorize a large number of details of laws and regulations at a set rate. He adopted this method and told me that it had made a big difference; now he was often looking forward to reading instead of dreading the seemingly insurmountable tasks of memorizing material read at a great speed.

The treatment lasted for two more weekly sessions, and I saw the patient on two follow-up sessions 2 and 4 months later. He had resumed playing squash regularly, which he enjoyed. He was dating and looking forward to the future, and he told me that sometimes after an evening out or after returning from the movies, he would look up with keen interest some points of law that had passed through his mind. Some nights he had to discipline himself to go to bed in order to get enough sleep. He now felt he had regained his former energy and zest.

Comment

The first patient had a viral infection with some evidence of laboratory abnormalities. Psychiatric treatment was ineffective. In the second case, fatigue was apparently caused by psychological factors. Improvement coincided with his attendance for psychotherapy and with the major changes he had made in his life.

Prognosis

The prognosis of the chronic fatigue syndrome apparently differs widely from one individual to the next and differs with the site of the study. There are numerous patients who have episodes of fatigue of various durations while convalescing from a physical illness, particularly after viral infections (Morrison 1980). In some patients, the disorder is chronic and lasts for many years. In a study of fatigue conducted in a medical outpatient clinic, the mean duration at the time of the first attendance was 13 years (Manu et al. 1988). About 60% of the patients in a general medical practice who could be followed up by a telephone interview were still fatigued (Valdini et al. 1988). In a family practice clinic, 72% had not improved after 1 year. The Sickness Impact Profile was similar to that reported for patients with a major medical illness (Kroenke et al. 1988). In Wessely et al.'s (in press) study of patients with a severe chronic fatigue syndrome (see pp. 37–38 of this chapter), 72% of those who agreed to undergo psychiatric treatment improved, and the improvement was largely maintained on a brief follow-up. A follow-up from an internal medicine outpatient clinic showed persistence of psychiatric diagnoses in most patients (Manu et al. 1988).

Discussion

Dawson (1987), in summarizing a report of the Myalgic Encephalitis Study Group, concluded that "there is no definite answer as to what causes this perplexing syndrome, but further controlled trials and applications of gene probes and monoclonal antibodies may provide one" (p. 328). Reporting on a meeting on the postviral fatigue syndrome, Dawson (1988) further concluded that "the advances achieved with the up to date methods will disappoint anyone looking for a cut and dried differential diagnosis or a realisation of Koch's postulates" (p. 1151).

There is evidence to suggest that people who are psychologically vulnerable have a tendency to overreport symptoms of an illness. Studies by Imboden et al. (1961) and Cluff et al. (1966), in which psychological test scores were available for a group of people before an influenza epidemic, showed that subjects with neurotic traits were more likely to report infections. (See Chapter 10, pp. 207–208, of this volume for a discussion of the interplay of neurotic traits and physical symptoms.)

David et al. (1988) discussed the concept of the postviral fatigue syndrome and its virology, immunology, neurophysiology, and histopathology. The authors listed studies to show that the postviral fatigue syndrome is frequently accompanied by psychological disturbances, predominantly depression and anxiety. They also noted that several studies suggest that viral and immunological changes are found in some patients with chronic fatigue. Kennedy (1988) and White (1989) surveyed studies on fatigue and fatigability that include epidemiology, physiology, and pathology. The reviews indicated that fatigue can be a symptom of abnormal psychological states and psychiatric disorders. Persistent viral infections are apparently rare. In some patients, a syndrome persists beyond the stage of infection, and this may be an immunological complication of viral infections (Straus 1988).[3]

Studies of symptoms of psychiatric patients suggest that some patients with chronic fatigue are depressed or neurotic, although the proportion that have no immunological contributing factor has not been determined with certainty. The patient may explain that his or her psychological distress is caused by fatigue and incapacity. In these patients, the symptoms, as well as the patient's belief in the nature of the disorder, are liable to act as links in a hypochondriacal reaction (see pp. 199–200, this volume).

I have interviewed several patients in whom, apparently, reinforcement by physicians contributed to the belief that they were suffering from a physical disease. In one instance, a physician found a laboratory abnormality such as evidence of EBV infection, and the patient was told that it was the cause of the fatigue; this was subsequently disputed by an expert in infectious diseases. Patients may belong to one of the support organizations such as the Chronic Fatigue Syndrome Society or the Chronic Fatigue and Immune Syndrome Association and frequently receive medical information about recent research; some of this research is difficult to interpret for experts and so must be confusing for

---

3

  White et al. (personal communication, 1991) carried out a prospective study of 249 patients with recent infectious illness, with the largest group having had EBV infections. The prevalence of a fatigue syndrome at 2 months was 39%, with a median duration of 9 weeks. The prevalence decreased to 10% after 6 months. The independent variables were physical, virological, immunological, and psychological. These associations changed with the passage of time; close to the onset of infection, the associations were mainly physical, and after 6 months they were a mixture of physical and psychological.

lay people. If patients attend a support group, their beliefs may be reinforced by the other members who hold similar beliefs. Patients who are fatigued because of a psychiatric disorder such as depression may become trapped by their conviction of having a physical disease and the resulting search for a physical cure, and they may not get appropriate treatment for their psychiatric illness. In patients who do have persistent infections or an immunological complication that causes fatigue, the physical symptoms tend to interact with the processes of somatization (see Chapter 10, p. 207, of this volume).

David et al. (1988) concluded that the dichotomy of organic versus functional is fruitless and should be replaced by a "multi-factorial approach." In his survey of chronic fatigue, Kennedy (1988) commented that there is no reliable method of distinguishing between psychological and physiological aspects of fatigue and that perhaps the distinction remains artificial. Similarly, Komaroff et al. (1989) recommended that "with the chronic fatigue syndrome, as with other illnesses, it may be more productive to avoid the kind of mind-body dualism that has characterized much of past thinking about the pathogenesis of illness" (p. 407).

Research clearly shows that chronic fatigue can be caused by concurrent disease; in other individuals, it appears to be caused by an immunological response to a previous viral infection that can be difficult to detect. If detected, the extent to which this infection contributes to chronic fatigue in a particular patient remains uncertain. Some authors who found biochemical abnormalities in muscles did not control for the effects of muscle disuse (White 1989).

Some patients have a viral infection that causes the inception of the syndrome. Postviral lassitude induces these patients to avoid physical activity (D. Goldberg, personal communication, 1991), and the excessive tiredness is eventually caused, in part, by inactivity and lack of fitness and, in part, by the psychological stresses of being disabled.

There is evidence that stress and psychiatric disorders make individuals more susceptible to some infections (Kellner, in press). In some patients, physical and psychological causes coexist and interact. Although the distinction is often difficult and sometimes impossible to make, it is desirable for the treating physician to distinguish between fatigue caused by a postviral immunological process with coexisting psychiatric ill health, and fatigue that is a symptom of a psychiatric disorder, because the choice of treatments should depend on the diagnosis. In many cases, the psychiatrist will need to proceed with treatment in spite of the uncertainty.

Summary and Main Conclusions

The chronic fatigue syndrome has several characteristic features that include chronic or recurrent debilitating fatigue aggravated after exertion. This syndrome needs to be distinguished from chronic fatigue as a symptom.

Fatigue, tiredness, and lack of energy are common symptoms. The prevalence of chronic fatigue syndrome varies with the method of study. In a questionnaire study in the general population, 14% of males and 24% of females responded and reported that they felt fatigued "some of the time." In another questionnaire study in random employees, the question "Have you felt tired or lacking in energy during the past week?" was affirmed by over 40% of the employees. The symptom of fatigue is unrelated to age. Although it is more common in people who are physically inactive, the cause of this association is unknown. Experimental studies with fatigued individuals show that in some there is an impairment in the rate of recovery after muscular exertion and that these patients appear to have an increased perception of effort. Three quarters of patients with chronic fatigue believe that there is a physical cause for their symptoms.

A few patients with chronic fatigue have physical diseases that are diagnosed by routine medical diagnostic procedures. The *chronic fatigue syndrome* is likely to be caused, at least in some patients, by an immunological complication of viral infections, but the evidence for such a process is inconclusive. Several infections have been implicated as the cause of such complications, for example, HHV-6. Some other studies suggest previous infections with CBV, whereas EBV appears to be an unlikely cause. A few studies suggest involvement of the central nervous system. Findings on neuropsychological deficits have been conflicting.

The symptom of fatigue is associated with depression as well as anxiety and is substantially more common in neurotic patients than in nonpatient control subjects. In a study of patients who were chronically fatigued, about two thirds had psychiatric disorders that were considered to be the main cause of their fatigue. In psychiatric patients a neurasthenic cluster of symptoms that included fatigue was shown in a cluster analysis. That depression can cause fatigue is demonstrated by the contrast of psychomotor retardation in the depressive phase and the endurance and energy in the manic phase of bipolar disorder. Some patients have a viral infection, and postviral fatigue induces them to avoid activity. This could lead eventually to impaired fitness and excessive tiredness caused in part by inactivity.

There is evidence to suggest that psychosocial stress can decrease immune competency as well as increase the susceptibility to infection. Incapacitating fatigue is stressful in itself, and this could conceivably contribute to a vicious cycle of stress, decreased immune competency, and more chronic fatigue. However, there is no direct evidence that such a cycle exists.

Thus, there are various causes for chronic fatigue. In some patients there appears to be an immunological complication of a previous viral infection; in others, a psychiatric disorder (usually depression) is found; and in yet others, physical disease and a psychiatric disorder coexist. Some patients have evidence of neither physical disease nor conspicuous psychiatric disorders, and fatigue and exhaustion are their main complaints. The proportion of patients in these categories has not been established with certainty and remains a controversial issue.

In a controlled study the effects of acyclovir on fatigue and laboratory findings did not differ from those of placebo. There was an association of improved mood and decrease in fatigue regardless of the treatment.

There are no published controlled studies on the psychological or psychiatric treatment of this syndrome. In a drug trial of anxious patients, self-rated vigor improved with administration of diazepam.

However, because there are various causes of the syndrome, it is unlikely that the same treatment will be effective for all patients. All recommendations, including the guidance in this chapter, depend on a physician's beliefs and bias.

After adequate examinations and investigations have reasonably excluded treatable physical disease, the patient should be persuaded not to pursue further medical treatment, but to begin a rehabilitation program that includes a realistic gradual increase in physical activity. The coexisting psychiatric disorder may be amenable to treatment. There is evidence from an uncontrolled study suggesting that such a rehabilitation program is helpful for a substantial proportion of patients.

The prognosis varies greatly and most likely depends on the predominant cause of the syndrome. The disorders range from, on the one hand, brief and mild episodes of fatigue during recovery from viral infections and adjustment disorders in patients who have neurasthenic features, to chronic and debilitating disorders on the other. Between 60% and 70% of patients with chronic fatigue were found to be unimproved on follow-up. In an uncontrolled study of patients with severe chronic fatigue syndrome, 72% improved after attending a rehabilitation program with psychiatric treatment, and the improvement was maintained during a brief follow-up.

References

Acheson ED: The clinical syndrome variously called benign myalgic encephalomyelitis, Iceland disease, and epidemic neuromyasthenia. Am J Med 26:569–595, 1959

Altay HT, Toner BB, Brooker H, et al: The neuropsychological dimensions of postinfectious neuromyasthenia (chronic fatigue syndrome): a preliminary report. Int J Psychiatry Med 20:141–149, 1990

American Psychiatric Association: Statistical and Diagnostic Manual of Mental Disorders, 3rd Edition, Revised. Washington, DC, American Psychiatric Association, 1987

Aoki T, Usuda Y, Miyakoshi H, et al: Low natural killer cell syndrome: clinical and immunologic features. Nat Immun Cell Growth Regul 6:116–128, 1987

Archard LC, Bowles NE, Behan PO, et al: Postviral fatigue syndrome: persistence of enterovirus RNA in muscle and elevated creatine kinase. J R Soc Med 81:326–329, 1988

Bannister BA: Post-infectious disease syndrome. Postgrad Med J 64:559–567, 1988

Bastien S: Neuropsychological deficits in chronic fatigue syndrome. Paper presented at the International Conference on Epstein-Barr Virus: The First 25 Years, Oxford University, Oxford, UK, April 1989

Beard GM: American Nervousness—A Practical Treatise on Nervous Exhaustion (Neurasthenia): Its Symptoms, Nature, Sequences, Treatment. Richmond, VA, 1880

Behan PO, Behan WMH, Bell EJ: The postviral fatigue syndrome: an analysis of the findings in 50 cases. J Infect 10:211–222, 1985

Bell EJ, McCartney RA, Riding MH: Coxsackie B viruses and myalgic encephalomyelitis. J R Soc Med 81:329–331, 1988

Buchwald D, Sullivan JL, Komaroff AL: Frequency of "chronic active Epstein-Barr virus infection" in a general medical practice. JAMA 257:2303–2307, 1987

Byrne E: Idiopathic chronic fatigue and myalgia syndrome (myalgic encephalomyelitis): some thoughts on nomenclature and aetiology. Med J Aust 148:80–82, 1988

Caligiuri M, Murray C, Buchwald D, et al: Phenotypic and functional deficiency of natural killer cells in patients with chronic fatigue syndrome. J Immunol 139:3306–3316, 1987

Chatel JC, Peele R: The concept of neurasthenia. Int J Psychiatry Med 9:36–49, 1970

Chen MK: The epidemiology of self-perceived fatigue among adults. Prev Med 15:74–81, 1986

Cluff LE, Canter A, Imboden JB: Asian influenza. Arch Intern Med 117:159–163, 1966

David AS, Wessely S, Pelosi AJ: Postviral fatigue syndrome: time for a new approach. Br Med J 296:696–701, 1988

Dawson J: Royal Free disease: perplexity continues. Br Med J 294:327–328, 1987

Dawson J: Brainstorming the postviral fatigue syndrome. Br Med J 297:1151–1152, 1988

DeFreitas E, Hilliard B, Cheney P, et al: Evidence of retrovirus in patients with chronic fatigue immune dysfunction syndrome. Paper presented at the Eleventh International Congress of Neuropathology, Kyoto, Japan, September 1990

Farmer M, Locke B, Moscicki E, et al: Physical activity and depressive symptoms: the NHANES 1 epidemiologic follow-up study. Am J Epidemiol 128:1340–1351, 1988

Glaser R, Kiecolt-Glaser JK, Speicher CE, et al: Stress, loneliness, and changes in herpesvirus latency. J Behav Med 8:249–260, 1985

Gold D, Bowden R, Sixdy J, et al: Chronic fatigue: a prospective clinical and virological study. JAMA 264:48–53, 1990

Hellinger WC, Smith TF, Van Scoy RE, et al: Chronic fatigue syndrome and the diagnostic utility of antibody to Epstein-Barr virus early antigen. JAMA 260:971–973, 1988

Holmes GP, Kaplan JE, Stewart JA, et al: A cluster of patients with a chronic mononucleosis-like syndrome. JAMA 257:2297–2302, 1987

Holmes GP, Kaplan JE, Gantz NM, et al: Chronic fatigue syndrome: a working case definition. Ann Intern Med 108:387–389, 1988

Hotchin NA, Read R, Smith DG, et al: Active Epstein-Barr virus infection in postviral fatigue syndrome. J Infect 18:143–150, 1989

Hughes JR, Crow RS, Jacobs DR Jr, et al: Physical activity, smoking, and exercise-induced fatigue. J Behav Med 7:217–230, 1984

Imboden JB, Canter A, Cluff LE: Convalescence from influenza. Arch Intern Med 108:393–399, 1961

Jamal GA, Hansen S: Electrophysiological studies in the post-viral fatigue syndrome. J Neurol Neurosurg Psychiatry 48:691–694, 1985

Jones JF, Ray CG, Minnich LL, et al: Evidence for active Epstein-Barr virus infection in patients with persistent, unexplained illnesses: elevated anti-early antigen antibodies. Ann Intern Med 102:1–7, 1985

Kellner R: Somatization and Hypochondriasis. New York, Praeger, 1986

Kellner R: Physical health, mental health, and exercise, in Sports Medicine, 3rd Edition. Edited by Appenzeller O. Baltimore, MD, Urban and Schwarzenberg, 1988, pp 73–81

Kellner R: Psychosocial stress and disease: a historical sketch, in Stress and Immunity. Edited by Plotnikoff NP, Murgo A, Faith D, et al. Caldwell, NJ, Telford Press (in press)

Kellner R, Sheffield BF: The one-week prevalence of symptoms in neurotic patients and normals. Am J Psychiatry 130:102–105, 1973

Kennedy HG: Fatigue and fatigability. Br J Psychiatry 153:1–5, 1988

Kiecolt-Glaser JK, Garner W, Speicher C, et al: Psychosocial modifiers of immunocompetency in medical students. Psychosom Med 46:7–14, 1984a

Kiecolt-Glaser JK, Ricker D, George J, et al: Urinary cortisol levels, cellular immunocompetency, and loneliness in psychiatric inpatients. Psychosom Med 46:15–23, 1984b

Komaroff AL, Straus SE, Gantz NM, et al: The chronic fatigue syndrome. Ann Intern Med 110:407, 1989

Kroenke K, Wood DR, Mangelsdorff D, et al: Chronic fatigue in primary care. JAMA 260:929–934, 1988

Kruesi M, Dale J, Straus S: Psychiatric diagnoses in patients who have chronic fatigue syndrome. J Clin Psychiatry 50:53–56, 1989

Lloyd AR, Hales JP, Gandevia SC: Muscle strength, endurance and recovery in the post-infection fatigue syndrome. J Neurol Neurosurg Psychiatry 51:1316–1322, 1988

Lobstein DD, Mosbacher BJ, Ismail AH: Depression as a powerful discriminator between physically active and sedentary middle-aged men. J Psychosom Res 27:69–76, 1983

Locke SE, Hurst MW, Heisel JS, et al: The influence of stress and other social factors on human immunity. Paper presented at the American Psychosomatic Meeting. Cited in Psychoneuroimmunology. Orlando, FL, Academic, 1981, pp 129–138

Manu P, Matthews DA, Lane TJ: The mental health of patients with a chief complaint of chronic fatigue. Arch Intern Med 148:2213–2217, 1988

Manu P, Lane TJ, Matthews DA: Somatization disorder in patients with chronic fatigue. Psychosomatics 30:388–395, 1989

Martinsen EW: Physical Fitness Training in the Treatment of Patients With Nonpsychotic Mental Disorders. Vikersund, Norway, The Research Institute Modum Bads Nervesanatorium, 1989

Mena I, Villanueva-Meyer J: Study of cerebral perfusion by neurospect in patients with chronic fatigue syndrome, in Proceedings of the First International Symposium on Myalgic Encephalomyelitis (Chronic Fatigue Syndrome). Cambridge, UK, April 1990

Montague T, Marrie T, Klassen G, et al: Cardiac function at rest and with exercise in the chronic fatigue syndrome. Chest 95:779–784, 1989

Montgomery GK: Uncommon tiredness among college undergraduates. J Consult Clin Psychol 51:517–525, 1983

Morrison JD: Fatigue as a presenting complaint in family practice. J Fam Pract 10:795–801, 1980

Phelps JR: Physical activity and health maintenance: exactly what is known? West J Med 146:200–206, 1987

Poteliakhoff A: Adrenocortical activity and some clinical findings in acute and chronic fatigue. J Psychosom Res 25:91–95, 1981

Schwartz GE, Davidson RJ, Coleman D: Patterning of cognitive and somatic processes in the self-regulation of anxiety: effects of meditation versus exercise. J Psychosom Med 40:321–328, 1978

Shoenfeld Y, Shapiro Y, Drory Y, et al: Rehabilitation of patients with NCA (neurocirculatory asthenia) through a short-term training program. American Journal of Physical Medicine 57:1–8, 1978

Slater E, Roth M: Meyer Grosz Clinical Psychiatry. Baltimore, MD, Williams & Wilkins, 1969

Southern P, Oldstone MBA: Medical consequences of persistent viral infection. Seminars in Medicine of the Beth Israel Hospital, Boston 314:359–367, 1986

Stokes MJ, Cooper RG, Edwards RHT: Normal muscle strength and fatigability in patients with effort syndromes. Br Med J 297:1014–1017, 1988

Straus SE: EB or not EB?—that is the question. JAMA 257:2335–2336, 1987

Straus SE: The chronic mononucleosis syndrome. J Infect Dis 157:405–412, 1988

Straus SE, Tosato G, Armstrong G, et al: Persisting illness and fatigue in adults with evidence of Epstein-Barr virus infection. Ann Intern Med 102:7–16, 1985

Straus SE, Dale JK, Tobi M, et al: Acyclovir treatment of the chronic fatigue syndrome. N Engl J Med 319:1692–1698, 1988

Tobi M, Morag A, Ravid Z, et al: Prolonged atypical illness associated with serological evidence of persistent Epstein-Barr virus infection. Lancet 1:61–64, 1982

Uhlenhuth EH, Turner DA, Purchatzke G, et al: Intensive design in evaluating anxiolytic agents. Psychopharmacology (Berlin) 52:79–85, 1977

Valdini AF: Fatigue of unknown aetiology: a review. Fam Pract 2:48–53, 1985

Valdini AF, Steinhardt S, Valicenti J, et al: A one-year follow-up of fatigued patients. J Fam Pract 26:33–38, 1988

Verhaest S, Pierloot R: An attempt at an empirical delimitation of neurasthenic neurosis and its relation with some character traits. Acta Psychiatr Scand 62:166–176, 1980

Wessely S, Butler S, Chalder T, et al: The cognitive and behavioural management of the chronic fatigue syndrome. J Neurol Neurosurg Psychiatry (in press)

White P: Fatigue syndrome: neurasthenia revived. Br Med J 298:1199–1200, 1989

World Health Organization: Draft of the 10th Revision of the International Classification of Diseases. Geneva, World Health Organization, 1988

Yousef GE, Bell EJ, Mann GF, et al: Chronic enterovirus infection in patients with postviral fatigue syndrome. Lancet 1:146–150, 1988

Chapter 3

Globus and Fear of Choking

> I had a lump in my throat.
>> Erica, a fellow student,
>> commenting years ago on the
>> film *The Diary of Anne Frank*

Globus

There are various disorders of swallowing that are discussed in this chapter and in Chapter 4. *Globus* (the Latin word for lump) is a sensation of a ball or lump in the throat. It should be distinguished from *dysphagia,* which is a difficulty in swallowing. There are several terms in the literature describing this complaint: globus, globus hystericus, globus pharyngeus, and globus syndrome.

Development of the Concept

As the term *globus hystericus* implies, the complaint has been regarded as one of the symptoms of hysteria (Merskey 1986). Hippocrates described this symptom as a consequence of the wandering uterus exerting pressure on the neck (Adams 1849), which was one of the astonishing feats of that mischievous organ.

Malcomson (1968, p. 219) quotes Purcell (1707), who describes globus patients as follows: ". . . they have difficulty in breathing and think they feel something in the throat ready to choke them. . . . Women . . . feel a hard ball pressed against the outside of their throat; sometimes as if it were a stick thrust down their throats . . . [or] a rising of something up their throats." Purcell believed that the sensation was due to the contraction of the strap muscles of the neck pressing on the thyroid cartilage.

A brief history of the concept was described by Malcomson (1968). Glaser and Engel (1977) believed it to be a manifestation of repressed crying. Ferenczi (1926) believed that it was a "peripheral materialization of a repressed idea and a subconscious desire for oral sexual activity" (p. 92). In DSM-III-R (American

Psychiatric Association 1987), difficulty in swallowing is one of the symptoms listed in the category of somatization disorder.

Symptoms and Signs

The globus sensation is described as a lump in the throat or as a feeling of something sticking in the throat. The symptom is either relieved or not affected by swallowing (Bradley and Narula 1987).

Thompson and Heaton (1982) found that only 3% of subjects with globus related it to eating, 75% experienced it between meals, and 22% experienced it between times, as well as at times, of eating; thus, dysphagia and fear of swallowing or fear of choking are usually not related to the globus sensation.

Prevalence

About 45% of a nonpatient population have reported to have had globus sensation, and between 3% and 4% of attendances in ear, nose, and throat clinics are because of this symptom. Globus sensation is more common in women, and the largest proportion that seek help at an ear, nose, and throat clinic is in the 41-to-50 age group (Moloy and Charter 1982; Thompson and Heaton 1982).

Etiology

There are several controversies in the literature about the causes and physiological concomitants of globus, or at least about the proportion of cases with globus in which an organic abnormality or physiological disturbance can be demonstrated. For example, Cohen (1973) believes that various organic pathologies are responsible for globus symptoms, whereas Wilson et al. (1987b) claim that the incidence of organic pathology is "extremely low."

Malcomson (1966, 1968), in a study of 307 patients, found that in only 20% of these patients was there a "completely negative clinical and radiological examination" (p. 584). Among the patients who had physical abnormalities, local lesions were found in 38%, and 62% of the patients had distal lesions. Among those with distal findings, the largest proportion had a hiatal hernia (69%). It is unknown whether the lesions were causing globus or were coincidental. The other abnormalities found by the author were osteophytes of the cervical spine, overactive cricopharyngeus muscle, goiter, postcricoid web, and distal lesions, including duodenal ulcers and gastric lesions. In a subsequent study (Malcomson 1968), 112 more patients with globus were enrolled. In the total of 419 globus patients, the distributions of pathologies remained essentially the same.

Weisskopf (1981) reported cases of reflux esophagitis in which the patient had a globus sensation; he described case histories in which treatment of the cause of reflux abolished the globus sensation. Because this was an uncontrolled study, it is uncertain whether a placebo effect or the passage of time contributed to the recovery. Ardran (1982) found evidence of reflux in a substantial proportion of patients and reproduced the globus sensation with hydrochloric acid. Thompson and Heaton (1982) questioned 301 subjects from various populations as to whether they suffered from heartburn, and asked about one half of the subjects whether they experienced a globus sensation (a question added in the course of the study). One third of the subjects said that they had experienced heartburn at least once a year. Forty-six percent of the subjects who had been asked about globus reported that they had experienced occasionally a lump in their throat; this was equally common in those patients with and those without heartburn. There was no relationship between symptoms of lower bowel functions, such as symptoms of the irritable bowel syndrome, and globus. The author concluded that globus, a dysfunction of the upper esophagus, is extremely common and tends to occur independently of heartburn, which is a symptom dysfunction of the lower esophagus, and that globus is not associated with bowel dysfunction. Yet, Watson et al. (1978), in a study of patients with the irritable bowel syndrome, found a higher prevalence of globus symptoms than was found in age-matched patients attending a gynecology clinic. The discrepancy between these results may be explained by self-selection of the clinic patients with irritable bowel syndrome in Watson's study (see Chapter 6, this volume).

On radiological examination of patients with globus, Malcomson (1966) found evidence of hiatal hernia and gastric and duodenal ulcers; he concluded that esophageal reflux was responsible for globus in a large proportion of patients. Freeland et al. (1974) identified acid sensitivity in over 77% of globus patients and found that their symptoms were relieved by antacid treatment. Mair et al. (1974) found distal pathology in 47% of patients with globus, but the coexistence of hiatal hernia was unrelated to recovery from globus. Wilson et al. (1987a), using a more accurate method of detecting reflux (i.e., prolonged ambulatory monitoring), found that abnormal degrees of reflux were present in only 15% of globus patients.

Gray (1983) expressed the view that the globus sensation can be explained as swallowing initiated from the lingual tonsil–epiglottis area involving mainly the inferior constrictor muscle, a mechanism termed the *inferior constrict swallow*. The author described the two groups of patients as follows:

> [One group gave] "a positive statement—it feels like a 'cake crumb,' a 'fish bone,' 'a pea,' a 'hair.' They will localize their sensation accurately with one finger. . . . Anesthetization of this trigger area with an application of local anesthetic causes them to lose the lump in the throat. . . . The other group are more vague . . . a lump in the throat . . . a feeling of something there . . . a tightness . . . a constricting feeling. . . . They localize the sensation by grasping the throat with the whole hand at the level of the hyoid bone or point to the suprasternal notch or just below it. (p. 608)

The author expressed the view that the set of symptoms described by the first group is caused by local irritation in the region of the lingual tonsil, and the other set of symptoms, described by the second group, is caused by a vicious cycle of increased cricopharyngeus muscle tension and strain in swallowing. (See Gray 1983 for a more detailed description of these syndromes.) Gray recommends the terms *hypopharyngeal syndrome* or *strain swallow syndrome,* instead of globus.

There are controversies about the role of the cricopharyngeal sphincter. Watson and Sullivan (1974) compared cricopharyngeal sphincter pressure in patients with globus (n = 9) to that of other patients (n = 22) who did not experience this sensation. There were striking differences between the two groups; only one patient in each group had the same pressure. The mean for the globus group was 175.6 mm Hg (SD = 26.0) and for the control group, 96 mm Hg (SD = 15.6).

Bonington et al. (1988) concluded from histological studies of the cricopharyngeus that the findings are consistent with a sphincteric role in deglutition, vomiting, and control of aerophagia. Yet Calderelli et al. (1970) could not find elevated cricopharyngeal pressure in globus patients compared with control subjects. Flores et al. (1981) measured esophageal manometric changes in 12 patients who had persistent globus. In 10 patients there was increased resting pressure in the body of the esophagus. The authors concluded that their data failed to confirm the observation by Watson and Sullivan (1974) that hypertonicity of the cricopharyngeus is one cause of globus. They quoted the findings of Jones (1938) and Kramer and Hollander (1955), that suprasternal choking or pressure discomfort can be elicited by inflating balloons at different levels of the esophagus. Flores et al. concluded that globus is caused largely by a hypertonic and incoordinated esophagus. Because intermittent nonperistaltic motor responses may be associated with emotional stress (Nagler and Spiro 1961), the authors hypothesize that emotion may cause a derangement of neuromuscular control.

Cook et al. (1987) found that there was a significant increase in upper esophageal sphincter pressure in healthy subjects when they were exposed to experimental stress. In a later study, however, Cook et al. (1989) examined upper esophageal sphincter pressure in 7 patients with globus and 13 control subjects under basal condition and experimental stress. Resting pressure and response to stress did not differ significantly in both globus patients and healthy control subjects.

Other abnormalities that have been suggested as being responsible for globus are functional disorders or disease of the upper cervical spine, pharyngeal pouch, mucosal web, sinusitis (Biesinger et al. 1989; Bradley and Narula 1987), pathology in stomach or duodenum (Mair et al. 1974), and malocclusion. (The last hypothesis was tested in a blind study of treatment of malocclusion, as described later in this chapter [Puhakka and Kirveskari 1988].) Adour et al. (1980a, 1980b) suggested that globus may sometimes be caused by acute laryngeal superior nerve palsy as part of a polyneuritis arising from herpes simplex virus reactivation.

In contrast to numerous other authors, Wilson et al. (1988) concluded that globus is often recognizable clinically after a few minutes consultation and after the patients undergo extensive investigations to exclude pathological lesions that are reported to produce symptoms. The authors noted that organic lesions "are extremely rare and if they exist they almost always produce other significant symptoms. When globus occurs in isolation, the incidence of positive finding is extremely low" (Wilson 1988, p. 335).

Psychological Studies

Lehtinen and Puhakka (1976) compared the results of psychological inventories of 20 patients with globus (11 females and 9 males) with those of a control group. The Middlesex Hospital Questionnaire, the Taylor Manifest Anxiety Scale, and the Holmes-Rahe Schedule of Recent Events did not show significant differences between the two groups. The authors' clinical impressions were that the patients did not show hysterical personality traits; males with globus resem bled control subjects, whereas the female patients had depressive and obsessive traits. Pratt et al. (1976) administered the Minnesota Multiphasic Personality Inventory (MMPI) to patients with globus who had attended a private clinic. They found that males had a higher incidence of depression and elevation of the hypochondriasis (Hs) scale.

Cook et al. (1989) administered the Eysenck Personality Inventory, the Spielberger State-Trait Anxiety Scale, and the Beck Depression Inventory. They found that clinic patients with globus were more anxious, depressed, and introverted than healthy control subjects.

Wilson et al. (1988) examined 37 females and 9 males with globus who attended the ear, nose, and throat department of the Royal Infirmary in Edinburgh. All patients had the clinical diagnosis of globus hystericus, and physical causes for difficulty in swallowing had been carefully excluded. Most of the patients also underwent esophageal manometry and 23-hour ambulatory pH monitoring to assess the extent of gastroesophageal reflux. Esophageal acid exposure time (AET) was calculated as the total percentage time the esophageal pH was less than 4 at the site of the probe, which was 3 cm above the lower esophageal sphincter.

The authors administered the General Health Questionnaire, 60-Item Version (GHQ-60) and the Eysenck Personality Inventory (EPI). Female patients had significantly higher N (neuroticism) scores than did a healthy group matched by age and sex, whereas male globus patients had significantly lower N scores than did the control subjects. The E (extroversion) scores in male patients were similar to those in control subjects, but female patients were found to be significantly more introverted than control subjects. Fourteen of the patients scored above 12 on the GHQ-60, which the authors regarded as a score for psychiatric morbidity. There was an inverse relationship between the neuroticism scores and the AET, which suggests that patients with gastroesophageal reflux probably had less psychological disturbance. The EPI scores clustered in the neurotic introverted range (the dysthymic quadrant) that includes patients with various neuroses, such as phobic, depressive, and anxiety neuroses. The authors also commented that male globus patients had low N scores and concluded that male patients with globus may be psychologically more abnormal than females.

Based on their study, Wilson et al. (1988) concluded that globus is a conversion disorder, thus hysterical, and they also argued that globus should be included among the dysthymic disorders. (The authors used the term *dysthymic disorder* in accord with the concept proposed by Eysenck, who regards individuals with this disorder as having high N scores and low E scores; this definition is unrelated to the later DSM-III category of the same name.) The controversies about the meaning of extroversion scores in hysteria are discussed in Chapter 11, pp. 231–232, this volume. The authors believe that their data may help to resolve a debate on the nature of conversion disorder. They consider two main possibilities: 1) that patients report "normal physiological stimuli as symptoms (the 'symptom monitoring' hypothesis)"; or 2) that patients "are converting emotional concerns into a physical manifestation (the 'materialization' hypothesis)" (p. 337). The authors quote Gray (1983), who postulated that minor pharyngeal irritation imitated the globus sensation, with a subsequent increase in dry swallowing, thus perpetuating a vicious cycle. Wilson et al. argue that no materialization has been demonstrated so far in globus; they could not find convincing cricopharyngeal abnormality by a manometric study in globus patients. Although abnormal esophageal contractions have been shown to be produced by stress, these contractions may represent "relatively normal stimuli that become a globus symptom only in pre-disposed individuals" (p. 338).

This study was discussed by Mace et al. (1989), who criticized the method as well as the conclusion on several counts. For example, according to Mace et al., the authors had not described selection criteria and chose the EPI to make a psychiatric diagnosis. Wilson and colleagues (1989) replied and defended their conclusion that globus was indeed "hystericus."

Diagnosis

The patient's description of the symptoms is usually characteristic (see pp. 54–56). Physical diseases that may cause the globus sensation as well as true dysphagia (see Chapter 4) need to be excluded. The diagnoses of 145 patients with globus symptoms are listed in Table 3-1.

There are no guidelines in the current diagnostic manuals on the classification of an isolated globus sensation. The diagnoses that appear to be appropri-

Table 3-1. **Diagnoses of patients with globus sensation**

Diagnoses	No.	% Age (approx.)
No diagnosis	74	51
Acid reflux	19	13
Pharyngitis	10	7
Cancer phobia/bereavement	9	6
Mucosal web	4	3
Sinusitis	5	3.5
Pharyngeal pouch	4	3
Oral/dental infection	4	3
Vallecular polyp/cyst	5	3.5
Goiter	3	2
Motor neuron disease	1	1
Squamous carcinoma	7	5
Failed follow-up	5	3.5

Source. Reprinted from Bradley and Narula 1987, p. 691, with permission.

ate are undifferentiated somatoform disorder in DSM-III-R (American Psychiatric Association 1987) and somatoform autonomic dysfunction in the ICD-10 draft (World Health Organization 1988).

Treatment

Physical disease contributing to or causing globus sensation needs to be excluded. If such disease is found, it needs to be, of course, appropriately treated. To my knowledge, there is only one published controlled study of globus, and the authors used a new treatment. Puhakka and Kirveskari (1988) carried out a double-blind study with 22 patients with globus symptoms. One group had occlusal adjustment, whereas the control group had mock adjustment. The effect of treatment on globus symptoms was assessed after 2 to 3 months as part of the double-blind study. Among the patients who had occlusal adjustment, a significantly larger proportion reported a disappearance of globus than was found among patients who had mock adjustment.

There is evidence from a follow-up study that explanation and reassurance constitute adequate treatment in most cases (Gray 1983). If the symptoms persist, or perhaps as the initial treatment, antacid and head elevation in bed should be tried for 1 month, because 15% or more of the cases have esophageal reflux (Wilson et al. 1988). Most patients will recover or substantially improve with this treatment (Bradley and Narula 1987).

Patients referred to psychiatrists usually suffer from anxiety or depression, which is the main cause for consultation because most of the patients are managed by the primary physician or the nonpsychiatric specialist (Wilson et al. 1988). Coexisting psychiatric disorders should, of course, be appropriately treated. A few published case histories (Rosenthal 1987; Weinstein 1987), including the case history in the next section, suggest that in most patients, globus remits when the psychiatric disorder is appropriately treated. If the globus symptom persists, explanation and reassurance are usually adequate. In the rare cases in which the patient is firmly convinced that an undiagnosed physical disease is causing the symptoms and the symptoms and the false belief persist despite explanation and reassurance, the strategies as outlined in Chapter 10 on the treatment of hypochondriasis may be used.

Case Histories

Case 1

The patient was a 50-year-old female who had a part-time job as a salesperson; her husband was a bank manager. I had treated her for almost 20 years with lithium as maintenance for an atypical bipolar disorder. She became depressed on two occasions shortly after stopping the lithium.

Her lithium blood level had been maintained at around 0.8 meq/ml and had remained fairly stable, and I tried to decrease the dose and maintain the patient at a lower blood level. I reduced the dose from 600 mg lithium carbonate to 450 mg daily, and the level subsequently decreased to 0.5 meq/ml. The patient said that she felt more nervous since the dose had been decreased. She said that she had a feeling of constriction in her throat unrelated to eating that had started since the dose of lithium was reduced. She had had these sensations many times before and had consulted ear, nose, and throat surgeons, but she had never mentioned the sensations to me previously because she believed that her symptoms were not in the realm of psychiatry. She noticed also that these symptoms were particularly troublesome when she was excited about some problem at work or concerning her family. Conversely, when she was in the movies or when she was preoccupied, she did not notice the sensation. At about the same time that the dose was reduced, she inhaled inadvertently an insecticide spray that made her cough. She believed that this had aggravated her throat symptoms, but her physician did not find evidence of damage.

I explained to the patient that this was a typical symptom of no consequence, and because there was no evidence that she had a disease, she should try to ignore it. Over the years the patient had also been taking chlordiazepoxide intermittently for anxiety. She also noticed when she took 10 mg of chlordiazepoxide that it relieved anxiety as well as her feeling of constriction in her throat.

Comment. I was unaware of the patient's globus symptoms, although I had treated her for almost two decades. The patient mentioned the throat constriction to me only because she wondered whether the decrease in the dose of lithium could be associated with her symptom.

Case 2

The patient, a 56-year-old insightful professional woman, had been having moderate intermittent episodes of anxiety. (I was writing the present chapter on globus at the time, so I asked patients and acquaintances about globus sensations.) The patient replied, "I had it a few times; I had it when my mother was ill and I used to get it before exams." When I asked her whether she associated it with any emotions, she replied, "It is as predictably linked to anxiety as trembling."

Prognosis

Bradley and Narula (1987) found that in about one half of patients referred with globus to an ear, nose, and throat clinic, the symptoms resolved before the cause was investigated. On a 15-year follow-up by Gray (1983), 10% of the patients still had symptoms, 43% had had minor recurrences during the follow-up period, and 43% had had no further symptoms.

In a random population, 46% of patients admitted to globus symptoms (Thompson and Heaton 1982). So, apparently, a large proportion of people do not report these symptoms to physicians, and the symptoms are either short-lived or cause little distress. There is no evidence of weight loss—the globus sensation does not interfere with eating—and there is no evidence that there is any risk to the patient's physical health. In some patients the globus sensation reccurs intermittently at times of stress.

Discussion

There are wide disagreements among the results of studies on the physical concomitants of globus. Evidence on the role of increased tension in the cricopharyngeus, as well as on the extent of the role of gastroesophageal reflux, has been conflicting. In some patients the coexistence of other pathology is coincidental; in others it appears to cause globus symptoms.

Patients who seek help from ear, nose, and throat surgeons tend to score higher on psychological tests, including the depression (D) and the hypochondriasis (Hs) scales of the MMPI, than do healthy control groups; women score higher on the neuroticism (N) scale of the EPI than do men, and are also significantly introverted.

Thompson and Heaton (1982) found no relationship between globus and symptoms of the irritable bowel syndrome, whereas Watson et al. (1978) found globus significantly more often in patients with the irritable bowel syndrome than in other patients. Because the former study was a community survey, the discrepancy between the results of these two studies may be explained by the selective referral, or self-selection, of patients with irritable bowel syndrome attending a clinic. The higher prevalence of neuroses in patients with irritable bowel syndrome who attend clinics (compared with those individuals in the community) may have been responsible for the higher prevalence of globus sensation.

Wilson et al. (1988) expressed the view that globus patients are hysterical and based this view on psychological test scores, mainly the EPI. The finding that patients with globus attending an ear, nose, and throat clinic score in the introverted-neurotic quadrant of the EPI is insufficient to conclude that these patients are hysterical. This quadrant is shared by patients with other neuroses, and authors have not tried to distinguish between hysteria and other somatoform disorders. To my knowledge, there is no study using personality inventories that succeeded in distinguishing between patients with conversion disorder and patients with other somatoform disorders. The authors also expressed the view that the hysterical nature of globus is suggested because the symptom is reinforced by attention from physicians. This observation does not necessarily support the view that globus is a hysterical symptom. The role of reinforcement as a cause for somatic symptoms in general, and conversion symptoms in particular, is discussed in Chapters 10 and 11 of the present volume.

Still unresolved is the question of whether globus is a conversion or a "materialization"—that is, whether psychological distress is converted to a physical disorder, or whether it is a manifestation of somatization with the etiological components described in Chapter 10. Schatzki (1964) believes that it is caused in part by selective perception and excessive swallowing:

> The patient under tension may start to observe himself more intensely than he would otherwise. He becomes aware of the swallowing of saliva, becomes interested in it, and swallows several times in quick succession. He may swallow repeatedly for other reasons, not just because he observes his swallowing act. In any event, an inability to swallow results, since no more saliva is available. A peculiar sensation of a lump in the hypopharynx results, as anyone can easily confirm by trying to swallow repeatedly. (p. 676)

Judging from the available studies, the evidence points to somatization processes rather than to conversion. Gray (1983) hypothesized that a minor pharyngeal irritation can initiate the globus sensation, which is followed by a subsequent increase in dry swallowing, thus perpetuating a vicious cycle. Patients who are anxious or depressed, particularly those who attend to bodily sensations, will more likely become aware of discomfort and unpleasant sensations in their body, including their throat. The patients may or may not believe or fear that they have a disease—several authors have commented that some of the patients feared that they had cancer (Bradley and Narula 1987)—and the vicious cycle can be explained as a chain of sensations, anxiety, selective perception, and false beliefs (see Chapter 10, pp. 198–199, this volume).

To my knowledge, there has been no systematic study of personality disorders of patients with this syndrome except for the studies summarized above that included the administering of psychological inventories. Yet, there is agreement among authors that, clinically, patients with globus do not have hysterical or histrionic personalities (Malcomson 1968; Wilson et al. 1988).

Several authors have recommended that the term globus hystericus should be abandoned in view of the large number of coexisting anatomical and physiological abnormalities and the lack of evidence for hysteria. Some of the other terms that have been suggested, as mentioned in the opening of this chapter, are *globus, globus syndrome, hypopharyngeal syndrome* (Gray 1983), and *globus pharyngeus.*

Some authors have commented on the relationship between anxiety and globus. In a study of healthy subjects who, on questioning, admitted to globus symptoms (Thompson and Heaton 1982), 95 patients said that these had occurred with strong emotions, and "many volunteered that ... [they] disappeared on crying" (p. 47). Weinstein (1987) has expressed the view that the inability to cry is a causative factor. Puhakka et al. (1976) has expressed the view that "the globus mechanism is a part of normal bodily function and that symptoms can be provoked as a result of strong emotional mechanisms in almost any person." Flores et al. (1981) found high esophageal resting pressure and disordered motor activity among globus patients. The evidence that emotions can alter esophageal motor activity (Nagler and Spiro 1961) might explain the link of anxiety and globus.

The proportion of globus patients with cancer phobia or hypochondriasis is unknown. Apart from Thompson and Heaton's and Weinstein's observations discussed above, Glaser and Engel's (1977) view—that globus is a manifestation of repressed crying—has not been systematically studied. Ferenczi's view that globus represents a subconscious desire for oral sexual activity has not had to date empirical support, but this explanation would lend itself to one of the more interesting epidemiological surveys.

Fear of Choking, or Pseudodysphagia

The patients with this syndrome complain of difficulty with swallowing or of an inability to swallow with no physical disease to account for these symptoms.

Symptoms and Signs

The usual complaint of *pseudodysphagia* is an inability to swallow. On questioning, most patients admit that they are afraid that they will choke. The difficulty is usually limited to solids, but the nature of the difficulty varies: most patients are able to swallow soft foods or semisolids, whereas others are able to swallow only small pieces of solid food or only when the food is thoroughly lubricated. In some others, the fear is limited to certain items such as pills; a minority of patients are more afraid to drink liquids. In a few patients, there is a substantial loss of weight.

Patients with pseudodysphagia are usually anxious and concerned about not being able to eat. In the case histories summarized below, many of the patients had conspicuous psychiatric disorders, including depression, obsessions, hypochondriasis, agoraphobia, and panic attacks.

Prevalence

The prevalence of pseudodysphagia is not known. The condition is sometimes listed in conjunction with the globus sensation, although the the two are different phenomena. Judging by the number of patients seeking treatment from ear, nose, and throat surgeons because of the inability to swallow as compared with patients with globus sensation, the latter condition is far more common.

Etiology

Little is known about the etiology of pseudodysphagia. Most of the published reports are case histories of patients with the main emphasis on methods of treatment and outcome. These studies are described below. Physiological correlates of pseudodysphagia are not known.

Psychological and Psychiatric Studies

The section above on symptoms and signs is based on published case histories. These suggest that most patients with severe pseudodysphagia also have other psychiatric disorders.

To my knowledge, there is no controlled study with adults, and there is only one controlled study with children. Di Scipio and Kaslon (1982) examined children who had had surgery for cleft palate within 1 year after surgery. By means of a questionnaire, the authors compared the eating habits of these children with those of their siblings and a group of control children. The questionnaire dealt with 32 questions pertaining to eating, including questions pertaining to taste aversion to different foods. The questionnaire was administered to the adults who were in closest contact with the children while they were eating. The children who had had surgery had higher scores on the questionnaire of feeding difficulties than did the two control groups. The items that discriminated most between the groups were "Requires Assistance," "Small Bites," "Does Not Finish," and "Has To Be Prompted." Because of their cleft palate, two thirds of the children also had feeding difficulties such as nasal regurgitation and inability to eat solids before surgery. Parents of only two children reported new difficulties that arose immediately after surgery.

The authors concluded that the feeding difficulties were caused by classical (Pavlovian) conditioning. The physical trauma during surgery, the intrusive diagnostic procedures, or the nasal regurgitation or poor suckling prior to surgery were unconditional aversive stimuli that, when paired temporarily with swallowing, resulted in conditioned avoidance of swallowing.

Diagnosis

There are numerous diseases that can cause oropharyngeal dysphagia (see Chapter 4, this volume). The characteristic features of pseudodysphagia have been described in the section above on symptoms and signs. Several authors have used the terms globus and pseudodysphagia synonymously, whereas others distinguish between the two. Globus is a sensation of constriction of the throat that is only rarely present while eating and with which there is no difficulty in swallowing. In patients with pseudodysphagia, difficulty in swallowing is the main complaint, and most patients have no throat symptoms when not eating. There are rare case reports (see Brown et al. 1986) in which globus sensation has preceded the fear of choking.

Case Histories of Treatment

Behavior therapy. The psychology of fear of swallowing and the psychological treatments have been surveyed by Whitehead and Schuster (1985) and Klinger and Strang (1987). Summaries of published case histories follow that illustrate the psychological treatments that have been used.

Solyom and Sookman (1980) described four patients with swallowing difficulty treated with various methods of behavior therapy. The first patient was a 21-year-old male college student who would not swallow in public because of his conviction that swallowing produced an unpleasant noise. Explanation and reassurance were ineffective. After one session of flooding in which swallowing noises were greatly amplified, the patient dropped out of therapy.

The second patient was a 75-year-old retired accountant who had lost 20 pounds in 3 months. He took 2 1/2 hours to eat half a bowl of cereal and had difficulty swallowing water. He had had various psychiatric disorders since the age of 20. The patient was treated with aversion relief therapy; finger shock was initiated and increased gradually in intensity until the patient started to swallow. A feeling of relief due to cessation of the finger shock was paired with the swallowing movement. Within a week the patient was eating at a normal rate in the laboratory. The initial total reinforcement was followed by a partial reinforcement schedule. Upon discharge from the hospital he was drinking with some caution. He had by that time regained his weight and had no anxiety swallowing solid food.

The third case involved a 47-year-old patient who experienced a recurrent nightmare in which he was choking on an inedible object. He would awaken terrified. He avoided candy and peanuts and would eat meat very cautiously. His nightmares were treated with desensitization in imagery. Eventually, the nightmares occurred infrequently, and he no longer feared choking or avoided eating.

The fourth case was a 60-year-old male who feared choking, experienced great difficulty in swallowing, and had lost 20 pounds. He was described as extremely hypochondriacal and had been agoraphobic for 20 years. He had some mild swallowing difficulties with liquids when he was 15, and his present inability to swallow started 2 months previously. The patient was treated with relaxation training that he practiced three times a day before eating. He was also treated with an aversion relief paradigm similar to that of the patient in the second example above. Desensitization to his throat symptoms was achieved by putting a large tongue depressor at the back of his throat. At the end of nine sessions his anxiety was less intense. On follow-up at 1 year he had lost his fear of swallowing and choking.

Di Scipio et al. (1978) treated three children under the age of 2 1/2 years for inability to swallow. The children were being fed by a gastrostomy. Two of the children had previously undergone oropharyngeal surgery. In the third child, the diagnosis was uncertain, but the difficulty was considered to be a congenital neurological disorder and probable pseudobulbar palsy. The dysphagia was unexplained but may have been aggravated after a traumatic experience of a barium swallow.

The treatment of the three cases consisted of the following elements:

1. Positive reinforcement of the psychomotor component of oral feeding was shaped.
2. Tube feeding was contingent on oral feeding; the child was fed by a tube when the child attempted to swallow.
3. The treatment further consisted of massed learning trials over 72-hour periods. Treatment took between 1 and 2 years.

In all cases the treatment led to removal of the gastrostomy tube and reestablishment of oral feeding.

Haynes (1976) reported a case of a 25-year-old female who had a feeling of continuous constriction of throat muscles. This constriction occurred especially during stressful periods in her life such as upcoming examinations and during family conflicts. This sensation, although nearly constant, was a particular problem during meals. Under stress, swallowing became so aversive that the patient was frequently unable to eat. She had been treated with "several types of minor tranquilizers and had received a series of relaxation training sessions. Both had resulted in noticeable but only temporary improvement" (p. 122).

After a 2-month baseline phase the patient had 20 half-hour sessions of frontalis electromyographic feedback. She was instructed to employ techniques she had learned in the laboratory and to practice relaxing at home at least once a day. She was also instructed to attempt to relax whenever she felt her throat becoming tense or tight. The symptoms decreased in severity as treatment progressed, and the patient gained an increased sense of control over the feeling of tension during stressful situations. The improvement was maintained over a 6-month follow-up period.

Walco (1986) reported a case of a 13-year-old boy who was treated for acute lymphocytic leukemia. He was unable to swallow pills. When he tried to do so, it resulted in him gagging and choking, but he had no difficulty in swallowing other substances. Ice chips were chosen for graded practice over pieces of candy because they melted rapidly and they were less threatening. Initially the ice was placed on the back of the patient's tongue and swallowed after it had melted. The patient was encouraged to swallow when the ice chunk had almost completely melted and later encouraged to swallow larger pieces. When the patient started to choke, the whole procedure was repeated. On the third day the patient gleefully informed the therapist that he had swallowed his pills that morning because the pills were so much smaller than the large chunks of ice he had mastered. Although he had never been able to swallow pills previously and had only 2 days of treatment, he had no recurrence in an 8-month follow-up.

Black (1980), using hypnosis, treated a 14-year-old boy for fear of choking and swallowing difficulty who had developed pseudobulbar palsy after a bicycle accident. He was only hypnotizable to a light trance, and he was treated with 78 sessions of hypnosis over 6 months. After treatment he was eventually able to swallow.

Cerny et al. (1988) carried out a study of treatment of dysphagic functional disorders located in the region of the cricopharyngeus with hypnosis ($n = 21$). (Patients with esophageal dysphagia were also included in this study, and those results are summarized in Chapter 4 of the present volume). The patients were selected from a larger group based on their apparent susceptibility to hypnosis, which in turn was based on a score of 3 through 12 on the Stanford Hypnotic Susceptibility Scale. The authors included a small group of healthy individuals to examine the physiological effects of the treatment on esophageal functioning. Treatment consisted of suggestion under hypnosis followed by posthypnotic suggestion that a specific behavior (e.g., clinching of the fist) before and during eating would abolish spasm. The number of sessions ranged from 5 to 20. About 85% of the patients improved or recovered at the end of treatment. In about 66% of the patients the improvement was maintained on follow-up.

Kaplan and Evans (1978) treated a woman who had difficulty swallowing in public places, which started after she witnessed a gun battle in a restaurant. She was treated with systemic desensitization, which led to a marked improvement in her symptoms.

Drug treatment. Brown et al. (1986) treated with antidepressant drugs three patients who had severe difficulty in swallowing. The first patient was treated successfully with imipramine, which was gradually increased to 250 mg a day; she maintained her improvement on follow-up. The second patient, a 40-year-old woman, was admitted with "anorexia." She refused to eat because of the fear that she would not be able to breathe while swallowing food. She also had a history of agoraphobia. She was treated with phenelzine, 60 mg a day, which led to a remission of her symptoms. One-year follow-up showed no recurrence of swallowing difficulties. The third case was a 78-year-old woman with moderate Alzheimer's disease who was afraid of swallowing and had lost 30 pounds in 2 months. She failed to improve with neuroleptics and benzodiazepines; she was treated with tranylcypromine, 30 mg daily, and her symptoms remitted after 7 days, at which time she resumed eating. The medication was discontinued, and she remained symptom free. These patients were described as suffering from globus hystericus syndrome, but the descriptions of these cases suggest that the patients were actually afraid of choking.

Greenberg et al. (1988) reported three cases in which patients with fear of choking were treated with alprazolam. A 28-year-old woman developed fear of swallowing after she choked on a fish bone. She was hungry but ate only small amounts of solid food. She was treated with alprazolam, 1 mg four times a day, and recovered, at which time the alprazolam was successfully tapered. In another case, a 43-year-old man with metastatic rectal carcinoma stopped eating when he choked on pills and developed a fear of eating solid food. Administration of alprazolam, 0.5 mg four times a day, led to resolution of his fears, and he gained weight in spite of his cancer; he died of respiratory failure 6 weeks later. A final example is a 36-year-old woman who experienced a sudden onset of choking sensation while driving. This sensation had subsequently become frequent. Later feelings of anxiety, palpitations, and tachypnea became associated with these episodes. She became frightened of eating solid foods and was frightened to go to restaurants. She lost 15 pounds over 2 years. The patient was treated with alprazolam, 1 mg twice a day, which relieved both her fear of choking and the associated anxiety symptoms. Her symptoms recurred when she attempted to withdraw from the drug. Reinstitution of alprazolam again led to a resolution of her symptoms.

Discussion

Di Scipio and Kaslon (1982) make a strong case for their view that the feeding difficulties in children who had had corrective surgery for a cleft palate were caused by classical conditioning. Most of these children, however, had various eating disorders, and, except for one child who had a brief episode immediately after surgery, none had obvious fear of choking. The authors' explanation of an acquired conditioned response would have had stronger support if they had included control groups of children who had had surgery in other parts of the body unrelated to the alimentary tract or a control group of children who had abnormalities that caused parental concern and unusual parental attention to the child's eating. The explanation, however, of a classically conditioned response appears likely in view of the case histories they had reported previously (Di Scipio et al. 1978), as well as those reported by other authors. Patients with fear of choking date the onset of symptoms to a traumatic event that occurred while eating, such as choking on food.

The physiological processes that are responsible for pseudodysphagia are unknown. The two most likely explanations are 1) conditioned contractions of oropharyngeal muscles at times of eating brought on by the fear of choking, and 2) an inhibition of the swallowing reflex at times of fear. Examples of the latter are reports by patients with social phobia who are unable to eat in public but have no difficulty when eating alone or with family members. The problem may be aggravated by insufficient salivation caused by fear. A combination of these processes may be responsible for pseudodysphagia, and there may be differences among individuals in the relative contribution of these mechanisms. Another process may be involved: the idea that the patient may choke actually induces fear while eating, leading to selective perception of sensation from the throat, which in turn aggravates the fear. By frequent repetition the association in this chain becomes overlearned. A method of desensitization or diminution of the fear with the aid of antipanic drugs removes a link in this vicious cycle.

Recommended Treatments

Various methods of desensitization have been used in the treatment of pseudodysphagia. The case histories are inadequate to recommend one treatment method in preference to another. Treatments that appear to be the least time consuming, simplest, and least uncomfortable should be the first choice. More elaborate treatments should be introduced only when the simpler methods have failed. For example, teaching a patient to swallow gradually larger chunks of ice may be the most efficient method for a patient who has difficulty in swallowing pills, and perhaps other solids as well. Systematic desensitization of eating in a threatening situation is probably the most effective treatment if the difficulty is associated with social phobic elements such as being unable to eat in public. Other methods may include relaxation training or distraction while eating, shaping steps that gradually diminish the associated anxiety in order to reestablish reflex swallowing without the patient paying attention to the process.

If the symptom occurs in conjunction with another psychiatric disorder such as depression or panic disorder, treatment of the primary disorder may be adequate in most cases. A few case histories suggest that pseudodysphagia can be effectively treated with drugs that have antipanic effects, such as tricyclic antidepressants, monoamine oxidase inhibitors, and alprazolam. The administering of these drugs should be tried in conjunction with psychological treatments if the former alone has not achieved the desired result.

Prognosis

Several of the patients described in the literature had had long-standing difficulties with weight loss before they sought help, yet treatment was successful. The proportion of patients with this syndrome who recover spontaneously is unknown. The few published case histories and small series suggest that behavior therapy as well as treatment with antipanic drugs is successful in a substantial proportion of patients. Only successful cases, however, are usually submitted for publication; so without reports, larger series estimates of the success rates of treatment are often inaccurate.

Summary and Main Conclusions

Globus

Globus is a sensation of a lump or ball in the throat that, in most cases, disappears temporarily while eating. It should be distinguished from dysphagia—difficulty in swallowing—and from the fear of choking. About 45% of random subjects report that they have experienced globus. The syndrome ranges from the mild and transient to the persistent and distressing. About 3% to 4% of patients in ear, nose, and throat clinics attend because of globus symptoms.

Pathology found in some patients with globus includes gastroesophageal reflux, abnormal contractility of the esophagus, vertebral disease, and malocclusion. One study showed strikingly increased cricopharyngeal sphincter pressure in globus patients, but two studies failed to confirm this finding.

There is conflicting evidence about the cause of globus. The findings suggest that in a small minority of patients, the globus sensation is caused by physical disease or anatomical abnormalities, although there are widely varying estimates on how large this proportion is. In some other patients, coexisting physical pathology is unrelated to the complaint and is an accidental finding.

There are only a few systematic psychological studies on patients with globus. Patients who seek treatment for globus have, on the average, more psychopathology than do other medical patients. There is a consensus in the literature that patients with globus do not have hysterical or histrionic personalities. There is still some controversy about whether the syndrome should be regarded as "hysterical," with most authors concluding that it is not, meaning that it is not a conversion disorder. The psychopathology and psychophysiology of globus appear to be similar to those of somatization (see Chapter 10, this volume). Some of the patients fear or believe that they have cancer.

In a blind study of the treatment of malocclusion, results showed that globus can be abolished in some patients when appropriate occlusion is reestablished. There are several uncontrolled studies of various treatments, including the treatment of coexisting conditions such as gastroesophageal reflux.

In some patients, globus is caused by abnormal contraction of the lower part of the esophagus, the sensation being referred to the neck, with anxiety or other strong emotions being common precipitants. Preoccupation with and attention to the sensation form links in a vicious cycle of fear and selective attention and excessive swallowing. There are probably two syndromes: the first begins with a local irritation or lesion in the throat and consequent excessive swallowing; the second is the classical type of feeling a lump.

After physical disease has been excluded, explanation and reassurance usually constitute adequate treatments. Antacid treatment and other treatments of gastroesophageal reflux may be tried. If the symptoms persist, the patient may benefit from the methods of treatment outlined in Chapter 10.

The prognosis is good in the majority; there is no difficulty in swallowing food, no weight loss, and no evidence of risks to health. In a follow-up of globus patients who had attended an ear, nose, and throat clinic 15 years previously, 10% still had symptoms, 47% had had minor recurrences during the follow-up period, and 43% had remained symptom free.

Fear of Choking

Pseudodysphagia, or fear of choking, differs in several ways from the globus sensation. Globus is usually unrelated to eating, whereas pseudodysphagia is a difficulty in swallowing or an inability to swallow. The disorder may appear in various forms; the most common symptom is the inability to swallow solids. In some patients, there are social phobic features, and these patients' difficulty is typically limited to eating in public. Pseudodysphagia may become disabling and can cause severe loss of weight. The prevalence is not known; it appears to be far less common than that of globus.

In published case histories, many of the patients also experienced other phobic symptoms or other psychiatric disorders such as depression or panic attacks. A substantial proportion of patients date the onset of their symptoms to a traumatic event while eating, such as an episode of choking. Children who have had corrective surgery for cleft palate have more eating difficulties than do their siblings, which suggests that conditioning may have caused the onset of symptoms.

The psychophysiological processes that are responsible for pseudodysphagia are unknown. A plausible explanation is as follows: inhibition of the swallowing reflex occurs at times of fear and is aggravated by dryness of mouth; the idea that the patient may choke induces fear while eating, leading to selective perception of sensations from the throat, which in turn aggravates the fear. By frequent repetition, the associations in this chain become overlearned. It is not known whether conditioned constriction of pharyngeal muscles occurs.

There are several published case histories of patients with pseudodysphagia who were treated successfully by various methods of behavior therapy, including desensitization, aversion relief, electromyographic biofeedback, and shaping. In an uncontrolled study, retraining with the aid of hypnosis was effective in a substantial proportion of patients. There are several case reports and two small series of patients who were treated effectively with antipanic drugs that included tricyclic antidepressants, monoamine oxidase inhibitors, and the minor tranquilizer alprazolam.

The few published case histories and small series suggest that the prognosis of treated pseudodysphagia is good in a substantial proportion of patients. However, because only successful cases are usually submitted for publication, this estimate of success rate of treatment may be inaccurate. The prognosis in untreated patients is unknown.

References

Adams F (transl): The Genuine Works of Hippocrates. London, The Sydenham Society, 1849

Adour KK, Hilsinger RL Jr, Byl FM: Herpes simplex polyganglionitis. Otolaryngol Head Neck Surg 88:270–274, 1980a

Adour KK, Schneider G, Hilsinger RL Jr: Acute superior laryngeal nerve palsy: analysis of 78 cases. Otolaryngol Head Neck Surg 88:418–424, 1980b

American Psychiatric Association: Diagnostic and Statistical Manual of Mental Disorders, 3rd Edition, Revised. Washington, DC, American Psychiatric Association, 1987

Ardran GM: Feeling of a lump in the throat: thoughts of a radiologist. J R Soc Med 75:242–244, 1982

Biesinger E, Schrader M, Weber B: Osteochondrosis of the cervical spine as a cause of globus sensation and dysphagia. HNO 37:33–35, 1989

Black S: Dysphagia of pseudobulbar palsy successfully treated by hypnosis. N Z Med J 91:212–214, 1980

Bonington A, Mahon M, Whitmore I: A histological and histochemical study of the cricopharyngeus muscle in man. J Anat 156:27–37, 1988

Bradley PG, Narula A: Clinical aspects of pseudodysphagia. J Laryngol Otol 101:689–694, 1987

Brown SR, Schwartz JM, Summergrad P, et al: Globus hystericus syndrome responsive to antidepressants. Am J Psychiatry 143:917–918, 1986

Calderelli BD, Andrews AH, Derbyshire AJ: Esophageal motility studies in globus sensation. Ann Otol Rhinol Laryngol 79:1098–1100, 1970

Cerny M, Setka J, Jarolimek M, et al: Self-regulation of esophageal activity. Act Nerv Super (Praha) 30:181–183, 1988

Cohen BR: Emotional considerations in oesophageal diseases, in Emotional Factors in Gastrointestinal Illness. Edited by Linder AE. Amsterdam, Excerpta Medica, 1973, pp 37–44

Cook IJ, Dent J, Collins SM: Measurement of upper esophageal sphincter pressure: effect of acute emotional stress. Gastroenterology 93:526–532, 1987

Cook IJ, Dent J, Collins SM: Upper esophageal sphincter tone and reactivity to stress in patients with a history of globus sensation. Dig Dis Sci 34:672–676, 1989

Di Scipio WJ, Kaslon K: Conditioned dysphagia in cleft palate children after pharyngeal flap surgery. Psychosom Med 44:247–257, 1982

Di Scipio WJ, Kaslon K, Ruben RJ: Traumatically acquired conditioned dysphagia in children. Ann Otol Rhinol Laryngol 87:509–514, 1978

Ferenczi S: The phenomena of hysterical materialization, in Further Contributions to the Theory and Technique of Psychoanalysis (Intl Psychoanalytical Library No 11). Translated by Suttie JI, et al. London, L & V Woolf, 1926, pp 89–104

Flores TC, Cross FS, Jones RD: Abnormal esophageal manometry in globus hystericus. Ann Otol Rhinol Laryngol 90:383–386, 1981

Freeland AP, Ardran GM, Emrys-Roberts E: Globus hystericus and reflux oesophagitis. J Laryngol Otol 88:1025–1031, 1974

Glaser JP, Engel GL: Psychodynamics, psychophysiology, and gastrointestinal symptomatology. Clinics in Gastroenterology 6:507–537, 1977

Gray LP: The relationship of the "inferior constrictor swallow" and "globus hystericus" or the hypopharyngeal syndrome. J Laryngol Otol 97:607–618, 1983

Greenberg DB, Stern TA, Weilburg JB: The fear of choking: three successfully treated cases. Psychosomatics 29:126–129, 1988

Haynes SN: Electromyographic biofeedback treatment of a woman with chronic dysphagia. Biofeedback Self Regul 1:121–126, 1976

Jones CM: Digestive Tract Pain. New York, Macmillan, 1938

Kaplan PR, Evans IM: A case of functional dysphagia treated on the model of fear of fear. J Behav Ther Exp Psychiatry 9:71–72, 1978

Klinger RL, Strang JP: Psychiatric aspects of swallowing disorders. Psychosomatics 28:572–573, 1987

Kramer P, Hollander W: Comparison of experimental esophageal pain with clinical pain of angina pectoris and esophageal disease. Gastroenterology 29:719–743, 1955

Lehtinen V, Puhakka H: A psychosomatic approach to the globus hystericus syndrome. Acta Psychiatr Scand 53:21–28, 1976

Mace C, Ron M, Deahl M, et al: Is globus hystericus? Br J Psychiatry 154:727, 1989

Mair IWS, Schroder KE, Modalsli B, et al: Aetiological aspects of the globus symptom. J Laryngol Otol 88:1033–1040, 1974

Malcomson KG: Radiological findings in globus hystericus. Br J Radiol 39:583–586, 1966

Malcomson KG: Globus hystericus vel pharyngis. J Laryngol Otol 82:219–230, 1968

Merskey H: The importance of hysteria. Br J Psychiatry 149:23–28, 1986

Moloy PH, Charter R: The globus symptom: incidence, therapeutic response, and age and sex relationships. Arch Otolaryngol 108:740–744, 1982

Nagler R, Spiro HM: Serial esophageal motility studies in asymptomatic young subjects. Gastroenterology 41:371–379, 1961

Pratt LW, Tobin WH, Gallagher RA: Globus hystericus: office evaluation by psychological testing with the MMPI. Laryngoscope 86:1540–1551, 1976

Puhakka HJ, Kirveskari P: Globus hystericus: globus syndrome? J Laryngol Otol 102:231–234, 1988

Puhakka HJ, Lehtinen V, Aalto T: Globus hystericus: a psychosomatic disease? J Laryngol Otol 90:1021–1026, 1976

Purcell J: A Treatise of Vapours or Hysteric Fits, 2nd Edition. London, 1707

Rosenthal SH: Letter. Am J Psychiatry 144:529, 1987

Schatzki R: Globus hystericus (globus sensation). N Engl J Med 270:676, 1964

Solyom L, Sookman D: Fear of choking and its treatment. Can J Psychiatry 25:30–34, 1980

Thompson WG, Heaton KW: Heartburn and globus in apparently healthy people. Can Med Assoc J 126:46–48, 1982

Walco GA: A behavioral treatment for difficulty in swallowing pills. Behav Ther Exp Psychiatry 17:127–128, 1986

Watson WC, Sullivan SN: Hypertonicity of the cricopharyngeal sphincter: a cause of globus sensation. Lancet 2:1417–1419, 1974

Watson WC, Sullivan SN, Corke M, et al: Globus and headache: common symptoms of the irritable bowel syndrome. Can Med Assoc J 118:387–388, 1978

Weinstein F: Letter. Am J Psychiatry 144:529, 1987

Weisskopf A: Reflux of esophagitis: a cause of globus. Otolaryngol Head Neck Surg 89:780–782, 1981

Whitehead WE, Schuster MM: Gastrointestinal Disorders. New York, Academic, 1985

Wilson JA, Maran AGD, Pryde A, et al: Globus sensation is not due to gastroesophageal reflux. Clin Otolaryngol 12:271–275, 1987a

Wilson JA, Murray JAM, von Haacke NP: Rigid endoscopy in ENT practice: appraisal of the diagnostic yield in a district general hospital. J Laryngol Otol 101:286–292, 1987b

Wilson JA, Deary IJ, Maran AGD: Is globus hystericus? Br J Psychiatry 153:335–339, 1988

Wilson JA, Deary IJ, Maran AGD: Is globus hystericus (reply). Br J Psychiatry 154:727, 1989

World Health Organization: Draft of the 10th Revision of the International Classification of Diseases. Geneva, World Health Organization, 1988

Chapter 4

Dysphagia and Esophageal Motility Disorders

There are numerous causes of difficulty in swallowing. Fear of choking was discussed in the previous chapter; the present chapter deals with dysphagia and esophageal motility disorders.

Symptoms and Signs

Dysphagia is usually divided into two types: oropharyngeal and esophageal. In *oropharyngeal dysphagia,* the patient complains that the food sticks at the level of the suprasternal notch, and this dysphagia may be associated with nasopharyngeal regurgitation and aspiration. Congenital abnormalities and local pathology usually cause difficulty in swallowing solids only, whereas muscular weakness caused by systemic disease or neurological disease may cause difficulty in swallowing liquids as well.

In *esophageal dysphagia,* the food sticks in the middle or lower sternal area. There may be pain on swallowing, regurgitation of food and fluids, and aspiration. The patient may concurrently complain of heartburn if there is also esophageal reflux such as in peptic strictures or scleroderma. Some of the motility disorders of the esophagus are associated with substernal pain.

Pseudodysphagia was described in the previous chapter. The difficulty is usually limited to solids, and there is no nasopharyngeal regurgitation and no aspiration.

Motor Disorders of the Esophagus

The many reviews of esophageal motility disorder include those by Whitehead and Schuster (1985), Müller-Lissner (1987), Nelson and Castell (1988), Traube and McCallum (1985), and Buchin (1988). A brief summary of the various types of motility disorders of the esophagus follows. More detailed descriptions and controversies about their classification lie beyond the scope of this chapter, and they are discussed in textbooks of medicine and gastroenterology.

There are various kinds of motility disturbances of the esophagus ranging from absent peristalsis to excessive peristalsis. These kinds of disturbances can be combined with abnormal functioning of either the upper or the lower esophageal functions. The manometric findings consist either of nonspecific abnormalities or characteristic syndromes.

Aperistalsis. This condition is the absence of motor activity of the esophagus as determined by motility and manometric studies. It is usually associated with physical diseases such as scleroderma and systemic lupus erythematosus, but it can also occur in elderly individuals. Aperistalsis may be combined with abnormal functioning of the lower esophageal sphincter.

Achalasia of the esophagus. Achalasia is a disorder of motility that consists mainly of an inadequate relaxation of the lower esophageal sphincter causing obstruction, and there is a loss of primary peristalsis in the smooth muscle portion of the esophagus. Dysphagia is initially intermittent. There is often dilation of the esophagus, which has a smooth, tapered distal end. Sometimes the circular muscle of the esophagus is hypertrophied. In vigorous achalasia, contractions of the esophagus resemble diffuse esophageal spasm (see below).

Diffuse esophageal spasm. In this disorder there are multiple intermittent contractions in the distal end of the esophagus that may be either spontaneous or induced by swallowing. These contractions are simultaneous in onset, of long duration, and repetitive. There is often chest pain and dysphagia. Diagnosis is made by manometry.

Nutcracker esophagus. This is a disorder in which manometry shows abnormally high-amplitude peristaltic contractions. There is dysphagia and substernal pain, and particularly cold or hot food may precipitate spasm. There is usually high lower esophageal sphincter pressure, but the sphincter relaxes normally.

Gastroesophageal reflux. Regurgitation of the gastric contents into the esophagus can lead to esophagitis with substernal burning or pain. The symptoms are usually aggravated by recumbency or an increase in abdominal pressure, or an incompetent lower esophageal sphincter. The various contributory causes include an increased gastric volume, acid hypersecretion, bending and lying flat, obesity, pregnancy, ascites, or wearing tight clothes. Regurgitation is sometimes associated with a hiatal hernia, but a hernia is of no significance if it does not cause reflux (Navab and Dexter 1985; Richter and Castell 1982).

Hypertensive lower esophageal sphincter. The resting pressure of the sphincter is increased, but relaxation and peristalsis are normal. Some of the patients with nutcracker esophagus have a hypertensive lower esophageal sphincter (Richter et al. 1989).

Relationship to Other Gastrointestinal Disorders

There are controversies about the way motor disorders are related to one another (Blackwell and Castell 1984). Some of the disorders change their character with the passage of time (Dalton et al. 1988). There is also an association of contraction abnormalities of the esophagus with symptoms of the irritable bowel syndrome, so some of the contraction abnormalities represent a diffuse neuromuscular derangement of the gastrointestinal tract (Clouse and Eckert 1986). This would explain why patients with the irritable bowel syndrome complain of upper gastrointestinal symptoms.

Chest Pain and Esophageal Motor Disorders

Between one quarter and one third of patients who were investigated for cardiac pain were diagnosed to have pain not of cardiac origin, but of motor disorders of the esophagus (Brand et al. 1977; Clouse et al. 1983; Katz et al. 1987). These figures have been challenged because of other causes of cardiac pain such as insufficiency of coronary microcirculation (see Chapter 9, this volume).

In a substantial proportion of patients referred because of noncardiac chest pain, esophageal manometry is abnormal; in others, abnormal motility can be detected by other methods such as videoradiography with barium swallow, radionucleotide transit studies, and acid profusion testing. The most common abnormality detected by such methods is the nutcracker esophagus; others are nonspecific esophageal motility disorder, diffuse esophageal spasm, and, less frequently, achalasia (Cargill et al. 1987; Chobanian et al. 1986; Dupin et al. 1984; Katz et al. 1987). If only one method is used, for example, videoesophagography, a large proportion of abnormalities of motor function can be missed (Benjamin et al. 1983; Chobanian et al. 1986; Linsell et al. 1987).

The type of motor abnormality is associated with symptoms, but the findings are complex and inconsistent across studies, and the correlations are low (Blackwell and Castell 1984). In a group of over 900 patients with noncardiac chest pain, 28% had abnormal esophageal motility disorder, with nutcracker esophagus being the most common. In patients who presented with dysphagia, manometric abnormalities were more common (53%); of these, achalasia and nonspecific esophageal motility disorders comprised 74%, whereas nutcracker esophagus accounted for only 10% (Katz et al. 1987).

There is evidence to suggest that in many cases the pain is not caused by smooth muscle spasm. Clouse et al. (1983) studied nine patients with intermittent chest pain that was believed to be secondary to esophageal spasm. These patients also developed typical pain while being studied with an intraluminal transducer probe placed in the esophagus. No differences in manometric changes were found during periods when the patients reported pain and during control periods when the patients had no pain. The authors concluded that in patients who are suspected of having esophageal spasm as the source of the chest pain, the pain is seldom caused by spasm even when motility abnormalities are found on conventional esophageal manometric studies.

In a subsequent study, Reidel and Clouse (1985) administered a symptom questionnaire to patients referred for manometry. Chest pain did not vary with the number of manometric abnormalities, whereas dysphagia tended to increase in prevalence with such abnormalities. Heartburn was reproduced by acid instillation in less than half of those patients studied. The authors concluded that symptoms are poor predictors of manometric abnormalities.

MacKenzie et al. (1988) found that the rewarming rate of the esophagus after a standardized cold challenge was significantly slower in patients with nutcracker esophagus than in healthy control subjects. The authors expressed the opinion that these results are consistent with the hypothesis that the esophagus is ischemic in these patients because rewarming time in other sites of the body correlates with blood flow.

Distension of the esophagus by means of a balloon causes discomfort or pain. Kramer and Hollander (1955) found that distension at different levels causes different symptoms. When the upper esophagus was distended, there was a close correlation between the area of discomfort and the position of the balloon. "Pressure" was the most common complaint regardless of the position of the balloon; other patients described their discomfort as choking, bloating, or burning.

Edwards (1982) described a syndrome that he termed "tender esophagus." He observed 65 patients who had an abnormal sensitivity to stretch of parts of the esophageal wall. Subsequently, the author found another 35 patients with this syndrome (D. A. W. Edwards, personal communication, 1990). Endoscopy showed mucosa that was normal in appearance and biopsy. The pain simulates a sensation of obstruction, and patients with tender esophagus present with painful dysphagia, living on liquids and sometimes regurgitating food. Descent of an opaque semibolus identifies the site of induction of the pain, and this is confirmed by inflating and deflating a balloon. A liquid diet in these patients is comfortable. The author reported that spontaneous recovery is common, but the duration of the disorder ranges from a few weeks to many years.

Barish et al. (1986) and Richter et al. (1986a) studied esophageal pain perception in patients with esophageal chest pain. Fifty patients with chest pain and negative coronary arteriograms and 30 healthy volunteers participated. A balloon was positioned above the esophageal sphincter and was gradually inflated in a placebo-controlled design. Pain occurred in 56% of the patients and in 20% of the volunteers; pain resolved immediately with decompression of the balloon. Patients experienced pain at significantly lower degrees of distension. Intraesophageal acid perfusion and intravenously administered edrophonium chloride reproduced the pain in a smaller proportion of patients and thus were less sensitive provocative tests for esophageal chest pain. During pain, esophageal contractions above the balloon and esophageal tone did not differ significantly between the groups. The authors concluded that the mechanism of chest pain in these patients may be related to lowered pain threshold to distension that is independent of esophageal contractions.

When heart disease and esophageal motility disorders occur together, only the results of thorough laboratory evaluations allow an estimate of the contribution of the two pathologies to the chest pain. Particularly, the coexistence of ischemic heart disease can pose problems in diagnosis and management (Lee et al. 1985).

Prevalence

The exact prevalence of esophageal motility disorders is unknown. Esophageal motility disorders, often presenting with chest pain, are common. It has been estimated that between 25,000 and 75,000 of new cases are diagnosed yearly (Richter and Castell 1984).

Psychological Studies

Whitehead and Schuster (1985), Richter et al. (1986b), and several other authors have reviewed the relationship among psychological stress, other psychological factors, and esophageal motility. Earlam (1975) and Henderson (1980) have noted that the esophageal spasm occurs more frequently when the patient is tired or anxious.

Numerous early studies—for example, Faulkner (1940) and Jacobson (1927)—have shown that stress from interviews can cause esophageal spasm. Some of the important studies are summarized in this section.

Wolf and Almy (1949) studied 14 patients who complained that swallowed food seemed to stick in the retrosternal region. The authors examined these patients by means of barium swallows. Cardiospasm, an obstruction at the lower end of the esophagus with hypermotility in the lower two thirds, became more pronounced during noxious stimuli such as heat and cold and emotionally charged topics, while relative security and relaxation were associated with diminutions. The patients' symptoms were correlated with periods of stresses in their lives. (Cardiospasm is no longer regarded as a diagnostic entity; some of these patients may have had vigorous achalasia.)

Rubin et al. (1961) recorded changes in motility and pressure in the esophagus of five volunteers who had no major psychiatric difficulties. Each subject was studied three times, and they were encouraged to talk about their problems. In two of the subjects there was a significant association of nonpropulsive activity with emotionally charged topics in all three interviews. These responses tended to recur repetitively and continuously as long as these subjects remained involved in the discussion of the highly charged material. One subject showed such association only in two of the interviews and another, only in the first interview, and the fifth subject did not show such an association.

Stacher et al. (1979b) carried out a study in 16 healthy subjects measuring esophageal pressure in response to acoustic stimuli. They found that nonpropulsive esophageal contractions were evoked by intense acoustic stimuli regardless of the rise time and the signal content of the stimuli. The authors concluded that contractile responses of the esophagus to intense exogenous stimuli are normal reactions in healthy individuals. In another study, Stacher et al. (1979a) found that a minimum intensity of an acoustic stimulus was required in order to produce tertiary esophageal responses. On repetitive stimulation, a habituation effect occurred; there was a significant decrease in the number and amplitude of esophageal responses.

Cook et al. (1987) found that in healthy individuals experimental stress of a dichotic listening task increased upper esophageal sphincter pressure from control levels. This increase coincided with alterations in heart rate, blood pressure, and skin conductance.

Richter et al. (1986a) administered the Millon Behavioral Health Inventory (MBHI) to 20 patients with recurrent noncardiac chest pain and a nutcracker esophagus and to 20 patients with the irritable bowel syndrome. Twenty patients with benign symptomatic abnormalities (peptic strictures or Schatzki rings) served as one of the control groups; these patients had various symptoms such as dysphagia or regurgitation that were troubling enough to seek medical care. There were two additional control groups of 20 healthy subjects, each with normal manometric findings.

The MBHI consists of 150 items divided into 20 scales that are based on clusters compiled from a consensus of experts. The results of six of these scales were examined in the present study: chronic tension, recent stress, somatic anxiety, premorbid pessimism, future despair, and gastrointestinal susceptibility. The last scale is highly correlated with the somatic anxiety scale ($r = .91$); the authors expressed the opinion that this scale measures many of the same patient attributes as does the somatic anxiety scale, but that the two are not equivalent to each other. The authors claim that the MBHI has construct validity supported by a factor analysis.

Patients with irritable bowel syndrome and nutcracker esophagus scored significantly higher on the gastrointestinal susceptibility scale and the somatic anxiety scale than did subjects in the control groups. These patients were also seeking more medical care. The difference between the nutcracker esophagus patients and patients in the structural abnormality group approached significance. On the scales of chronic tension, recent stress, and premorbid pessimism, the scores of the patients with irritable bowel syndrome were significantly greater than those of all other groups, whereas on the future despair scale, the scores of the patients with irritable bowel syndrome were significantly greater than the scores from only two of the healthy control groups.

Clouse and Lustman (1983) found that among 50 patients referred for esophageal motility testing, 25 had various esophageal contraction abnormalities. The patients were divided into three groups. Group 1 consisted of patients with the following contraction abnormalities: increased mean wave duration and amplitude, increased frequency of abnormal motor responses, and presence of triple-peaked waves; these were further subdivided into subgroups according to the patterns observed. Group 2 were patients with aperistalsis—that is, no normal peristaltic sequences were observed. The patients in Group 3 were unclassified; the tracings in these patients for various reasons could not be further classified. Diagnoses were carried out independently using the Diagnostic Interview Schedule. Of the patients in group 1, 84% (21 patients) had a lifetime prevalence of psychiatric diagnoses; 31% of patients with normal manometric findings and 33% of patients in other categories of esophageal motility disorder had such diagnoses. The most common diagnoses were depression (13), anxiety disorder (16), and somatization disorder (5). The Social Adjustment Rating Scale, Beck Depression Inventory, and Visual Analogue Scales of anxiety and depression did not discriminate significantly among the manometric tracings. Some patients had more than one diagnosis. The study showed that a history of psychiatric illness was in fact associated with a specific cluster of esophageal abnormalities.

Clouse and Lustman (1989) administered in a subsequent study the Symptom Checklist-90–Revised (SCL 90-R) to 86 patients with contraction abnormalities, 14 with aperistalsis, and 36 with normal peristaltic patterns. There were only minor differences among the groups, and most of these differences failed to reach significance levels. Thus, self-ratings of recent emotional distress did not effectively differentiate those patients with esophageal symptoms and contraction abnormalities from those patients who had symptoms but other manometric diagnoses.

Anderson et al. (1989) compared esophageal pressure in patients with non-cardiac chest pain and healthy volunteers. Among 19 patients with chest pain, 10 had nutcracker esophagus, and 9 had normal baseline manometry. The stressors administered were intermittent bursts of white noise and difficult discrimination tasks interposed with unsolvable cognitive problems. The patients were administered the abbreviated state anxiety scale portion of the Spielberger State-Trait Anxiety Inventory and were rated by observers at the end of each baseline and stressor period. The motility tracings were coded and read by an investigator who did not know the experimental condition from which the tracing was made. Esophageal contraction amplitudes, self-rated state anxiety, and observer-rated anxiety were significantly greater during stressors than during the baseline period. All patients showed significantly greater responses during the cognitive problem solving than during the noise stressor (Figure 4-1).

Patients with nutcracker esophagus showed greater increase in contraction amplitude during problem solving than did control subjects, whereas measurements of chest pain patients with normal baseline manometry were not significantly different from those of control subjects. Four of the patients with chest pain developed high-amplitude contractions during the cognitive problem stressor; however, this response was not observed among the control subjects.

There were no significant changes in heart rate. Changes in systolic blood pressure from baseline to stressor periods were greater in patients than in control subjects. Only one patient experienced pain during the stressor studies; he had normal baseline manometry, and there were only minimal increases in esophageal pressure. In contrast to previous studies (Rubin et al. 1961; Stacher et al. 1979a, 1979b; Wolf and Almy 1949), Anderson et al. did not find an increased frequency of nonpropulsive (simultaneous) contractions in response to stressful stimuli. The authors proposed that various factors may be responsible for these differences, including a more reliable procedure for measuring nonpropulsive contractions.

The authors emphasized that the changes in contraction amplitudes were small and that the stressor was not severe enough to change heart rate. In parallel with other studies, there was no correlation of pressure changes with chest pain. In a previous study by the same authors (Peters et al. 1988), abnormal esophageal motility had been observed to have occurred subsequent to the onset of chest pain, rather than preceeding it. The authors concluded that an increase in contraction amplitude is a primary esophageal response to stress and that the nutcracker esophagus may be an epiphenomenon resulting from an exaggerated response to various stressors, including chest pain.

Diagnosis of Dysphagia

The pharyngeal causes include anatonomical abnormalities such as a congenital web, aberrant vessels, Zenker's diverticulum, local pathology such as carcinoma of the pharnyx and eye strictures, and muscular dysfunction such as amyotrophic lateral sclerosis, multiple sclerosis, bulbar and pseudobulbar palsy, myasthenia gravis, steroid myopathy, thyrotoxic myopathy, and cricopharyngeal achalasia.

The pharyngeal causes of dysphagia were summarized in Chapter 3. The numerous physical diseases that cause dysphagia of esophageal origin include carcinoma, peptic stricture, a lower esophageal ring, scleroderma, various infections such as *Candida albicans* and herpes, and esophagitis caused by drugs such as tetracycline, aspirin, or ferrous sulfate.

Some patients with mitral valve prolapse (MVP) have chest pain. In one study a substantial proportion of patients who had chest pains with MVP also had esophageal motility disorders, whereas in patients with MVP without pain, no such disorders were found. These findings suggest that in a substantial proportion of patients with MVP and chest pain, the pain is caused by abnormal esophageal motility and not by MVP (Koch et al. 1989).

If emotions induce or exacerbate a motility disorder causing symptoms, in DSM-III-R (American Psychiatric Association 1987) the disorder is classified under "psychological factors affecting physical conditions" (316.00), and the corresponding code in the ICD-10 draft (World Health Organization 1988) is

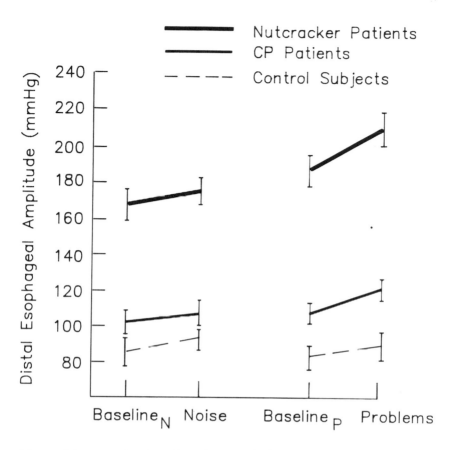

Figure 4-1. Mean distal esophageal amplitude (±SE) in mm Hg for each stressor and baseline period for the groups of 10 nutcracker esophagus patients, nine chest pain (CP) patients with normal baseline manometry, and 20 healthy control subjects (Anderson et al. 1989). Reprinted from Anderson et al. 1989, with permission from the author and Plenum Publishing Corporation. Copyright 1989, Plenum.

F45.31. If emotions are unrelated to disordered motility, the disorder should not have a psychiatric classification.

Treatment

Various treatments have been proposed in esophageal motility disorders. These have included drugs, bouginage, various surgical operations, and psychological treatments (Buchin 1988; Nelson and Castell 1988; Traube and McCallum 1985).

Drug Treatment

Traditionally, anticholinergic drugs have been used in the treatment of motility disorders, but, to my knowledge, there are no controlled studies that have evaluated the efficacy of these drugs. Animal studies have shown that calcium channel blockers decrease lower esophageal sphincter pressure and inhibit contraction amplitude and duration (Andersson 1986). In a single-dose placebo-controlled study, Richter et al. (1984) compared diltiazem in various doses in 10 patients with nutcracker esophagus and in 5 healthy volunteers. Amplitude and duration of peristaltic contractions decreased in the patients, but not in the volunteers. The difference between the effects of drug and placebo, however, did not reach significance because placebo also had a substantial effect. Richter et al. (1985) examined the effect of nifedipine, another calcium channel blocker, on contraction of the esophagus in 5 volunteers and 10 patients with nutcracker esophagus. The distal amplitude decreased significantly in the control subjects and in the patients, and this agent also had a significant dose-dependent depressant effect on distal duration; this decrease showed a plasma-level response correlation. Nasrallah et al. (1985) performed a crossover study of orally administered nifedipine and placebo in patients with primary esophageal motor disorders ($n = 20$), 10 of whom had a hypertensive lower esophageal sphincter. The chest pain or dysphagia improved significantly with nifedipine compared with placebo. Richter et al. (1987) examined the effect of orally administered nifedipine in 20 patients with noncardiac chest pain and nutcracker esophagus in a 14-day double-blind crossover study. Nifedipine significantly decreased esophageal contraction, amplitude, and duration, and also lowered esophageal sphincter pressure, but was no better than placebo in the relief of chest pain as assessed by patient diaries. The authors commented that the patients improved on long-term follow-up and decreased the use of drugs and physician visits for chest pain. There was a poor correlation between the decrease in contraction pressure and improvement in chest pain; the authors suggested that identification of the esophagus as the cause of the chest pain coupled with supportive intervention may be more effective in reducing visits to doctors than the specific effects of the drug in improving the patient's pain. Davies et al. (1987) found no significant effects of nifedipine on chest pain in a placebo-controlled crossover study with 8 patients.

The treatment of gastroesophageal reflux differs from that of motility disorders. Apart from decreasing reflux by simple methods such as not sleeping flat and avoiding large meals, histamine (H_2) blockers improve symptoms of reflux. Of these, ranitidine has been shown to be effective in several studies (Robertson et al. 1987; Sherbaniuk et al. 1984; Sontag et al. 1987).

Comment. The controlled studies with nifedipine show conflicting results, with one study showing improvement in chest pain that was superior to that of placebo, whereas in others no such difference could be demonstrated. There is, however, evidence that nifedipine decreases amplitude of esophageal contractions in healthy individuals as well as in subjects with motility disorders. There is, however, poor correlation between the decrease in amplitude and relief from chest pain. No definite conclusions can be reached from the studies to date. Judging from similarly conflicting data, it seems likely that some patients will get relief from chest pain with nifedipine, and perhaps relief from the effects of other disorders using calcium channel blockers (perhaps mainly those patients who have microvascular angina), whereas the effects of nifedipine will be no better than those of placebo in a substantial proportion of patients. The long-term effects of calcium channel blockers on esophageal motility disorders cannot be assessed from the available studies.

Psychological Treatments and Psychotropic Drugs

Jacobson (1927), who introduced the method of progressive muscular relaxation into medicine, described two cases of chest pain treated by his method. (This method was subsequently incorporated by Wolpe [1958] into his technique of systematic desensitization for the treatment of neuroses.)

The first patient had chest pain that coincided with increased pressure in the esophagus as detected by an inflated balloon. Within 1 hour of progressive muscular relaxation, the pain disappeared: "as he [the subject] became trained to habitual relaxation in the course of weeks or months, the subjective symptoms diminished or disappeared and the roentgen-ray examination revealed no spasm" (p. 437).

The second case was a 19-year-old university student who had daily severe pain in the epigastrium and in whom "esophageal spasm was plainly revealed as the source of the spasm by fluoroscopy" (p. 437). Pain coincided with esophageal spasm as revealed by an inflated balloon. After treatment with progressive muscular relaxation three times a week, the patient learned to relax his esophagus. Jacobson noted that "[a]fter 6 months, pain was reduced to about one half of its original duration and severity" (p. 438). Fluoroscopic tests no longer revealed spasm.

Ward et al. (1985) examined the outcome of patients who had chest pain and in whom cardiac pain had been excluded. The patients were divided into two groups. The first group included those patients in whom esophageal disease had been definitely identified; these were then subdivided into those who remembered that they had been told and others who did not remember having been told. The remainder of the patients, forming the second group, were judged to have chest pain for which neither a cardiac nor a definite esophageal cause had been found. The patients in whom esophageal disease had been identified and who remembered having been told had a significantly smaller proportion of those who believed that the pain came from their heart. In addition, fewer felt disabled by their pain and fewer attended physicians because of their pain. The authors concluded that reassurance may represent a crucial aspect of therapy once the diagnosis of esophageal chest pain has been identified. No such reassurance could be given to the patients of chest pain of unknown origin.

Latimer (1981) reported a case history of a female patient with severe diffuse esophageal spasm. She was treated with relaxation training, after which the spasm decreased in frequency. During a biofeedback session, the author noted that when the patient swallowed twice in rapid succession, the symptoms of spasms at the lower esophageal sphincter decreased. After treatment, manometry continued to show diffuse esophageal spasm, but the patient was able to prevent dysphagia and pain by having acquired new skills.

Shabsin et al. (1988) reported a female patient with vigorous achalasia who had chest pain and dysphagia for 12 years. This patient had previously been treated with pneumatic dilation, myotomy, and various drugs. She was treated by a combination of behavioral and psychotherapeutic strategies. Manometric tracings remained unchanged; however, there was a complete remission of symptoms.

There are a few published case histories of treatment of dysphagia with hypnosis (Klumbies 1977; Langen 1972). Cerny et al. (1988) treated with hypnosis a series of 30 patients having achalasia and two patients having diffuse esophageal spasm. The selection of patients (choosing those who appeared to be susceptible to hypnosis) and the method of treatment are summarized in Chapter 3 of the present volume (see p. 67). At the end of treatment, 55% showed "significant or full improvement." In at least 28% of the patients the results were maintained without severe relapse. In several of the patients and in four of the five healthy control subjects, a prompt change of LES activity was observed in response to the self-induced signal.

Gastroesophageal reflux depends on anatomical factors and is not a psychophysiological disorder. Schuster et al. (1973) examined the effects of biofeedback on gastroesophageal reflux. Six patients who had esophageal reflux and three healthy volunteers learned to increase the pressure in the lower esophageal sphincter. This finding suggests that some patients may be able to learn to increase lower esophageal pressure and to decrease reflux.

There are no controlled studies of psychological treatments or biofeedback of primary motor disorders of the esophagus, only a few case histories. Explanation and reassurance constitute adequate treatment in most patients. Training in systematic desensitization has been used; it is an entirely safe and inexpensive treatment and should be the next treatment of choice.

Clouse et al. (1987) carried out a controlled study of administration of a low dose of trazodone (100–150 mg/day). Patients on trazodone reported significantly greater improvement and were less distressed than those on placebo; however, manometric changes during the course of the trial were not influenced by treatment or by clinical response. Remarkable reduction in ratings of chest pain was reported by both treatment groups. The authors emphasize that manometric abnormalities in these patients were not solely responsible for the symptoms and suggested that low-dose trazodone therapy could be of benefit in the management of these patients.

Surgical Treatment and Bouginage

There are several studies of myotomy in the treatment of primary motor disorders of the esophagus (Brown et al. 1987; Henderson 1987; Jamieson et al. 1984). Henderson et al. (1987) followed up 34 patients for 5 years or longer who had been treated with myotomy for diffuse esophageal spasm. Of these patients, 82% were eating without dysphagia and spontaneous pain, and 6% had mild dysphagia. The authors claim that good results have been achieved in 94% of patients on follow-up from 5 to 10 years. Jamieson et al. (1984) reported similar results of myotomy in treating achalasia, and Traube et al. (1987) also reported similar results in four patients with severe nutcracker esophagus. Various other successful surgical procedures have been reported (Wright and Cuschieri 1987).

Bouginage has been recommended for patients with painful esophageal motility disorders. In eight patients in whom either therapeutic bouginage was performed or a "placebo bouginage" with a smaller-sized bougie was used, no differences could be shown between the two (Winters et al. 1984). This study may, however, have been too small to evaluate the effect of this treatment. The authors concluded that the close physician-patient interaction may have been more important than the actual size of the bougie.

Case History

D.B. is a 66-year-old professional woman who became widowed 3 years previously. She had a stressful life; her father suffered from recurrent depression and committed suicide when the patient was 22. The patient regarded herself as anxious and excessively worried most of her life. She had had psychoanalytical psychotherapy on two occasions.

Throughout her adult life she had pain and discomfort in the epigastrium, and sometimes she had symptoms suggestive of an irritable bowel syndrome with diarrhea. For the past 4 years she also had lower sternal chest pain. When the pain started, no cardiac cause was found, and manometry showed diffuse esophageal spasm. Some of her symptoms, particularly the epigastric discomfort, she associated with worry, mainly when she had some cause to worry about her children. She always had regarded herself as highly anxious and overly conscientious. Clinical assessment and the Symptom Rating Test showed her to be moderately anxious but not depressed.

The patient wanted to try medication because she believed that she had had adequate psychotherapy in the past. Because she also had symptoms of an irritable bowel syndrome, I treated her initially with amitriptyline. The patient could not tolerate doses higher than 30 mg because the drug made her too sedated. This dose relieved, to a large extent, her diarrhea and intestinal symptoms and, to a lesser extent, the epigastric discomfort and chest pain. I changed the medication to imipramine, but therapeutic serum levels also caused side effects; she could tolerate 50 mg at night, which appeared to relieve episodes of anxiety. Desipramine also diminished her intestinal symptoms and, to a lesser extent, her epigastric discomfort and chest pain. I treated her next with progressive muscular relaxation, which seemed to improve her symptoms further. She later agreed that she might benefit from supportive psychotherapy, which she continued weekly for 1 year. All her symptoms improved with the passage of time. Her bowel symptoms became rare and only slight. She still had epigastric discomfort, and chest pain came on at times that she found to be stressful, but both conditions became less frequent and less severe.

The patient appeared to have benefited from psychiatric treatment, because she claimed that she felt better than she had most of her adult life. It is not possible to judge which of the ingredients of the various treatments had contributed to the improvement.

Prognosis

The results of studies on prognosis vary with the criteria and length of followup. Ward et al. (1985) sent a questionnaire to 119 patients who had been referred for manometry 12 to 43 months previously. Over 86% of the patients still had recurrent pain. Patients in whom an esophageal cause for the noncardiac chest pain had been identified had a better prognosis (in that 30% reported they were disabled) than did patients with noncardiac chest pain for which no definite esophageal cause had been found (50% disabled). Burns et al. (1985) found that in some patients, there was a spontaneous resolution of chest pain, and pain decreased in the remainder on a follow-up of over 4 years and rarely interfered with daily activities. Richter and Castell (1987) concluded that failure of all regimens, including drugs, psychotherapy, and reassurance, is quite unusual.

Discussion

In a review of swallowing disorders, Stacher et al. (1979a, 1979b) argued against the contribution of emotional stress to abnormal esophageal motility and claimed that it is not justifiable to label dysphagic symptoms, achalasia, or esophageal spasm as psychosomatic disorders. He also recommended that these patients should not be treated by psychotherapy, but by appropriate surgical and medical means. Cohen (1973) concluded that the psychological factors in diffuse esophageal spasms were trivial.

Overall studies do show an association of stress with esophageal contractions and at least some of the motility disorders. Patients who have chest pain and abnormal contractility have a substantially larger percentage of lifetime prevalence of psychiatric diagnoses (made by observers who are unaware of the results of manometric studies) than do patients with chest pain and normal manometric results. Patients with nutcracker esophagus show greater increase in contraction amplitude while solving difficult cognitive problems, or while being subjected to other stressors, than do control subjects.

Psychological inventories and scales have yielded conflicting results. Richter et al. (1986b) administered the MBHI to patients with nutcracker esophagus and found higher scores on self-rating scales that measure anxiety, depression, and somatic concerns than were found in control subjects, including patients with structural abnormalities of the esophagus.

Clouse and Lustman (1983) administered the Beck Depression Inventory and Visual Analogue Scales of anxiety and depression, and these did not discriminate between patients with chest symptoms who had manometric abnormalities and patients without such abnormalities. In their subsequent study, Clouse and Lustman (1989) found that the SCL-90-R also largely failed to discriminate between such groups.

The authors suggested various possibilities that explain their conflicting results. Because lifetime prevalence of psychiatric diagnosis, but not current distress as measured by self-rating scales, discriminated between these groups, a psychiatric disorder may have initiated the esophageal motility disorder, which persisted, whereas the psychiatric disorder may have waned. (Fewer patients in their study had a *current* psychiatric disorder.) The authors studied patients with various manometric abnormalities, whereas the patients in Richter et al.'s study (see above) were limited to those with nutcracker esophagus. Richter et al. have suggested that the MBHI is more suitable than standard psychological inventories; there are substantial differences among rating and self-rating scales in sensitivity—that is, in the property to discriminate between groups or between the effects of treatments—and the scales in Clouse and Lustman's studies may have been less sensitive (Kellner et al. 1978). The control groups in Clouse and Lustman's studies may have shown abnormal illness behavior, and patients with this behavior tend to show psychological distress (see Chapter 10, pp. 210–211, this volume).

The studies that show psychopathology to be associated with esophageal motility disorders were carried out in patients who attended for diagnosis or treatment because of chest pain. These patients may have been self-selected or selectively referred for esophageal motility evaluations. To my knowledge, there are no published psychological studies of subjects with these disorders who have not sought treatment. Moreover, in most of the studies summarized herein, the pain was judged to be not of cardiac origin, but cardiac causes such as microvascular angina (see Chapter 9, this volume) had not been excluded by the use of current diagnostic methods.

Thus, there is an association between noncardiac chest pain and esophageal motility disorders, yet several studies have shown that pain and contractions do not coincide. The source of chest pain at times of stress or chest pain in psychiatric patients has not been definitely determined; this pain is likely to be caused by a low pain threshold or perhaps esophageal ischemia.

Apart from one study with trazodone, there have been, to my knowledge, no controlled studies of psychotropic drugs. Judging by the effects of tricyclic antidepressants in treatment of the irritable bowel syndrome, the high proportion of patients with noncardiac chest pain who are depressed, and the antidepressant as well as antianxiety effects of tricyclic antidepressants, it might be worthwhile to try the effects of this class of drugs.

There are several reviews in the literature on the effects of surgery in primary esophageal motor disorders, and the authors claim good results (Brown et al. 1987; Henderson 1987). Blackwell and Castell (1984) concluded that, in view of the good prognosis, the need for these treatments arises only rarely.

Summary and Main Conclusions

In 10% to 30% of patients who are investigated for cardiac pain and in whom no cardiac abnormality is found, motility disorders may be detected in the esophagus. Disorders encountered include aperistalsis, achalasia, diffuse esophageal spasm, nutcracker esophagus, hypertensive lower esophageal sphincter, and gastrointestinal reflux. In some patients, it takes elaborate laboratory investigations to determine the kind of esophageal motility disorder. There is evidence to suggest that these disorders are not all distinct and may change their character with the passage of time.

Dysphagia is associated with manometric abnormalities of the esophagus. Some abnormalities (most commonly the nutcracker esophagus) are associated with chest pain. Although there is a statistical association between chest pain and esophageal motor abnormalities, chest pain and contractions do not usually coincide. In many of the studies of chest pain, some of the causes of cardiac pain such as microvascular angina were not excluded by current diagnostic methods.

Several studies have examined the relationship of esophageal motility and psychological factors. Measurable changes in contraction of the esophagus can be demonstrated in the laboratory with stressful stimuli such as complicated cognitive tasks. Patients with abnormal manometric findings who complain of chest pain have a significantly larger proportion of lifetime prevalence of psychiatric diagnoses than do patients with chest pain who have normal manometric findings. Psychological tests that measured psychopathology in patients with chest pain and esophageal motor abnormalities have yielded conflicting findings when the results were compared with those of control groups, including patients who had symptoms due to esophageal disease. There are, to date, too few studies to reach definite conclusions on the reasons for these discrepancies; the scales used may not have been equally suitable or current distress may have been associated only with certain kinds of motility disorder.

Lifetime prevalence of psychiatric disorders is higher in patients with motility disorders than in other subjects, but current distress as measured with self-rating scales is not. The psychiatric disorder may have initiated the motility disorder, which then persisted; conversely, the esophageal dysfunction may have led to introspection and anxiety. The psychopathology was found in patients with motor abnormalities who sought treatment for chest pain, but the findings may have been biased by patients' self-selection. There are no published psychological studies of subjects with these abnormalities who did not seek treatment.

The source of chest pain at times of stress has not been determined. One study has suggested that the pain may be caused by esophageal ischemia, because rewarming after cooling takes longer in patients with nutcracker esophagus than in healthy control subjects. Another study has suggested that an increase in contraction amplitude is a primary esophageal response that can occur in response to various stressors, including chest pain. Two studies showed a subgroup of patients who had a low threshold for esophageal pain in response to distention by a balloon (i.e., a "tender esophagus").

There are no controlled studies of psychological treatments of esophageal motor abnormalities. In an uncontrolled study of achalasia, treatment with hypnosis led to improvement in about one half of the patients; in about one quarter, improvement or recovery was maintained on follow-up. There are only a few published case histories of psychological treatments of or biofeedback in esophageal motility disorders. Explanation and reassurance constitute adequate treatment for the majority of patients. The few case histories suggest that progressive muscular relaxation has perhaps helped some patients.

Various drug treatments have been used in the treatment of motility disorders. Many patients respond to placebo, which confounds the evaluation of specific drug effects. Results from the studies with nifedipine are conflicting; in a clinical study, nifedipine was superior to placebo in some patients, but not in others; overall, the evidence suggests that nifedipine is an effective treatment in some patients. Other calcium channel blockers have been recommended, but there are, to date, no adequate controlled studies. In a controlled study of trazodone in patients with chest pain and esophageal motility disorders, the patients' pain became less severe, but trazodone had no effect on manometric abnormalities.

Bouginage has been recommended in patients with severe and painful esophageal motility disorders. In one controlled study, both groups improved, but there was no difference between therapeutic bouginage and a placebo procedure. Good results have been claimed in uncontrolled studies of myotomy in carefully selected cases of severe motility disorders of the esophagus, and the results were maintained on follow-up. In view of the good prognosis for the majority of patients with these disorders, the need for surgery arises only rarely.

The treatment of gastroesophageal reflux differs from that of other motility disorders. Apart from decreasing reflux by various methods, such as not sleeping flat and avoiding large meals, H_2-receptor antagonists improve symptoms of reflux; for example, ranitidine was found to be effective in several studies. Gastroesophageal reflux is not a psychosomatic disorder; a small uncontrolled study has suggested that the tone of the lower esophageal sphincter may be improved with biofeedback. However, it is unknown whether biofeedback can diminish reflux.

References

American Psychiatric Association: Diagnostic and Statistical Manual of Mental Disorders, 3rd Edition, Revised. Washington, DC, American Psychiatric Association, 1987

Anderson KO, Dalton CB, Bradley LA, et al: Stress induces alteration of esophageal pressures in healthy volunteers and non-cardiac chest pain patients. Dig Dis Sci 34:83–91, 1989

Andersson KE: Calcium channel blockers and motility disorders of the esophagus. Acta Pharmacol Toxicol 58 (suppl 2):201–204, 1986

Barish CF, Castell DO, Richter JE: Graded esophageal balloon distention: a new provocative test for noncardiac chest pain. Dig Dis Sci 31:1292–1298, 1986

Benjamin SB, Richter JE, Cordova CM, et al: Prospective manometric evaluation with pharmacologic provocation of patients with suspected esophageal motility dysfunction. Gastroenterology 84:893–901, 1983

Blackwell JN, Castell DO: Oesophageal chest pain: a point of view. Gut 25:1–6, 1984

Brand DL, Martin D, Pope CE II: Esophageal manometrics in patients with angina-like chest pain. American Journal of Digestive Diseases 22:300–304, 1977

Brown M, Taxier MS, May ES: Esophageal myotomy and treatment of "nutcracker esophagus." Am J Gastroenterol 82:1331–1333, 1987

Buchin PJ: Swallowing disorders. Otolaryngol Clin North Am 21:663–676, 1988

Burns RW, Kellum WC, Bienvenu L, et al: Esophageal motor disorders and atypical chest pain: long-term clinical follow-up (abstract). Am J Gastroenterol 80:833A, 1985

Cargill G, Aumont MC, Juliard JM, et al: Esophageal motility in cases of chest pain with normal coronarography. Ann Med Intern 138:407–410, 1987

Cerny M, Setka J, Jarolimek M, et al: Self-regulation of esophageal activity. Act Nerv Super (Praha) 30:181–182, 1988

Chobanian S, Benjamin SB, Curtis DJ, et al: Systematic esophageal evaluation of patients with noncardiac chest pain. Arch Intern Med 146:1505–1508, 1986

Clouse RE, Eckert TC: Gastrointestinal symptoms of patients with esophageal contraction abnormalities. Dig Dis Sci 31:236–240, 1986

Clouse RE, Lustman PJ: Psychiatric illness and contraction abnormalities of the esophagus. N Engl J Med 309:1337–1342, 1983

Clouse RE, Lustman PJ: Value of recent psychological symptoms in identifying patients with esophageal contraction abnormalities. Psychosom Med 51:570–576, 1989

Clouse RE, Staiano A, Landau DW, et al: Manometric findings during spontaneous chest pain in patients with presumed esophageal "spasms." Gastroenterology 85:395–402, 1983

Clouse RE, Lustman PJ, Eckert TC, et al: Low-dose trazodone for symptomatic patients with esophageal contraction abnormalities: a double-blind, placebo-controlled trial. Gastroenterology 92:1027–1036, 1987

Cohen BR: Emotional considerations in esophageal disease, in Emotional Factors in Gastrointestinal Illness. Edited by Lindner AE. Amsterdam, Excerpta Medica, 1973, pp 37–44

Cook IJ, Dent J, Shannon S, et al: Measurement of upper esophageal sphincter pressure. Gastroenterology 93:526–532, 1987

Dalton CB, Castell DO, Richter JE: The changing faces of the nutcracker esophagus. Am J Gastroenterol 83:623–628, 1988

Davies HA, Lewis MJ, Rhodes J, et al: Trial of nifedipine for prevention of oesophageal spasm. Digestion 36:81–83, 1987

Dupin B, Bory M, Moro P, et al: Esophageal spasm: a common cause of spontaneous precordial pain. Arch Mal Coeur 77:1390–1396, 1984

Earlam R: Clinical Tests of Esophageal Function. New York, Grune & Stratton, 1975

Edwards DAW: "Tender oesophagus": a new syndrome (abstract). Gut 23:A919, 1982

Faulkner WB Jr: Severe esophageal spasm: an evaluation of suggestion-therapy as determined by means of the esophagoscope. Psychosom Med 2:139–140, 1940

Henderson RD: Motor Disorders of the Esophagus, 2nd Edition. Baltimore, MD, Williams & Wilkins, 1980

Henderson RD: Esophageal motor disorders. Surg Clin North Am 67:455–474, 1987

Henderson RD, Ryder D, Marryatt G: Extended esophageal myotomy and short total fundoplication hernia repair in diffuse esophageal spasm: five-year review in 34 patients. Ann Thorac Surg 43:25–31, 1987

Jacobson E: Spastic esophagus and mucous colitis: etiology and treatment by progressive relaxation. Arch Intern Med 39:433–445, 1927

Jamieson WRE, Miyagishima RT, Carr DM, et al: Surgical management of primary motor disorders of the esophagus. Am J Surg 148:36–42, 1984

Katz PO, Dalton CB, Richter JE, et al: Esophageal testing of patients with noncardiac chest pain or dysphagia: results of three years' experience with 1,161 patients. Ann Intern Med 106:593–597, 1987

Kellner R, Sheffield BE, Simpson GM: The value of self-rating scales in drug trials with nonpsychotic patients. Prog Neuropsychopharmacol Biol Psychiatry 2:197–205, 1978

Klumbies G: Psychotherapie in der Inneren und Allgemein-medizin. Leipzig, S Mirzel Verlag, 1977

Koch KL, Davidson WR Jr, Day FP, et al: Esophageal dysfunction and chest pain in patients with mitral valve prolapse: a prospective study utilizing provocative testing during esophageal manometry. Am J Med 86:32–38, 1989

Kramer P, Hollander W: Comparison of experimental esophageal pain with clinical pain of angina pectoris and esophageal disease. Gastroenterology 29:719–743, 1955

Langen D: Kompendium der medizinischen Hypnose. London, S Karger, 1972

Latimer PR: Biofeedback and self-regulation in the treatment of diffuse esophageal spasm: a single-case study. Biofeedback Self Regul 6:181–189, 1981

Lee MG, Sullivan SN, Watson WC, et al: Chest pain: esophageal, cardiac, or both? Am J Gastroenterol 80:320–324, 1985

Linsell J, Owen WJ, Mason RC, et al: Edrophonium provocation test in the diagnosis of diffuse oesophageal spasm. Br J Surg 74:688–689, 1987

MacKenzie J, Belch J, Land D, et al: Oesophageal ischaemia in motility disorders associated with chest pain. Lancet 2:592–595, 1988

Müller-Lissner S: Motility disorders of the esophagus. Leber Magen Darm 17:19–27, 1987

Nasrallah SM, Tommaso CL, Singleton RT, et al: Primary esophageal motor disorders: clinical response to nifedipine. South Med J 78:312–315, 1985

Navab F, Dexter EC Jr: Gastroesophageal reflux: pathophysiologic concepts. Arch Intern Med 145:329–333, 1985

Nelson JB, Castell DO: Esophageal Motility Disorders. Chicago, IL, Year Book Medical, 1988

Peters L, Maas L, Petty D, et al: Spontaneous noncardiac chest pain: evaluation by 24-hour ambulatory esophageal motility and pH monitoring. Gastroenterology 94:878–886, 1988

Reidel WL, Clouse RE: Variations in clinical presentation of patients with esophageal contraction abnormalities. Dig Dis Sci 30:1065–1071, 1985

Richter JE, Castell DO: Gastroesophageal reflux: pathogenesis, diagnosis, and therapy. Ann Intern Med 97:93–103, 1982

Richter JE, Castell DO: Diffuse esophageal spasm: a reappraisal. Ann Intern Med 100:242–245, 1984

Richter JE, Castell DO: Surgical myotomy for nutcracker esophagus: to be or not to be? Dig Dis Sci 32:95–96, 1987

Richter JE, Spurling TJ, Cordova CM, et al: Effects of oral calcium blocker, diltiazem, on esophageal contractions: studies in volunteers and patients with nutcracker esophagus. Dig Dis Sci 29:649–656, 1984

Richter JE, Dalton CB, Buice RG, et al: Nifedipine—a potent inhibitor of contractions in the body of the human esophagus: studies in healthy volunteers and patients with the nutcracker esophagus. Gastroenterology 89:549–554, 1985

Richter JE, Barish CF, Castell DO: Abnormal sensory perception in patients with esophageal chest pain. Gastroenterology 91:845–852, 1986a

Richter JE, Obrecht WF, Bradley LA, et al: Psychological comparison of patients with nutcracker esophagus and irritable bowel syndrome. Dig Dis Sci 31:131–138, 1986b

Richter JE, Dalton CB, Bradley LA, et al: Oral nifedipine in the treatment of noncardiac chest pain in patients with the nutcracker esophagus. Gastroenterology 93:21–28, 1987

Richter JE, Bradley LA, Castell DO: Esophageal chest pain: current controversies in pathogenesis, diagnosis, and therapy. Ann Intern Med 110:66–78, 1989

Robertson DAF, Aldersley MA, Sherherd H, et al: H_2 antagonists in the treatment of reflux oesophagitis: can physiological studies predict the response? Gut 28:946–949, 1987

Rubin J, Nagler R, Spiro HM, et al: Measuring the effect of emotions on esophageal motility. Psychosom Med 24:170–176, 1961

Schuster MM, Nikoomanesh P, Wells D: Biofeedback control of lower esophageal sphincter contraction. Rendiconti di Gastroenterologia 5:14–18, 1973

Shabsin HS, Katz PO, Schuster MM: Behavioral treatment of intractable chest pain in a patient with vigorous achalasia. Am J Gastroenterol 83:970–973, 1988

Sherbaniuk R, Wensel R, Bailey R, et al: Ranitidine in the treatment of symptomatic gastroesophageal reflux disease. J Clin Gastroenterol 6:9–15, 1984

Sontag S, Robinson M, McCallum RW, et al: Ranitidine therapy for gastroesophageal reflux disease: results of a large double-blind trial. Arch Intern Med 147:1485–1491, 1987

Stacher G, Schmierer G, Landgraf M: Tertiary esophageal contractions evoked by acoustical stimuli. Gastroenterology 77:49–54, 1979a

Stacher G, Steinringer H, Blau A, et al: Acoustically evoked esophageal contractions and defense reaction. Psychophysiology 16:234–241, 1979b

Traube M, McCallum RW: Primary oesophageal motility disorders: current therapeutic concepts. Drugs 30:66–77, 1985

Traube M, Tummala V, Baue AE, et al: Surgical myotomy in patients with high-amplitude peristaltic esophageal contractions: manometric and clinical effects. Dig Dis Sci 32:16–21, 1987

Ward BW, Wu WC, Richter JE, et al: Non-cardiac chest pain: is diagnosis of esophageal etiology helpful? (abstract) Gastroenterology 88:1627, 1985

Whitehead WE, Schuster MM: Gastrointestinal Disorders. New York, Academic, 1985

Winters C, Artnak EJ, Benjamin SB, et al: Esophageal bougienage in symptomatic patients with the nutcracker esophagus: a primary esophageal motility disorder. JAMA 252:363–366, 1984

Wolf S, Almy TP: Experimental observations on cardiospasm in man. Gastroenterology 13:401–421, 1949

Wolpe J: Psychotherapy by Reciprocal Inhibition. Stanford, CA, Stanford University Press, 1958

World Health Organization: Draft of the 10th Revision of the International Classification of Diseases. Geneva, World Health Organization, 1988

Wright C, Cuschieri A: Jejunal interposition for benign esophageal disease: technical considerations and long-term results. Ann Surg 205:54–60, 1987

Chapter 5

Non-Ulcer Dyspepsia

Various definitions have been proposed for the term *non-ulcer dyspepsia* (NUD). The common meaning of the term—symptoms suggesting disease of the upper gastrointestinal tract in which physical diseases have been excluded by the usual gastrological investigations—has been adopted for the present chapter.

Symptoms, Signs, and Etiology

Non-ulcer dyspepsia is a disorder that manifests itself with one or more symptoms of the upper gastrointestinal tract, including epigastric or retrosternal discomfort or pain, a burning sensation in the epigastrium, and nausea and vomiting without evidence of organic pathology. Less frequently, the term has been used to describe dyspepsia from any cause except that caused by peptic ulceration (Dotevall et al. 1982).

Non-ulcer dyspepsia can occur with the irritable bowel syndrome and with gastroesophageal reflux. The true relationship of NUD to food and the effect of food on this condition vary, among which are the various types described below. There are several clinical features that distinguish NUD from other pathology of the upper gastrointestinal tract, but the diagnosis cannot be made without careful exclusion of other causes of dyspepsia ("Data Base on Dyspepsia" 1978). Various types of NUD, as summarized below, have been proposed by a working party of gastroenterologists (Colin-Jones 1988).

Gastroesophageal-reflux–like dyspepsia. In this type of NUD there are symptoms of regurgitation, but there is no endoscopic evidence. Esophageal pH monitoring shows that regurgitation occurs in some patients in this group (Johnsen et al. 1987).

Ulcer-like dyspepsia. In this group the symptoms appear to be typical of a peptic ulcer, but no crater or scar is found on endoscopy. In ulcer-like dyspepsia there is usually relief during eating, and the pain may recur 1 to 3 hours after meals as in duodenal ulcer disease (Dotevall 1985, p. 47).

Dysmotility-type dyspepsia. This form of NUD often coexists with the irritable bowel syndrome and is typically associated with the symptoms of bloating and distension. About half of the patients with dyspeptic symptoms have some delay in gastric emptying (Malagelada and Stanghellini 1985) and postcibal antral hypomotility (Camilleri et al. 1986).

Dyspepsia with aerophagia. The typical features of this type of NUD include repetitive belching and gulping. Aerophagia is described in detail in Chapter 8 of this volume.

Idiopathic dyspepsia. Some patients do not fall into any of the above categories; this may in fact be up to one third of the patients with NUD (Colin-Jones 1988). In some patients discomfort appears soon after eating (Edwards and Coghill 1968). Spiro (1974) has argued that dyspepsia, duodenitis, erosions, and duodenal ulcer constitute a spectrum, and that the dividing line among these syndromes depends frequently on the definition and on the method of study. The distinction among these disorders, however, has been traditionally made, exists in current diagnostic systems, and thus has implications for treatment.

Colin-Jones (1988), in a review on the etiology of NUD, concluded that it is a group of heterogeneous conditions. Gastric acid may play a role in a few cases (e.g., those associated with reflux), whereas in others, abnormal motility, infection with *Campylobacter pylori,* and personality are more important. The role of diet is unknown.

Prevalence and Severity

The prevalence of non-ulcer dyspepsia varies across studies, depending on the definition, the exclusion criteria (such as brief duration), and the method of study. Thompson (1984) concluded in a review that no abnormalities are found in the upper gastrointestinal tract in about 45% of cases of dyspepsia.

In general practice in Sweden, 2% of all clinical diagnoses were gastritis or duodenitis (Adami et al. 1984). In a questionnaire study of symptoms experienced during the past week, about 20% of random employees in two countries (England and New Mexico) affirmed the items "stomach pains" and "sick, nauseated" (Kellner and Sheffield 1973). (The prevalence, of course, would have been substantially lower if short episodes of illness had been excluded.) The prevalence of peptic ulcers in the United States is about 1.7% (Kurata and Haile 1982). In Uppsala, Sweden, the prevalence of NUD that lasts for 2 months or longer was only slightly higher than that for peptic ulcer (Nyrén et al. 1986b), whereas in the U.S. Army, the prevalence of peptic ulcers was found to be higher than the combined diagnoses of gastritis, duodenitis, and "disorders of functions of the stomach" (Almy et al. 1975). In the United States, 27% of subjects take two or more doses of antacids each month (Graham et al. 1983).

Thus, gastric symptoms as detected by questionnaire are substantially more common than peptic ulcer, but most of the gastric complaints appear to be short-lived. Differences in prevalence among countries are unknown because methods of study have differed.

Incapacity

The incapacity from dyspepsia as opposed to other abdominal complaints has been investigated by Nyrén and his colleagues (1986b) in Sweden. Over an 18-month period the family physicians (general practitioners) in a county with a population of about 200,000 were requested to refer all patients suspected of having a peptic ulcer for endoscopy. Eighty-eight patients had ulcer-like complaints for at least 2 months, and upper endoscopy showed no evidence of ulcer disease or other pathology except for gastric mucosal reddening in 24 patients. There was no other explanation for the symptoms, such as irritable bowel syndrome or gall bladder disease. Unlike epidemiologic studies by questionnaire in which other disorders such as minor physical disease and irritable bowel syndrome could not be excluded with certainty, this prevalence study was truly limited to NUD.

The patients with NUD took more sick leave than the patients with peptic ulcer. When the sick leave was standardized for age, absenteeism was 1.7 times higher in the NUD patients than in the ulcer patients. The reasons for absence from work were different in the two groups; the majority of those ulcer patients who reported sick presented with abdominal complaints, whereas the NUD patients reported sick for numerous other complaints, especially musculoskeletal symptoms, infections, psychiatric problems, and injuries. The amount of sick leave taken for nonabdominal complaints was significantly greater in the NUD group than in the ulcer group (111 days vs. 50 days).

Scandinavian countries and some western European countries have generous national health and sickness disability programs, and it is conceivable that in other countries the absence from work because of dyspepsia and other costs to the community are less than in Sweden. The study by Nyrén et al. shows, however, that absence from work, the cost in sickness benefits, and the cost to the economy in loss of production are greater from NUD than from the common and distressing ulcer disease.

Psychological Factors

Goldberg et al. (1976) examined hospital charts for comments about emotional disturbances in patients with gastritis. They found that patients with gastritis who had no known predisposing factors such as alcoholism and salicylates had more comments about emotional disturbance than did patients with duodenal ulcer.

Magni and his colleagues carried out three studies in northern Italy on the psychological features of patients with dyspepsia in the absence of peptic ulcers. The first study was with patients with acute gastroduodenitis, and the other two involved patients with NUD in which patients with gastroduodenitis had been excluded.

Magni et al. (1982) administered the Symptom Rating Test (a self-rating scale of symptoms) to 25 patients with duodenal ulcer and to 36 patients with acute gastroduodenitis (NUD with gastroduodenitis confirmed by endoscopy and biopsy). Both patient groups had higher scores on the anxiety scale and higher total distress scores than did nonpatient control subjects. Depression and somatization were higher in patients with acute gastroduodenitis than in patients with duodenal ulcer. In the second study, Magni et al. (1985) administered the Middlesex Hospital Questionnaire to 27 people with dyspepsia and to matched neurotic psychiatric patients. The responses to the questionnaire were similar in the two groups. In Magni et al.'s third study (1987), 15 men and 15 women who were consecutive outpatients with NUD at a university gastroenterology unit were interviewed. All had dyspepsia, pain, nausea or discomfort for 1 month or longer. Excluded were patients who had serious physical disease as well as patients with esophagitis, gastritis, and duodenitis, and patients who had a history of peptic ulcer disease, clinical evidence of gastroesophageal reflux, and/or irritable bowel syndrome. All patients were interviewed by a psychiatrist, and DSM-III diagnoses were made based on a DSM-III flow sheet. A comparison group of 20 matched patients from the same gastroenterology unit were also interviewed (12 had gallstones and 8 had hiatal hernia). There were significant differences between the two groups. In the dyspepsia groups, 26 patients (86%) had a psychiatric diagnosis, whereas in the organic group, only 5 patients (25%) had one. The most common diagnoses in the NUD group were various anxiety disorders, and predominantly generalized anxiety disorder; the only depressive diagnosis in the dyspepsia group was a patient with dysthymic disorder, which often has an anxiety component.

Malagelada and Stanghellini (1985) examined manometric abnormalities in 104 patients with nausea, vomiting, and upper abdominal pain in the absence of structural gut abnormalities. No manometric abnormalities were found in 21 of the patients. Patients who had an abnormal Minnesota Multiphasic Personality Inventory (MMPI) were evaluated by a psychiatrist. Psychiatric diagnoses were made for 13 patients (62%) without manometric abnormalities, a substantially higher number than in those patients with manometric abnormalities.

Talley et al. (1986a) compared 76 patients with NUD and 66 patients with duodenal ulcer as well as community control subjects from which individuals with symptoms of NUD and ulcer symptoms had been excluded. They administered the Eysenck Personality Inventory (EPI), the Costello-Comrey Personality Questionnaire, the Beck Depression Inventory, and the Spielberger State-Trait Anxiety Inventory. Except for the extroversion scale of the EPI, which did not differentiate among the groups, all scores were significantly higher in the NUD group than in the community control subjects; the scores of patients with NUD and peptic ulcer were similar. The patients were followed for 2 to 7 months; although 36% were symptom free on follow-up, the psychological test scores remained essentially unchanged. The authors emphasized that the numerical differences on the psychological tests were small and that factors other than anxiety probably play more important roles in the etiology and symptomatology of non-ulcer dyspepsia.

Camilleri et al. (1986) examined postcibal antral motility under stress induced by experimental pain in 15 patients with NUD. The authors identified one group who had disordered gastric function under basal conditions resulting in antral hypomotility, and another group who had normal basal antral motility and had gastric motor responses to stress. The cause of the symptoms in the second group was undetermined, but it did not appear to be a motility disorder.

Johnsen et al. (1987) administered a questionnaire to over 14,000 people in Tromso, Norway. It included the questions "Do you often suffer from cramping abdominal pain?" and "Are you often bothered by bloating and abdominal rumbling?" Thus, the questionnaire dealt with abdominal symptoms in general, including irritable bowel syndrome. The prevalence of abdominal symptoms was 28% in men and 35% in women, and there was a weak negative association between age and prevalence. In a multiple regression analysis, abdominal symptoms were strongly associated with psychiatric symptoms. In both sexes, psychological factors (sleeping difficulties, depression, problems of coping, and use of analgesics) accounted for approximately 66% of the observed variance; social conditions and various other factors such as lack of education, for roughly 30%; and diet, for only 3% to 4%. There was an association between abdominal symptoms and frequency of alcohol intoxication and cigarette smoking. Associations with diet were weak and inconsistent. Those individuals who described their financial state as "very difficult" had the largest prevalence of abdominal symptoms in adult life. Further, there was a negative correlation between years of education and prevalence of symptoms. The authors concluded that the social factors may indicate that sufferers are less capable of coping with problems, and that these difficulties at least enhance symptoms. Subjects who had X-ray studies did not differ materially from the other patients on any of the variables.

Creed et al. (1988) found that severe life events, especially the breaking up of a close relationship, preceded the onset of functional abdominal pain significantly more often than before the onset of abdominal organic illness. Severe life events preceded functional abdominal pain as often as in patients who took deliberate overdoses of drugs.

Comment

Goldberg et al. (1976) found that physicians' comments about emotional problems were more frequent in the hospital charts of patients with gastritis than in those of patients with duodenal ulcer. The patients with gastritis in this study, however, may have been different from those with NUD. Moreover, this study may have been biased, because, as the authors point out, patients with duodenal ulcer may have had more severe illness and the physicians may have paid less attention to anxiety and depression.

In the other studies discussed above, patients with NUD had more anxiety and more neurotic symptoms than did other patients. All the NUD patients, however, sought treatment, and, therefore, these studies share the bias with many other studies of treated patients. Patients who are anxious or have other neuroses are more likely to seek medical treatment than patients with similar symptoms who have less psychopathology. The association of NUD with anxiety and other neurotic symptoms in people who do not seek treatment is not known. In Johnsen et al.'s (1987) and Creed et al.'s (1988) studies, abdominal symptoms in subjects in the community (thus not necessarily medically treated individuals) were clearly associated with psychosocial stress, but the symptoms were probably caused in part by other disorders, including the irritable bowel syndrome.

Diagnosis

Numerous physical diseases can cause dyspepsia, acute or chronic peptic ulcer, carcinoma, esophagitis, gastritis, hiatal hernia with gastroesophageal reflux, gallstones, chronic cholecystitis, and some rare conditions (some of which may be difficult to detect on a routine investigation) such as cholesterolosis (Jacyna and Bouchier 1987). NUD is associated with other psychosomatic disorders such as the irritable bowel syndrome and aerophagia (Talley and Piper 1985). There are many physical agents that can either induce or aggravate NUD; these include alcohol and smoking and numerous drugs such as aspirin and nonsteroidal anti-inflammatory drugs. A minority of patients with NUD have gastroduodenitis on endoscopy, but it remains uncertain whether such mucosal lesions cause symptoms (Talley et al. 1986a). In many cases endoscopy without biopsy is inadequate to make the correct diagnosis (Vaira et al. 1989). Food intolerance and allergy are rare causes of dyspepsia; patients with these conditions usually develop allergic symptoms such as urticaria, and these symptoms are limited to specific foods (Royal College of Physicians 1984).

One of the causes of peptic ulceration, active chronic gastritis, and, perhaps, NUD is infection by *Campylobacter pylori* (Marshall et al. 1988). The extent of the role of *C. pylori* is at present not known (Graham 1989; Talley and Phillips 1988), and it will remain a topic for study and perhaps controversy for some time to come.

There are no clear guidelines in DSM-III-R that apply to all cases of NUD, because the exact nature of the disorder is often uncertain. The guidelines can be interpreted as follows: if it is one of the kinds of dyspepsia in which organic factors probably play a role (see pp. 97–98, this volume), and if there are clearly emotional factors contributing, the psychiatric diagnosis should be "psychological factors affecting physical condition" (316.00; American Psychiatric Association 1987, pp. 333–334) on Axis I and NUD on Axis III. In the ICD-10 draft (World Health Organization 1988), the corresponding code is F45.31. In the idiopathic variety of NUD, the classification should be "undifferentiated somatoform disorder" (300.70; American Psychiatric Association 1987, pp. 266–267) on Axis I and, in parentheses, NUD. In the ICD-10 draft, the corresponding code is F45.1.

Treatment

Psychological Treatments

Bates et al. (1988) examined the effects of a behavioral treatment program in NUD; the treatment consisted in part of applied relaxation. The patient is first trained in deep muscle relaxation (Jacobson 1938), is later taught to relax without prior tensing of muscles, and is finally trained to relax rapidly in situations that are stressful or frightening. The development of the technique has been reviewed by Clark (1988) and Ost (1988).

Fifty-two patients were randomized to the treatment group and about the same number to the control group. Twenty patients dropped out for reasons such as spontaneous recovery, poor attendance, or the patient was not given time off work. Twenty-nine patients who refused to participate in the study were not randomized but agreed to record their epigastric pain; these patients served as an additional control group (see Figure 5-1).

The treatment lasted for 3 months and was carried out in groups. The patients were made aware of the situations in which their pain occurred, as well as the consequences of the pain. They were asked to fill in a pain diary that included places in which the pain occurred, person present, and thoughts or activities preceding the pain. Throughout the treatment, patients were trained in applied relaxation. Based on the information contained in the diary, the therapist, as well as group members, helped the patient to analyze the situation and suggested alternative ways of behaving. Problem-solving approaches, assertiveness training, and cognitive restructuring were suggested to the patients, and they then were advised to practice these behaviors.

Pain was assessed by self-recording that included the number of occasions the pain occurred, the self-rated intensity of the pain, the total duration of pain during the week (which averaged 25 hours a week), and the "pain index," which was the product of the intensity and duration of the pain.

At the end of treatment, pain intensity as well as frequency of pain was significantly less in the treated group than in the control groups. At 1-year follow-up, the treated group had significantly lower frequency of pain than did the additional control group (which consisted of patients who had declined treatment), but the difference between the treated group and the randomized control group was no longer significant.

The treated group was more successful in reducing the number of pain occasions between the end of the treatment and follow-up. The duration of pain did not significantly differ among the groups; this suggests that once the pain episode started, even treated patients had difficulty in cutting it short. It appeared that the patients learned to prevent some pain episodes either by actively avoiding precipitating circumstances or by correctly identifying precursors to the pain and taking active measures to counteract it.

Whitehead et al. (1975) found that visual feedback of gastric pH combined with money reinforcers substantially changed the rate of gastric acid secretion. Whitehead and Drescher (1980) found that healthy volunteers could learn to control gastric motility with biofeedback. However, it is unknown whether biofeedback would be effective in the treatment of NUD.

Drug Treatments

Antacids and H_2 receptor antagonists are widely prescribed in the treatment of NUD. In a controlled study, Norrelund et al. (1980) found antacids to be no more effective than placebo in the treatment of NUD. In three controlled studies, the effects of H_2 receptor blockers did not differ significantly from those of placebos (Bendtsen et al. 1983; La Broy et al. 1978; Lance et al. 1981). Nyrén et al. (1986a) described a controlled drug study of over 150 patients with NUD.

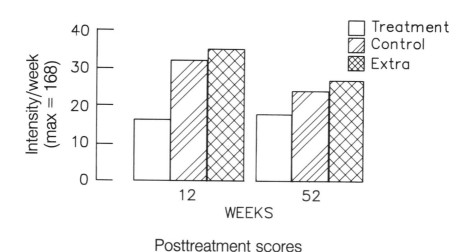

Figure 5-1. Outcome of group behavioral treatment of nonulcer dyspepsia (Bates et al. 1988). Pain intensity was measured at the end of treatment and on a 1-year follow-up. Reprinted from Bates et al. 1988, with permission of the authors and the editor in chief.

The authors compared placebo and two commonly prescribed medications for this disorder in a double-blind study: 400 mg of cimetidine twice a day and an antacid. Pain significantly decreased in all three groups, but there were no significant differences among the groups in any stage of the treatment.

Metoclopramide and domperidone were found to be more effective than placebo in a 4-week crossover study (DeLoose 1979). Talley et al. (1986b) compared cimetidine, pirenzepine, and placebo in a between-subjects (parallel) design as well as a crossover design. Cimetidine was superior to placebo in decreasing the number of pain episodes, but the absolute improvement was small.

The effect of drugs appears to depend on the type of dyspepsia. Johannessen et al. (1988) examined the effects of cimetidine in an intensive design (multiple crossover) study with 127 patients. Symptoms compatible with gastroesophageal reflux were more common in responders than in nonresponders. The opposite was true for those who had also symptoms of the irritable bowel syndrome. Gotthard et al. (1988) compared cimetidine, antacid, and placebo in a parallel study of 222 patients. Cimetidine was found to be superior to both placebo and antacid in relieving pain and nausea, but not bloating. Epigastric pain and symptoms relieved by food were associated in this study with a good response to cimetidine.

Baume et al. (1975) compared diazepam and lorazepam in a placebo-controlled crossover drug trial in patients with functional gastrointestinal disorders. Both drugs were found to be superior to placebo in these patients, who included a few patients with NUD.

Recommended Treatments

The working party on the management of NUD (Colin-Jones 1988) included the following recommendations: 1) general advice, 2) an explanation of the symptoms, and 3) firm reassurance. When necessary, patients should be counseled about risk factors contributing to their symptoms. The recommendations on drug treatment are divided in accord with the type of dyspepsia: for example, H_2-receptor antagonists in the gastroesophageal-reflux–like and ulcer-like dyspepsias. The authors also commented that some patients find antacids helpful. In the dysmotility-type dyspepsia, drugs such as metoclopramide may help. The report does not address systematic psychotherapy and psychotropic drugs.

No firm guidance can be given on the order of psychological treatments and psychotropic drugs because there are not enough data for such recommendations. If simple measures such as explanation and reassurance have not helped, in an anxious patient an antianxiety drug(s) should be tried. If symptoms persist, the patient should have brief counseling and psychotherapeutic support; although there are no controlled studies of supportive or nondirective psychotherapy in NUD, there are such studies with other gastrointestinal disorders (described in Chapter 6, this volume) that show such treatments to be effective. If the patient continues to have distressing symptoms, he or she should participate in a formal psychological treatment program such as the one described by Bates et al. (1988).

Case History

The patient, a 62-year-old male, was a senior research scientist in physical chemistry working at a national laboratory. He had distressing epigastric discomfort including intermittent pain for 5 months. He also had nausea with belching, and recently he had a change in bowel habits in that he had a few loose stools without apparent cause. Gastroenterological investigation, which included esophagoscopy and gastroscopy, did not reveal evidence of peptic ulcers or other physical pathology. About 20 years previously he had had a similar episode that had lasted about 3 months, and he was told at the time that he had no disease and that his symptoms were caused by stress. Food tended to relieve his symptoms; cimetidine did not appear to help, but antacids did somewhat. He made an appointment to see me because he wanted my opinion on whether his current symptoms could possibly be stress related.

The history revealed that he was working extremely hard. He had always enjoyed his work and had worked long hours by choice. Eight months previously he had started a new project; it was interesting original research that was likely to yield prestigious publications, and he felt flattered that he had been given this task. He had adequate research support, but the number of experiments his staff completed that he had to review was more than he could cope with. He had committed himself to complete the project within 18 months, but he had doubts now whether he could accomplish this in spite of the long hours he worked each day. He also felt that he was neglecting other work that was almost equally important. When I questioned him, he told me that a failure to meet the deadline would not hurt his career, and it would not slow down other work within the organization, because the results could not be applied in the near future. He said, however, that he would be ashamed if he had to break his promise and fail to complete the assignment on time. He worked during his vacation and worked also during weekends; he had stopped his hobbies but still was unable to keep up with his overambitious program. On questioning, he said that work had become a burden, that he was not enjoying it, and that frequently he felt so tense, particularly when facing complicated problems that required deliberation, that he had to leave his desk or bench and could not continue, but instead had to go for a brisk walk until he had calmed down.

I told the patient that judging by the history, his tension, unhappiness, and gastric symptoms were most likely caused by stress. I also asked him whether he thought it was worthwhile to attempt to meet the deadline that had been clearly overambitious and whether it would not be wiser to tell his director that the project might take longer than he anticipated.

At this point the patient said that he was convinced that the quality of the research would be better if he worked at a more reasonable pace, because some of the experiments had been poorly planned and time had been wasted.

I saw the patient 1 week later. He had decided to reduce the total number of hours he worked each week and to work at a pace that was comfortable. He said that he felt a great relief: he had taken two evenings off when he read newspapers and magazines unrelated to his work and thoroughly enjoyed the leisure. He said that his gastric symptoms were somewhat less troublesome. Two weeks later he said that he had about 4 days without any symptoms; after another 3 weeks the symptoms had ceased, except for 2 days when he worked longer hours than usual and felt under the same self-inflicted pressure.

The patient canceled a subsequent appointment. I saw him 2 months later and he had remained symptom free.

Prognosis

The prognosis for symptoms varies with the selection criteria, duration of the complaint, and length of follow-up. In a 6-year follow-up of 102 patients attending general practitioners offices in Wales, 76% of those who could be followed up had little or no dyspepsia, and 3% had developed peptic ulcer (Gregory et al. 1972). Spiro (1974) reported a substantially larger prevalence of peptic ulceration on follow-up. Weir and Backett (1968) found that about 9% of patients with NUD became symptom free in 1 year and that a similar number of new cases occurred in the same time period.

The mortality from NUD is almost the same as that for duodenal ulcer. In Denmark, Viskum (1977) found the ratio of observed to expected deaths in gastric disorders to be 1.92 for gastric ulcer, 1.34 for duodenal ulcer, and 1.32 for patients with ulcer-like symptoms of dyspepsia without an actual ulcer crater. The causes for the increased mortality in NUD are not known; perhaps this increased mortality is caused by behaviors that are associated with dyspepsia such as smoking or alcoholism (Pell and D'Alonzo 1970).

Summary and Main Conclusions

Non-ulcer dyspepsia is a common disorder that causes substantial distress and disability and involves great costs. The severity of symptoms and disability is as great or greater than that of duodenal ulcer.

Non-ulcer dyspepsia appears to be caused by various abnormalities, including gastroesophageal reflux, disorders of gastric motility, gastritis, duodenitis, aerophagia, and infection with *Campylobacter pylori*. There is evidence to suggest that neurosis, particularly anxiety, is more common in patients with this syndrome than in other patients.

In two controlled studies of the treatment of NUD with antacids and four controlled studies with H_2-receptor antagonists, drugs were no more effective than placebo. In some studies, however, specific types of NUD drugs were more effective than placebo: in the gastroesophageal-reflux–like NUD and in the ulcer-like NUD, cimetidine was found to be effective. In the dysmotility-type NUD, metoclopramide and domperidone were more effective than placebo. In a placebo-controlled crossover study, lorazepam and diazepam relieved functional gastrointestinal symptoms, including those in a few patients with NUD.

In a controlled study of a combination of psychological treatments that included applied relaxation as one of the treatment methods, the treated group had fewer episodes of pain than the control groups; treatment apparently hastened recovery from NUD.

The prognosis varies with the selection criteria. In a 6-year follow-up study of patients with NUD who sought treatment from a family practitioner, 76% had little or no dyspepsia. The estimates vary in the proportion of patients who develop peptic ulceration on follow-up. In one study, which so far has not been replicated, the mortality due to NUD was similar to that due to peptic ulcer. The increased mortality in NUD is, perhaps, caused by behaviors that are associated with dyspepsia, such as drinking alcohol and smoking.

References

Adami HO, Agenäs I, Gustavsson S, et al: The clinical diagnosis of "gastritis": aspects of demographic epidemiology and health care consumption based on a nationwide sample survey. Scand J Gastroenterol 19:216–219, 1984

Almy TP, Mendeloff AI, Rice D, et al: Prevalence and significance of digestive disease. Gastroenterology 68:1351–1371, 1975

American Psychiatric Association: Diagnostic and Statistical Manual of Mental Disorders, 3rd Edition, Revised. Washington, DC, American Psychiatric Association, 1987

Bates S, Sjödén PO, Nyrén O: Behavioral treatment of non-ulcer dyspepsia. Scandinavian Journal of Behaviour Therapy 17:155–165, 1988

Baume P, Tracey M, Dawson L: Efficacy of two minor tranquilizers in relieving symptoms of functional gastrointestinal distress. Aust N Z J Med 5:503–506, 1975

Bendtsen F, Dano P, Guldhammer B, et al: Cimetidinbehandling af rontgennegativ dyspepsi. Ugeskr Laeger 145:3090–3093, 1983

Camilleri M, Malagelada JR, Kao PC, et al: Gastric and autonomic responses to stress in functional dyspepsia. Dig Dis Sci 31:1169–1177, 1986

Clark DM: Applied relaxation: a new look at an old technique. Scandinavian Journal of Behaviour Therapy 17:79–82, 1988

Colin-Jones DG (Chairman): Management of dyspepsia: report of a working party. Lancet 1:576–579, 1988

Creed F, Craig T, Farmer R: Functional abdominal pain, psychiatric illness, and life events. Gut 29:235–242, 1988

Data base on dyspepsia (editorial). Br Med J 1:1163–1164, 1978

DeLoose F: Domperidone in chronic dyspepsia: a pilot open study and a multicentre general practice crossover comparison with metoclopramide and placebo. Pharmatherapeutica 2:140–146, 1979

Dotevall G: Stress and Common Gastrointestinal Disorders. New York, Praeger, 1985

Dotevall G, Sjödin II, Svedlund J: The peptic ulcer disease: a study of somatic and mental symptoms. Scand J Gastroenterol Suppl 79:50–57, 1982

Edwards FC, Coghill NF: Clinical manifestations in patients with chronic atrophic gastritis, gastric ulcer, and duodenal ulcer. Q J Med 37:337–360, 1968

Goldberg SJ, Smith CL, Connell AM: Emotion-related gastritis. Am J Gastroenterol 65:41–46, 1976

Gotthard R, Bodemar G, Brodin U, et al: Treatment with cimetidine, antacid, or placebo in patients with dyspepsia of unknown origin. Scand J Gastroenterol 23:7–18, 1988

Graham DY: *Campylobacter pylori* and peptic ulcer disease. Gastroenterology 96:615–625, 1989

Graham DY, Smith JL, Patterson DJ: Why do apparently healthy people use antacid tablets? Am J Gastroenterol 78:257–260, 1983

Gregory DW, Davies GT, Evans KT, et al: Natural history of patients with X-ray-negative dyspepsia in general practice. Br Med J 4:519–520, 1972

Jacobson E: Progressive Relaxation. Chicago, IL, University of Chicago Press, 1938

Jacyna MR, Bouchier IAD: Cholesterolosis: a physical cause of "functional" disorder. Br Med J 295:619–620, 1987

Johannessen T, Fjosne U, Kleveland PM, et al: Cimetidine responders in non-ulcer dyspepsia. Scand J Gastroenterol 23:327–336, 1988

Johnsen R, Jacobsen BK, Førde OH: Associations between symptoms of irritable colon and psychological and social conditions and lifestyle. Br Med J 292:1633–1635, 1987

Kellner R, Sheffield BF: The one-week prevalence of symptoms in neurotic patients and normals. Am J Psychiatry 130:102–105, 1973

Kurata JH, Haile BM: Racial differences in peptic ulcer disease: fact or myth? Gastroenterology 83:166–172, 1982

La Broy S, Lovell D, Misiewicz JJ: The treatment of non-ulcer dyspepsia, in Cimetidine: The Westminster Hospital Symposium. Edited by Wastell C, Lance P. London, Churchill Livingstone, 1978, pp 131–140

Lance P, Filipe MI, Schiller KFR, et al: Cimetidine for non-ulcer dyspepsia (abstract). Gastroenterology 80:1203, 1981

Magni G, Salmi A, Paterlini A, et al: Psychological distress in duodenal ulcer and acute gastroduodenitis: a controlled study. Dig Dis Sci 27:1081–1084, 1982

Magni G, Di Mario F, Aggio L, et al: Psychological distress in non-ulcerous dyspepsia (letter). Gastroenterol Clin Biol 9:86, 1985

Magni G, Di Mario F, Bernasconi G, et al: DSM-III diagnoses associated with dyspepsia of unknown cause. Am J Psychiatry 144:1222–1223, 1987

Malagelada JR, Stanghellini V: Manometric evaluation of functional upper gut symptoms. Gastroenterology 88:1223–1231, 1985

Marshall BJ, Warren JR, Blincow ED, et al: Duodenal ulcer: *Campylobacter pylori* key to etiology. Lancet 2:1437–1441, 1988

Norrelund N, Helles A, Schmiegelow M: Ukarakteristisk dyspepsi i almen praksis: in kontrolleret undersogelse med et antacidum (Alminox8R2). Ugeskr Laeger 142:1750–1753, 1980

Nyrén O, Adami HO, Bates S, et al: Absence of therapeutic benefit from antacids or cimetidine in non-ulcer dyspepsia. N Engl J Med 314:339–343, 1986a

Nyrén O, Adami HO, Gustavsson S, et al: Excess sick-listing in nonulcer dyspepsia. J Clin Gastroenterol 8:339–345, 1986b

Ost LG: Applied relaxation: description of an effective coping technique. Scandinavian Journal of Behaviour Therapy 17:83–96, 1988

Pell S, D'Alonzo CA: Sickness absenteeism of alcoholics. J Occup Med 12:198–210, 1970

Royal College of Physicians/British Nutrition Foundation: Food intolerance and food aversion: a joint report of the Royal College of Physicians and the British Nutrition Foundation. J R Coll Physicians Lond 18:83–123, 1984

Spiro HM: Moynihan's disease? The diagnosis of duodenal ulcer. N Engl J Med 291:567–569, 1974

Talley NJ, Phillips SF: Non-ulcer dyspepsia: potential causes and pathophysiology. Ann Intern Med 108:865–879, 1988

Talley NJ, Piper DW: The association between non-ulcer dyspepsia and other gastrointestinal disorders. Scand J Gastroenterol 20:896–900, 1985

Talley NJ, Fung LH, Gilligan IJ, et al: Association of anxiety, neuroticism, and depression with dyspepsia of unknown cause. Gastroenterology 90:886–892, 1986a

Talley NJ, McNeil D, Hayden A, et al: Randomized, double-blind, placebo-controlled crossover trial of cimetidine and pirenzepine in nonulcer dyspepsia. Gastroenterology 91:149–156, 1986b

Thompson WG: Nonulcer dyspepsia. Can Med Assoc J 130:565–569, 1984

Vaira D, Holton J, Osborn J, et al: Use of endoscopy in patients with dyspepsia. Br Med J 299:237, 1989

Viskum K: Ulcer disease: a comparison of some clinical and genetic aspects in patients suffering from duodenal ulcer, gastric ulcer, and the pseudo-ulcer syndrome. Dan Med Bull 24:213–235, 1977

Weir RD, Backett EM: Studies of the epidemiology of peptic ulcer in a rural community: prevalence and natural history of dyspepsia and peptic ulcer. Gut 9:75–83, 1968

Whitehead WE, Drescher VM: Perception of gastric contractions and self-control of gastric motility. Psychophysiology 17:552–557, 1980

Whitehead WE, Renault PF, Goldiamond I: Modification of human gastric acid secretion with operant-conditioning procedures. J Appl Behav Anal 8:147–156, 1975

World Health Organization: Draft of the 10th Revision of the International Classification of Diseases. Geneva, World Health Organization, 1988

Chapter 6

Irritable Bowel Syndrome

Sharp belchings, fulsom crudities, wind and rumbling in the guts, vehement gripings, suffocations, palpitations, heaviness of the heart, singing in the ears and unseasonable sweat all over the body ...

> Robert Burton (1611)
> *The Anatomy of Melancholy*

A general indisposition to action in the bowels accompanied with a degree of occasional uneasiness or pain within some part of the abdomen, in many instances brought on by a partial contraction in the intestine, the effect of excessive muscular action, not the consequence of disease.

> John Howship (1830)
> *Practical Remarks on the*
> *Discrimination and*
> *Successful Treatment of*
> *Spasmodic Stricture in the*
> *Colon*

The irritable bowel syndrome (IBS) is a common disorder that causes distress and sometimes incapacity. Gastrointestinal symptoms play an important role in somatization and are a common cause of bodily complaints.

Development of the Concept

The symptom complex of the IBS has been described for several centuries. Da Costa (1871) described membranous enteritis. Numerous other terms have been used to describe variants of this syndrome: mucous colitis, spastic colon, functional bowel disorder, nervous diarrhea, chronic catarrhal colitis, vegetative neurosis, and the irritable bowel syndrome. Early authors included cases that, in retrospect, appear to have been examples of infectious or idiopathic inflamma-

111

tory colitis, and only later was it generally appreciated that patients with this syndrome do not have inflammatory disease (Ruoff 1973).

Symptoms and Signs

The symptoms consist of an altered bowel habit, which may be diarrhea, constipation, or both; abdominal pain and gaseousness are present to a variable degree. Although exclusion of organic pathology is essential, "most experienced gastroenterologists can recognize this condition at the first clinical encounter" (Thompson 1985). Symptoms that occur more often in IBS than in organic disease are as follows (Manning et al. 1978):

1. Pain relieved by defecation
2. More frequent stools with pain onset
3. Looser stools with pain onset
4. Abdominal distension
5. Mucus in stool
6. Feeling of incomplete evacuation after defecation

The abdominal signs that have been described include an excessively palpable colon and an excessively tender colon, painful digital insertion on rectal examination, empty or nearly empty rectum, hard or firm feces, and the squelch sign (a crepituslike sensation, or a squelching sound, or both, on palpitation of the colon in the right iliac fossa) found in one third of patients with IBS (Fielding 1985).

For research purposes as well as for treatment, various subsyndromes need to be differentiated (Thompson 1984) as follows:

1. Spastic colon, in which pain is relieved by defecation and in which there is altered frequency and consistency of bowel movement with the onset of pain
2. Painless diarrhea
3. Atonic constipation
4. Lower gastrointestinal gaseousness
5. Chronic abdominal pain unrelated to meals, diarrhea, constipation, or defecation

The chronic abdominal pain subsyndrome has the least-understood physiology in that it sometimes occurs without any gut dysmotility (Thompson 1985).

Various noncolonic gastrointestinal symptoms have been reported and include nausea, vomiting, dyspepsia, esophageal symptoms, and early satiety (Thompson et al. 1979; Watson et al. 1978). The nonintestinal symptoms that occur significantly more frequently in patients with IBS than in random employees (Whorwell et al. 1986) are frequency and urgency of micturition, incomplete bladder emptying, nocturia, back pain, and tiredness and dyspareunia in women.

Signs that are unrelated to the gastrointestinal tract and that are indicative of stress, such as cool and clammy hands and flushing of skin of face and neck, are more common than in other patients. (In the epigraphs to this chapter, two subsyndromes are described: Howship [1830] describes the colonic symptoms of the IBS, whereas Robert Burton [1611/1883], when describing "hypochondriacal or flatuous melancholy," also includes several associated nonvisceral symptoms.)

Prevalence

There is incomplete agreement on the prevalence of IBS, and the prevalence depends in part on the inclusion criteria. In questionnaire studies, symptoms caused by other syndromes, such as non-ulcer dyspepsia and the pelvic pain syndrome in women, may have confounding effects by inflating the prevalence. Drossman et al. (1982) and Greenbaum et al. (1983) found that about 30% of the subjects in a population survey in the United States had abdominal complaints and that 17% of United States middle-class volunteers had symptoms of IBS. Thompson and Heaton (1980) found in interviews of various people that 21% had abdominal pain more than six times a year, 6% were constipated, and 4% had diarrhea (see Figure 6-1). The prevalence of symptoms was similar in the two sexes. The majority of people in these three surveys had not been to a physician for these symptoms (Thompson and Heaton 1980). In general, between 20% and 50% of outpatients' gastrointestinal consultations are because of IBS.

Etiology

There are numerous articles and chapters on the pathology and physiology of the IBS. See, for example, the comprehensive and authoritative review edited by Read (1985) and a shorter review by Whitehead and Schuster (1985). The studies on the etiology of IBS are summarized below.

Motility of the Colon

Stereotypic movement in the colon consists of coordinated contraction of the smooth muscle layer that occurs after meals and during periods of fasting. The slow wave activity in the distal colon is about six cycles per minute, although in some normal people three cycles per minute also are found. In patients with IBS, slow wave activity at three cycles per minute appears to predominate during both symptomatic and asymptomatic periods (Nostrand and Barnett 1989).

Numerous factors influence the motor activity of the colon. For example,

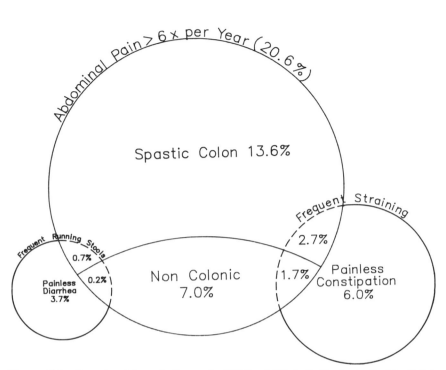

Figure 6-1. Functional bowel disease in 30.2% of 301 individuals studied in Britain (Thompson and Heaton 1980). The large circle indicates the 13.6% who have abdominal pain more than 6 times per year. It is divided to show 13.6% with irritable bowel syndrome and 7% with noncolonic pain. The small circles represent the 3.7% of the patients who have diarrhea and the 10.4% who have constipation. Overlap of these with the large circle indicates that some patients with diarrhea and constipation also have abdominal pain. Reprinted from Thompson and Heaton 1980, with permission of the authors and the W. B. Saunders Company. Copyright 1980, W. B. Saunders.

hypomotility of the sigmoid colon has been reported in humans after the parenteral administration of diarrhea-producing agents such as a prostaglandin or serotonin; hypomotility has also been noted after the administration of constipating drugs such as morphine. In contrast, a parasympathomimetic such as neostigmine induces heightened motility. Increased segmental activity has been found in constipation, but not in diarrhea, especially if painless, reduced segmental activity has been recorded. As Taylor (1985, p. 90) has noted, "in simplistic terms, the disorder of motility is considered to result in either excess segmentation, thus preventing movement of intraluminal content, or hypomotility, allowing bowel contents to run freely, unhampered by segmental contractions." In patients with IBS, motility changes have been found in relation to symptoms (Connell et al. 1965; Kock et al. 1968; Waller and Misiewicz 1972).

Patients with IBS were found to have abnormal motility of the small bowel (Thompson et al. 1979), as well as abnormal motility of the esophagus (Clouse and Eckert 1986; Watson et al. 1978; Whorwell et al. 1981).

Myoelectrical Abnormality

Several authors found evidence of myoelectrical abnormality in patients with IBS. Brief summaries of selected studies follow. (For more complete surveys of these studies and discussion of methodological problems, see Whitehead and Schuster 1985 and Taylor 1985.)

Constipated IBS patients show a significant increase in the incidence of short spike burst with no major changes in long spike burst compared to non-IBS control subjects. Patients with painless diarrhea, however, show few long spike bursts and a significant reduction in the incidence of short spike bursts (Bueno et al. 1980).

Recordings from the colon show continuous baseline fluctuations that have been described as electrical *slow waves*. These slow depolarizations depend upon sodium ion movement across the membrane. Rapid depolarization occurs because of calcium ion entry during some of the slow wave phases (Taylor et al. 1974, 1975). Snape et al. (1977) described the characteristic patterns of myoelectrical activity in the distal colons of patients with IBS who were compared to control subjects. There was a significantly higher incidence of slow-rate electrical activity at a lower frequency. This activity occurred in the symptomatic as well as the asymptomatic phases (Taylor et al. 1978). This abnormal rhythm tends to remain even though the incidence of other rhythms may return to normal (Taylor 1985; Taylor et al. 1978). Studies suggest that the low-frequency electrical rhythm is specific to patients suffering from IBS and not merely a reflection of altered bowel habit or abdominal pain, although how this abnormality relates to disordered motility is not clear (Taylor 1985). Latimer et al. (1981) found a greater number and duration of contractions in IBS patients than in non-IBS subjects at baseline, but the authors found no differences in electrical control activity or motor activity.

Comment. Several authors have found abnormal myoelectrical activity. The abnormality tends to be different between patients with diarrhea and those with constipation. The findings to date have not been uniform (Whitehead and Schuster 1985).

Increased Responsiveness to Stimulation

Whitehead et al. (1980) and Chasen et al. (1982) distended the rectosigmoid colon with an air-filled balloon in a stepwise fashion. This procedure is an experimental stimulus that simulates the physiological distension by gas or stool. Such a distension reliably elicited sigmoid motility in IBS patients that was significantly greater than the motility in non-IBS control subjects. There were no significant differences between patients and control subjects in regard to motility prior to the inflation. Faster contractions were related to bowel symptoms most commonly in patients with painless diarrhea and least commonly in patients with constipation (Whitehead et al. 1980). Chasen et al. (1982) found that injections of cholecystokinin increased colonic motility; this increase was significantly correlated with the magnitude of response to mechanical distension with balloon.

Lyrenas et al. (1985) compared the effects of the ß_2 agonist terbutaline, the ß_1 agonist prenalterol, and placebo. Sigmoid motility was decreased by ß_2-adrenoreceptor stimulation, whereas it was unaffected by ß_1-adrenergic receptor stimulation. Several other authors quoted in this chapter, including Burns (1980) and Taylor (1985), have discussed the factors that affect motility in IBS.

Increased Bowel Sensitivity

Several authors have examined the pain threshold of the colon and the sensitivity to distension in patients with IBS. Ritchie (1973) examined bowel sensitivity in IBS patients by inflating a balloon inserted in the sigmoid colon. A significantly larger proportion of patients with IBS reported pain than was reported by control subjects who were either normal or suffered from constipation. Whitehead et al. (1980) found that both normal and anxious subjects tolerated a greater distension of the rectum than did patients with IBS. A stepwise distension of the balloon in the bowel also showed greater sensitivity in IBS patients than in healthy control subjects (Figure 6-2) (Whitehead et al. 1980). Swarbrick et al. (1980) and Dawson (1985) distended balloons throughout the colon and small intestine and were able to identify in a substantial proportion of patients sites that reproduced the patients' usual pain. However, Latimer et al. (1979) failed to reproduce these results. The reason for the discrepancy is unknown; Whitehead and Schuster (1985) suggest that the results may have been confounded in Latimer et al.'s study, because the perception tasks were embedded in a study of the effects of stressful interviews and meal stimulation on colonic activity.

The sensitivity is limited to the bowel. In one study, patients with IBS had a higher pain threshold to electrocutaneous stimulation than did non-IBS patients (Cook et al. 1987).

Comment. Some studies, but not others, suggest that patients with IBS are abnormally sensitive to stimulation of the colon by distension (Barsky 1987). The nature of this sensitivity is not merely caused by higher levels of anxiety or neuroticism (Kullman and Fielding 1981). The causes of this increased sensitivity are not known and may constitute a physiological characteristic of patients with IBS.

Lactose Malabsorption (or Hypolactasia)

Low levels of lactase, an enzyme that breaks down milk sugar called lactose, lead to symptoms that are indistinguishable from IBS. It is an inherited disorder; the prevalence has been estimated to be between 60% and 70% in black Americans, but is under 10% in Caucasians (Johnson 1981). In a large proportion of patients with lactose malabsorption, the symptoms improve or remit when lactose is eliminated from the diet (Arvanitakis et al. 1977). This would suggest that the inclusion of patients with lactose malabsorption among IBS patients is a misdiagnosis and that hypolactasia is a deficiency syndrome that is separate from IBS (Whitehead and Schuster 1985). The psychological studies of patients with lactose malabsorption are described later in this chapter.

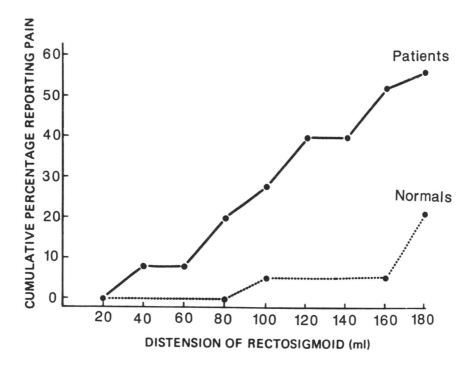

Figure 6-2. Pain complaints produced by stepwise distension of a balloon placed 15 cm into the bowel (Whitehead et al. 1980). The cumulative percentage of each group reporting pain is shown. Reprinted from Whitehead et al. 1980, with permission of the authors and Plenum Publishing Corporation. Copyright 1980, Plenum Publishing Corporation.

Noncolonic Findings and Symptoms

Various abnormal findings in sites other than the colon, as well as symptoms associated with these abnormalities, have been described. There is evidence of abnormal motility in other parts of the alimentary tract. Whorwell et al. (1981) found that patients with IBS had decreased lower esophageal sphincter pressure as well as other evidence of abnormal motility of the esophagus. The authors concluded that these findings help to explain complaints of upper gastrointestinal symptoms, including heartburn and dysphagia, and that the syndrome may be a widespread disorder of smooth muscle or of its innervation. Yunus et al. (1989) found a larger proportion of patients with IBS and chronic fatigue in a group of patients with fibromyalgia than could be expected by chance. (For the likely causes of this association, see Chapter 10, pp. 207–208, this volume.)

In patients with severe constipation or unexplained diarrhea, abnormal levels of motilin and pancreatic polypeptide and raised levels of prostaglandin have been reported. The significance of these increased levels is unknown. These and other abnormal findings have been surveyed by Lennard-Jones (1983).

Family History

Several studies have shown an increased prevalence of IBS among first-degree relatives. For example, Whorwell et al. (1986) found a family history of IBS in 32% of patients and in only 2% of control subjects. To my knowledge, there are no twin studies that have examined the genetic influences in IBS.

Stress and Psychosocial Factors

> Gut: adj Slang. Arousing basic emotions; visceral: a gut issue, a gut response
>
> *American Heritage*
> *Dictionary* (1976)

There are numerous psychological and psychiatric studies on IBS (Creed and Guthrie 1987; Langeluddecke 1985; Whitehead and Schuster 1985). In the following survey, the results of some of these studies are summarized and classified in accord with the aim of the inquiry rather than by describing the method and outcome of the individual studies.

Colonic pressure and motility. Several studies show that pressure in the colon and motility increase in experimental situations in response to emotionally charged topics and other stressors such as experimental pain. These responses occur in patients with IBS as well as in non-IBS individuals. Colonic pressure is higher in patients with IBS (Almy and Tulin 1947; Almy et al. 1949a,

1949b; Chaudhary and Truelove 1961; Wangel and Deller 1965). Motility and vascular changes vary with different emotions (Latimer 1981); for example, a series of studies during interviews that made the subject feel helpless and defeated led to hypomotility that coincided with weeping, whereas when the patient was hostile, dispirited, and defensive, there was an increase in sygmoid motility (Almy 1951).

Welgan et al. (1988) examined colon motor and spike potential activity in patients with IBS and healthy control subjects during resting and when exposed to two experimental anger stressors: during criticism of performance on an intelligence test and during a delay of assistance for a diagnostic procedure. Anger significantly increased colon motor and spike potential activity in both groups compared with the resting state; patients with IBS produced significantly higher motor and spike potential activity when angered. They reported themselves to be more hostile and appeared angrier than the control subjects, but did not report themselves to be more anxious or depressed, suggesting that the observed changes in colonic functioning in both groups were due to anger.

Stressful events. Four studies compared patients with IBS during stressful events with other patients or with subjects who had IBS and did not consult a doctor. In three studies, stressful events were more common in IBS patients than in other patients. The events were undesirable, beyond a person's control, and comprised losses or threats of losses, mainly those of "exits from the patient's social field" (Fava and Pavan 1976/1977a, 1976/1977b) such as marital discord, or death or severe illness of a relative (Hislop 1971). Psychiatric illness or anxiety-provoking situations preceded the onset of symptoms in two thirds of the patients with functional abdominal symptoms (75% of which had IBS and most of the others had non-ulcer dyspepsia) and in none of the patients with organic abdominal illness (Ford et al. 1987). Conversely, in a study in which the Life Experience Schedule was administered, IBS patients reported unexpectedly fewer unfavorable events but also fewer favorable events than did subjects with IBS who had not consulted a physician (Drossman et al. 1988).

Physiological indicators of stress. Urinary epinephrine secretion un-der stressful conditions is higher in patients with IBS who have predominantly diarrhea than it is in other medical patients (Esler and Goulston 1973). Basal forearm blood flow, an indicator of sympathetic-adrenergic arousal, is as high as that of psychoneurotic patients, and higher than that of nonpatients (Palmer et al. 1974).

Psychological inventories, rating, and self-rating scales. Numerous studies found higher self-ratings of anxiety in patients with IBS than in other patients when using the Institute for Personality and Ability Testing (IPAT) Anxiety Scale Questionnaire, the Spielberger State-Trait Anxiety Inventory, and the Middlesex Hospital Questionnaire, among others (Blanchard et al. 1986; Esler and Goulston 1973; Palmer et al. 1974; Richter et al. 1986). The patients with IBS also were found to be more depressed as measured by the Minnesota Multiphasic Personality Inventory (MMPI) (Whitehead et al. 1980), the States of Anxiety and Depression (SAD) scales (Arapakis et al. 1986), and the Zung Depression Scale (Heefner et al. 1978). Anxiety and depression decrease with improvement of IBS (Hillman et al. 1984). Neuroticism, as measured by the Eysenck Personality Inventory (EPI), was higher in IBS patients than in other patients in four studies; in two of these, IBS patients were also more introverted (Esler and Goulston 1973; Hill and Blendis 1967; Latimer et al. 1981; Palmer et al. 1974).

In studies with the MMPI, several of the clinical scales were elevated, usually those of the psychosomatic triad (hysteria [Hy], hypochondriasis [Hs], depression [D]); however, the elevation of various scales is not consistent across studies (West 1970; Whitehead et al. 1980; Wise et al. 1982a). Patients with IBS scored lower on social domineering attitudes and self-confidence and were more intrapunitive than other patients as measured by Fould's Personality Deviance Scale. Several studies that used the Johns Hopkins Symptom Checklist (SCL) (e.g., Whitehead et al. 1988), and studies in which other self-rating scales were administered, found more psychopathology in patients with IBS than in other patients.

Blanchard et al. (1986) administered several psychological inventories, including the Beck Depression Inventory (BDI), the State-Trait Anxiety Inventory, the MMPI, and the Psychosomatic Symptom Checklist. They also administered the Social Readjustment Rating Scale for the measurement of life events. Judging by the scores of these inventories, patients with IBS tended to be the most distressed; they were similar to patients with tension headaches and were significantly more distressed than patients with migraine and healthy control subjects on several measures.

Psychiatric diagnoses. Patients with IBS report more psychiatric illness than do other patients (Fava and Pavan 1976/1977a, 1976/1977b); in one study the prevalence of psychiatric illness was three times (and in another four times) more common in IBS patients than in those patients with organic illness (Ford et al. 1987; Young et al. 1976). In studies in which the authors used psychiatric Research Diagnostic Criteria (RDC) (Feighner et al. 1972), the diagnoses varied; a common diagnosis was hysteria, but the proportion varied from one study to another (Latimer et al. 1981; Liss et al. 1973; Young et al. 1976). In the studies in which the authors used the RDC, the diagnosis of hysteria was synonymous with that of Briquet's syndrome (see Chapter 11, pp. 227–228). In some patients, the onset of IBS coincides with the onset of panic disorder (Noyes et al. 1990).

Other psychiatric symptoms. Various symptoms such as self-blame, guilt, or suicidal ideation have been reported in patients with IBS that are indicative of stress or psychopathology (Hislop 1971). "Stress" scores are computed in part from stressful events and in part from indicators of psychopathology such as multiple marriages and multiple jobs (Young et al. 1976), nervousness, attacks of panic, insomnia, and tiredness (Whorwell et al. 1986). Johnsen et al. (1986) reported from a community study a strong association between abdominal symptoms and psychological and social conditions; in view of the nature of the study, these disorders were probably not limited to IBS.

Premorbid characteristics. In one study, patients with IBS reported significantly more often than those with peptic ulcer, that when they had a cold or flu as a child their parents gave them toys, gifts, or treat foods such as ice cream (Whitehead et al. 1982). Yet, there were no differences between subjects with IBS and peptic ulcer patients in the number who reported themselves to be anxious or depressed. The authors regarded this as compelling evidence that direct reinforcement of somatic complaints during childhood contributes to the etiology of IBS (Whitehead et al. 1982).

Patients with IBS report more visits to doctors, poorer general health, and more headaches in childhood, more parental attention to illness, and more frequent school absences than do individuals with IBS who did not seek medical care for their symptoms (Lowman et al. 1987).

Other indirect evidence of social learning comes from studies that show that abdominal pain is more common in the mothers of patients with chronic abdominal pain than in the fathers, because mothers typically spend more time with their children; also, patients with chronic abdominal pain tend to come from larger sibships (Hill and Blendis 1967; Whitehead and Schuster 1985).[1]

Subjects with irritable bowel syndrome who do not seek treatment. Several studies compared IBS clinic or office patients (IBS patients) with subjects in the community who had IBS but had not consulted a physician (IBS nonpatients) and other subjects in the community who had no abdominal symptoms (control individuals).

Approximately 50% to 60% of subjects with IBS did not seek treatment from a physician. Abdominal pain was three times more common in IBS patients; they also had more nausea, diarrhea, vomiting, and unexplained weight loss, and more nongastrointestinal symptoms such as headaches and back pain, and they visited doctors more often because of these symptoms than did IBS nonpatients (Drossman et al. 1982; Lowman et al. 1987; Sandler et al. 1984).

Drossman et al. (1988) found that among the three groups, IBS patients scored highest on several MMPI scales, including hypochondriasis (Hs), hysteria (Hy), and schizophrenia (Sc) scales, and on several scales of the Illness Behavior Questionnaire (i.e., health worry, illness disruption, and affective disturbance). Generally, IBS nonpatients were between IBS patients and control individuals on a psychosocial continuum, with many measures of IBS nonpatients being similar to those of the control individuals. The authors concluded that psychological factors previously attributed to IBS are associated with "pa-

---

[1] Since this chapter was written, Drossman and his colleagues completed a study of abdominal complaints. Women who had been sexually abused in childhood were more likely to report pelvic pain, multiple functional somatic symptoms, and more surgical operations (D. A. Drossman, in press).

tient status"; these factors influence how the illness is experienced and acted upon. IBS nonpatients were judged to have higher coping capabilities, experience illness as less disruptive, and exhibit less denial than IBS patients.

Whitehead et al. (1988) recruited a community sample of 149 middle-class women. Two sets of diagnostic criteria for IBS were compared: Manning's restrictive criteria and conventional criteria. Individuals with lactose malabsorption were included as one of the control groups (see p. 117, this chapter) to assess the causative effects of chronic bowel symptoms on psychological distress. Women who met Manning's restrictive criteria for IBS (see p. 112, this chapter) but had not consulted a physician had no more symptoms of psychological distress on the SCL than did control individuals. IBS patients as well as patients with lactose malabsorption had significantly more psychological symptoms than either IBS nonpatients or control subjects. Individuals who met only the conventional criteria for IBS reported more psychological distress than did control subjects regardless of whether these individuals had consulted a physician or not. The authors concluded that the results suggest that a) symptoms of psychologic distress are unrelated to IBS, but will influence which patient will consult a doctor, and b) conventional diagnostic criteria for IBS identify more psychologically distressed individuals than do the restrictive criteria.

Welch et al. (1984, 1985), in New Zealand, compared 26 IBS patients (6 men and 20 women) with blood donors who had symptoms of IBS but had not sought treatment (IBS nonpatients) and blood donors who had no abdominal symptoms (control subjects). The authors administered the Walkey-McCormick modification of the SCL that yields three factors: somatization, distress, and performance difficulty. Somatic distress was higher in IBS patients than in control subjects, but not higher than in IBS nonpatients. There was no difference between IBS patients and control subjects on the other two factors. The authors concluded that IBS patients and nonpatients do not differ in severity and that the preponderance of women may reflect sociological factors rather than the severity of the IBS.

Irritable bowel syndrome as learned behavior. Whitehead et al. (1982) examined whether chronic illness behavior results from early learning experiences in which somatic complaints are rewarded. The authors questioned over 800 people in a telephone survey in Cincinnati, Ohio. The diagnosis of IBS was made on the basis that the person had constipation or diarrhea in the past year and during the same period he or she also had abdominal pain. Peptic ulcer disease was assumed to be present if respondents replied that they had been told by a physician or a nurse that they had an ulcer. Subjects with IBS were more likely than people without this disorder to report that they had two or more colds during the past year. They stated the belief that their colds were more serious than those of most other people, and indicated that they were more likely to go to a doctor when they had a cold or flu than to treat it themselves. Individuals with IBS were twice as likely to indicate that they had two or more acute physical illnesses in the past year and twice as likely to have been hospitalized for acute illness in the past year as compared with people who did not have IBS. The IBS individuals reported that they had other chronic disorders at a significantly greater rate. They also showed more preoccupation with illness than did those with peptic ulcer disease. A larger proportion of IBS individuals reported that they had missed work or changed their activities because of illness in the preceding year. When asked, "Did your parents show special consideration for you when you had a cold or flu by giving you special foods, more toys, or other gifts?" subjects with IBS were significantly more likely to respond "Yes" to this question than were subjects with peptic ulcer disease and other individuals. Subjects with IBS and peptic ulcer disease reported more anxiety and depression than other subjects, but there was no difference between reports of patients with IBS and those of patients with peptic ulcer disease. The authors commented that social learning may contribute to the etiology of chronic illness behavior in patients with IBS but not in patients with peptic ulcer.

Self-ratings in irritable bowel syndrome and lactose malabsorption. Enck et al. (1984) administered the SCL to patients referred to a gastrointestinal clinic for lactose malabsorption. There were no significant differences in gastrointestinal symptoms nor in the levels of psychological distress between patients with lactose malabsorption and patients with IBS. In a subsequent study, Enck et al. (1988) examined 21 patients with lactose malabsorption and 20 patients with IBS and the irritable colon syndrome. Intestinal symptoms, intestinal motor activity, and psychopathology of patients with IBS were nonspecific and occurred equally as frequent in the lactose malabsorption patients. The authors concluded that this finding casts doubts on the view that psychological factors play a role in the pathogenesis of IBS. Whitehead et al. (1988), in the community study described above, found no difference in SCL scores between subjects who had lactose malabsorption but had not consulted a physician and control subjects who did not have abdominal symptoms.

Comment. The results of the comparison of IBS patients to IBS nonpatients are conflicting. Welch et al.'s study differed from the others in that it did not reveal differences between the two groups and, unlike other studies, it did not show an association between neurotic symptoms and IBS even among patients. The reasons for these findings are unknown. The authors explained their results by having used a psychometric instrument of greater clarity and reproducibility; they claimed that other authors failed to use an overall analysis of variance followed by pairwise comparisons, which increased the probability of detecting chance differences between pairs of groups. There may also be other explanations for the discrepancy than the one put forward by these authors. The discrepancy may be due to a difference in methodology; for example, blood donors may have differed from the control groups of other studies.

Among the various views on the relationship of psychosocial factors to IBS, the two main contemporary views are represented by Latimer (1981) and Whitehead and Schuster (1985). These are briefly summarized here.

Latimer describes four models of IBS:

1. The digestive disease model
2. The psychiatric disease model
3. The psychophysiological model
4. The behavioral model (as termed by Latimer to describe his model)

The author argues that there is inadequate evidence to support the first three and concludes that patients with IBS do not differ essentially from neurotic patients. Unadaptive physiological responses and symptomatic change in bowel habits are an unlearned response to stressful circumstances that IBS patients have in common with other neurotic individuals. For various reasons they choose to complain about symptoms of IBS; these reasons include having misconceptions about normal bowel habits and regarding symptoms of IBS as a socially more acceptable way to express distress. The extraversion scores that are midway between neurotic and control individuals facilitate the patient's tendency to voice symptoms.

Whitehead and Schuster (1985) conclude that patients with IBS show more motility in the colon than do control subjects in response to various stimuli such as pain caused by balloon distension, eating, and emotional arousal. The motility of the distal colon in patients with IBS is not qualitatively different from that of the control subjects. IBS patients are hyperactive to a variety of stimuli, and there is a biological predisposition to respond to any stimulus with exaggerated bowel motility. This biological predisposition interacts with the environmental stressors and psychological characteristics of the person to produce sustained colonic motility and bowel symptoms.

Emotional arousal is among the stimuli that provoke this response in predisposed individuals. Whitehead and Schuster hypothesize that the most likely explanation for both bowel symptoms and anxiety is Pavlovian conditioning, which refers to the tendency for a neutral stimulus that has been repeatedly paired with a stimulus that reflexively elicits an autonomic response to acquire the ability to elicit that response and present alone. The authors also associate IBS with learned illness behavior (Whitehead et al. 1982).

Latimer does not weigh adequately the evidence that points to a physiological disturbance of the alimentary tract in IBS. To my mind, Whitehead and Schuster's conclusions present a more balanced presentation of the current state of knowledge.

Diagnosis and Classification

After physical disease has been excluded, the diagnosis is made on the characteristic clinical picture. If psychosocial factors play a substantial role, the DSM-III-R classification on Axis I is *psychological factors affecting physical condition,* and on Axis III, *irritable bowel syndrome.* In the ICD-10 draft, the code is 45.32. If the syndrome is atypical, the diagnosis should remain the same if it fulfills at least some of Manning's criteria (see p. 112, this chapter). Only if there are no indications that the abdominal symptoms are caused by IBS should the conditions be classified as one of the somatoform disorders.

Treatments

Drug Treatments and Other Physical Agents

There are several published reviews of the controlled studies of medical treatments of IBS. (See, for example, Sullivan 1983, Whitehead and Schuster 1985, Holdsworth 1985, and Klein 1988.) The review by Klein (1988) is the most comprehensive; he critiques individual studies, and, unlike several other authors, he reaches pessimistic conclusions about the efficacy of the treatments.

Antispasmodic agents. In drug trials, antispasmodic agents have been used either alone or in conjunction with another drug and compared with placebo or with other drugs. Klein (1988) has reviewed these trials and has pointed out that many of the trials that showed some positive results had methodological flaws. Antispasmodics are widely used, but their status is controversial. Latimer (1983a) agrees with other authors that there is at least a theoretical justification for the use of these drugs in cases with pain and constipation. The evidence from controlled trials is inconsistent (Whitehead and Schuster 1985), perhaps because of the large placebo effect in patients with IBS.

Tricyclic antidepressants. Heefner et al. (1978) compared desipramine, 150 mg, with placebo. One of the four outcome measures (the degree to which symptoms interfered with daily activities) significantly favored 150 mg of desipramine over placebo.

Greenbaum et al. (1987) compared desipramine, atropine, and placebo in a crossover trial (each treatment lasting for a 6-week period) in 28 patients. In the diarrhea-predominant group, abdominal pain, stool frequency, and slow contractions on rectal sigmoid observation decreased more during desipramine treatment than during placebo and atropine treatments. Depression decreased also with desipramine treatment. The response was unrelated to the desipramine blood levels, and several of the favorable responses occurred with unusually low levels. The authors suggested that desipramine may be helpful because of its antimuscarinic effects as well as its antidepressant effects.

Myren et al. (1984) compared various dosage schedules of trimiprimine with placebo in a study of 428 patients in which over 100 physicians (largely general practitioners) participated. The authors used visual analogue scales to evaluate outcome. The results differed for different dosage schedules. Most drug groups showed a significant reduction of various abdominal symptoms when compared with placebo. There was also a significant decrease in depression in the group treated with trimiprimine. The results were somewhat better when most of the dose was given at bedtime.

Tranquilizers. A few studies with tranquilizers have shown these agents to be superior to placebo at least on some measures (Baume and Cuthbert 1973; Ritchie and Truelove 1979, 1980). As with tricyclic antidepressants, the mode of action is not fully understood; probably the relief of anxiety increases tolerance to abdominal symptoms or perhaps decreases bowel motility.

There are a few controlled studies of combinations of antianxiety agents with tricyclic antidepressants (Lancaster-Smith et al. 1982; Ritchie and Truelove 1980). These combinations generally produce a better result than antianxiety drugs alone, and it may be that the tricyclic drugs in these combinations are the effective agent.

Bulking agents and other drugs. Controlled studies suggest that bulking agents are effective when the main problem is constipation; other IBS symptoms are not improved when bulking agents are compared with placebo (Klein 1988; Lucey et al. 1987). Among other agents, opioids tend to be effective in the treatment of diarrhea, but there is no conclusive evidence that they are effective on the other symptoms of IBS. Evidence for dopamine agonists and several other drugs has been inconclusive (Klein 1988). The results with carminative agents have been conflicting; however, in two studies, peppermint oil was more effective than placebo (Dew et al. 1984; Rees et al. 1979). There are several other agents that have shown efficacy at least in one controlled trial; these include loperamide and leuprolide acetate (Cann et al. 1984; Lavö et al. 1987).

Two studies with phenytoin (Chadda et al. 1983; Greenbaum et al. 1973) yielded conflicting results. Greenbaum et al. (1973) had a negative outcome, whereas Chadda et al. (1983) showed some efficacy of phenytoin on some measures. Dicyclomine HCl, a smooth-muscle relaxant, was more effective than placebo in relieving symptoms (Page and Dirnberger 1981). Loperamide (a drug that acts on peripheral opiate receptors) was found to delay gut transit and was more effective than placebo in controlling diarrhea, pain, and unformed stools (Cann et al. 1984; Hovdenak 1987). Some combinations of drugs, such as an antidepressant and a bulking agent, were found to be more effective in some patients than other combinations or any of the agents given singly (Ritchie and Truelove 1979, 1980). A crossover study of diltiazem showed the drug to be more effective than placebo on some measures (Perez-Mateo et al. 1986). Timolol was found to be no more effective than placebo (Fielding 1981). In a recent open-label study, leuprolide acetate (a gonadotrophin-releasing hormone analogue agonist) showed promising results (Mathias et al. 1989) and was found to be more effective than placebo in a small study (Lavö et al. 1987). In an uncontrolled study of five patients with panic disorder and IBS, there was a rapid and dramatic relief of IBS symptoms upon effective treatment of panic attacks with alprazolam or lorazepam (Lydiard et al. 1986).

Comment. It appears that none of the drugs used in the treatment of IBS have been uniformly effective. One reason may be the high placebo response in IBS (Holdsworth 1985; Whitehead and Schuster 1985). There are several findings that suggest that drug treatment is more likely to be successful if it is chosen for a specific symptom such as constipation or diarrhea. Patients who are predominantly constipated may benefit from substances that increase bulk. Patients who predominantly have diarrhea are likely to benefit from small doses of tricyclic antidepressants that are gradually increased. There is no evidence at present that one tricyclic drug is better than another; drugs that have fewer side effects may be those of first choice. Because side effects tend to be idiosyncratic, several drugs may have to be tried. The doses needed appear to be substantially lower than those used for depression, and the rules of choice of drug and dosage schedules that apply to somatization in general (see Chapter 10, pp. 214–216, this volume) apply also to IBS. Antispasmodics that are widely used have a logical appeal, but their use has not been adequately supported in controlled studies and should not be the drugs of first choice. Overall, there is little evidence to date to support treatment with antianxiety agents unless they are needed for the treatment of coexisting anxiety. The evidence for other drugs at present is sparse, although some show promise.

Psychological Treatments

Numerous authors have reviewed and discussed psychological treatments in IBS. These include Latimer (1983a), Whitehead (1985), Drossman (1987), Whitehead and Schuster (1985), Creed and Guthrie (1989), and Walker et al. (E. A. Walker, P. P. Roy-Byrne, W. J. Katon, unpublished manuscript, 1990). Uncontrolled studies have shown substantial improvement in IBS symptoms after psychological treatments (Wise et al. 1982b). The section that follows is largely limited to descriptions of controlled studies and to brief summaries of some uncontrolled series.

Psychotherapy

Schonecke and Schüffel (1975) carried out a controlled study of psychotherapy in patients with functional abdominal complaints as a part of a drug trial with 78 patients. Psychotherapy lasted for 6 sessions of only 20 minutes each; it was found to be no more effective than other treatments in this study.

Giles (1978) compared four treatments in patients (n = 10) who had functional bowel complaints. It is not clear from the description what proportion had classical IBS. After receiving a personal communication from the author, Whitehead and Schuster (1985) expressed the view that most of the patients had IBS by the clinical criteria of altered bowel habits and abdominal pain. The treatments compared were psychotherapy alone (which focused on identifying stressors and solving personal problems), electromyographic biofeedback alone, combined psychotherapy with electromyographic biofeedback, and a control group that had no treatment. It was found that relaxation alone relieved the frequency of bowel movements and that the combined treatment was most effective in relieving the associated psychological symptoms.

Whorwell et al. (1984) carried out a controlled study of hypnotherapy in patients with IBS. The control group had psychotherapy. (This study is described in greater detail below in section on hypnosis.) The patients made small but significant gains with psychotherapy, but these gains were substantially less than those of patients treated with hypnosis.

Svedlund et al. (1983) carried out the largest study so far of psychotherapy in outpatients with IBS. All patients had either abdominal pain, changes in bowel habits (constipation or diarrhea), or some combination of these without demonstrable organic disease. In all cases, this disorder had lasted 1 year or longer. The 110 patients who agreed to participate were randomly allocated into two groups, unaware of the experimental design.

Both groups had routine medical treatments by their gastroenterologist. The psychotherapy group had, in addition, short-term dynamically oriented individual psychotherapy conducted by psychiatrists. The authors described this as follows:

> Psychotherapy, given in ten hour-long sessions spread over three months, aimed at modifying maladaptive behavior and finding new solutions to problems. The focus was on means of coping with stress and emotional problems. Sometimes a more educative or teaching strategy about relations between stressful life events and abdominal symptoms was used. All psychotherapeutic measures were tailored to suit individuals and took the patients' tolerance of anxiety into account. (Svedlund et al. 1983, p. 589)

Assessments were carried out prior to the study, after 3 months (at the end of therapy), and after 15 months. Unavoidably, raters became aware of which group the patients belonged to. Mental symptoms were rated on the Comprehensive Psychopathological Rating Scale and somatic symptoms, on a specially designed scale comprising 10 items, each rated on a 7-point scale. Patients also rated their somatic symptoms, and on follow-up they rated their improvement on a postal questionnaire.

There were only two early dropouts. In the remaining patients, the number of sessions ranged from 3 to 10 (mean = 7.4). Both experimental and control groups improved, but the improvement in the psychotherapy groups was significantly greater for abdominal pain and bowel dysfunction; this improvement continued after 15 months, whereas the control group had deteriorated slightly. Scores for the main psychopathological syndromes improved to a similar degree in the two groups during the first 3 months, with little further change on follow-up. Patients' self-ratings agreed with psychiatrists' ratings. The postal follow-up questionnaire also showed a significant degree of improvement in somatic symptoms and in "ability to cope with life in general."

Hypnosis

Whorwell et al. (1984) carried out the first controlled study of hypnosis in treating IBS. The results were impressive. Thirty patients with severe IBS who had been resistant to all previous treatment and had been treated by the authors for at least 1 year were randomly assigned to either hypnotherapy, or supportive psychotherapy and placebo. The mean number of previous treatments was six per patient. All patients were administered the General Health Questionnaire.

Before hypnosis the patient was given a simple account of intestinal smooth-muscle physiology. Hypnotherapy consisted of 7 half-hour sessions of decreasing frequency over a 3-month period. Patients were given a tape for daily auto-hypnosis after the third session. No subject proved to be unhypnotizable, and in all patients the trance was deep enough for arm catalepsy. Hypnotherapy was solely directed at general relaxation and control of intestinal motility, and no attempt was made at hypnoanalysis. Hypnosis was induced with an arm-levitation technique followed by a combination of several standard deepening procedures, depending on the patient's progress and visualization abilities. After general comments about improvement of health and well-being, attention was directed to the control of intestinal smooth muscle. The patient was asked to place his or her hand on the abdomen, feel a sense of warmth, and relate this to asserting control over gut function. Reinforcement by visualization was used if the patient had this ability. All sessions were concluded with standard ego-strengthening suggestions.

Patients in the control group received a placebo and 7 half-hour sessions of supportive psychotherapy by the same therapist. These sessions included discussion of symptoms and an exploration of any possible contributory emotional problems and stressful life events.

All patients were independently assessed and asked to keep a diary card, on which they recorded daily the frequency and severity of abdominal pain, abdominal distension, and bowel habits. Overall improvement of symptoms and well-being were scored weekly.

At the end of treatment the symptoms were either mild or absent in all 15 hypnotherapy patients. The changes were greater in the hypnotherapy group than in the psychotherapy-placebo group (see Figure 6-3). The control group showed small but significant improvement in all symptoms except bowel habits. There was no significant correlation between General Health Questionnaire scores and any improvement observed in either group. The General Health Questionnaire was not readministered after the treatment (P. J. Whorwell, personal communication, 1990).

The gains in hypnosis were maintained on an 18-month follow-up. Thirteen patients remained in remission, and two had a single relapse that was effectively treated by a single session of hypnotherapy.

The authors reported their subsequent experience of treating 35 IBS patients with hypnotherapy in an uncontrolled study. In typical cases of IBS, the success in atypical cases and those with "significant psychopathology" were 43% and 60%, respectively. Only 25% of those aged over 50 responded. In a total of over 200 patients, which included referrals of increasingly severe cases, the success rate was about 85%. Some patients required more than 12 sessions (Whorwell 1989; Whorwell et al. 1987).

Harvey et al. (1989) carried out individual and group hypnotherapy in 33 patients with IBS who had not responded to previous treatments. Hypnotherapy consisted of four 40-minute sessions over 7 weeks. Twenty patients improved, and the improvement was maintained on 3 months follow-up. Eleven lost almost all symptoms. Group hypnotherapy was as effective as individual therapy.

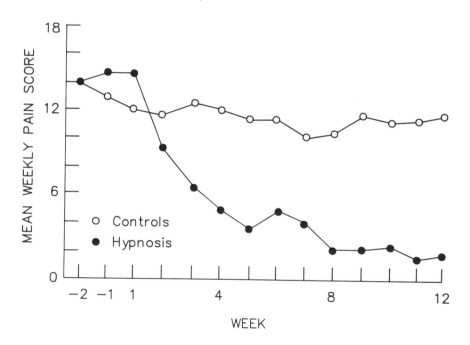

Figure 6-3. Change in mean weekly scores for abdominal pain during a controlled trial of hypnosis in patients with severe refractory irritable bowel syndrome (Whorwell et al. 1984). At the end of treatment, pain was mild or absent in all hypnotherapy patients. Reprinted from Whorwell et al. 1984, with permission of the authors and Lancet Ltd. Copyright 1984, Lancet Ltd.

Other Psychological Treatments

Voirol and Hipolito (1987) compared a special kind of relaxation treatment ("anthropo-analytical relaxation") in IBS patients with that of a selected control group that received conventional medical treatment. The authors describe the anthropo-analytic relaxation treatment (which is based on Schultz' autogenic training and adapted by Hipolito) as follows:

> [T]he monitor utilizes the "I" which allows the patient to use what he finds convenient; his freedom is therefore respected. After the first session that is more general the body is uncovered segment by segment and the emphasis put on the digestive system. . . . The relaxation techniques used are directed at the abdominal organs which are introduced in succession: stomach, liver, pancreas. . . . During the sessions the relaxed subject is invited to give free course to his fantasies and imagination, and to express his emotions and his internal self, remaining free to talk about them or not. (p. 1118)

Thus, the emphasis of the therapy appears to consist in a modification of autogenic training, with emphasis on concentrating on abdominal organs combined with nondirective group psychotherapy. The treatment lasted for 6 months. The number of consultations following treatment decreased from 74 to 6, whereas in the control group the decrease was from 53 to 41. The attacks of pain in a 2-month time period fell to zero in the treated group, and there was no change in the control group.

The MMPI showed significant decrease on several scales at the end of treatment, and this was maintained on a 40-month follow-up. Only a few of the scales did not show improvement, but these were scales that were in the normal range before the study started. The scores were significantly lower than those in the control group (M. W. Voirol, personal communication, 1990).

Berndt and Maercker (1985) compared the effects of individual psychotherapy combined with autogenic training to those of symptomatic treatment alone in 8 patients each. Two thirds of the patients also had neuroses. After 1 year, the group that had psychological treatment had improved significantly more, but the beneficial effect was limited to IBS patients who also had neuroses.

Bennett and Wilkinson (1985) compared psychological treatment alone with medical treatment; the medical treatment consisted of drug therapy as outlined by Ritchie and Truelove (1980). The psychological treatment consisted of a combination of methods as suggested by Latimer (1983a, 1983b) that consisted of stress management training such as relaxation and desensitization, cognitive therapy to change any misconception about bowel habits, and contingency management to reduce IBS-associated behavior such as complaints of pain. Unlike in previous controlled studies, the psychological treatment was given alone and was not combined with medical care.

Thirty-three patients with IBS who had not previously responded to reassurance and simple symptomatic treatment were randomly assigned to medical or psychological treatment for 8 weeks. Anxiety levels that were high in both groups were reduced in the psychological group but not in the medically treated group. IBS symptoms and associated behaviors were reduced equally with both treatments.

Whitehead (1985) compared biofeedback of colon pressure to a stress management procedure. Eight patients were assigned to two groups; one group was the stress management procedure consisting of systematic desensitization in imagery. The two types of treatment appear to have had specific effects, but the changes did not reach a level of statistical significance. The small number of patients may have been responsible for this result.

Neff and Blanchard (1987) evaluated the effects of a combination of treatments. Ten patients had 12 sessions of progressive muscular relaxation, thermal biofeedback, educational information, and training in stress-coping strategies. A control group was only used to monitor symptoms. Six of the 10 treated patients improved, and there was no change in the control group; there was also a significantly greater improvement in self-ratings in the treated group. When the monitoring group received treatment, there was an improvement similar to that in the treated group.

Comment

Svedlund and his colleagues (1983) showed a significant improvement in abdominal symptoms with a mere 7.4 sessions of psychotherapy for patients with IBS. The patients continued to improve on follow-up, whereas the symptoms became somewhat worse in the control group that had routine medical treatment. The study by Schonecke and Schüffel (1975) showed no effect of psychotherapy on functional somatic abdominal complaints; however, the patients had only six 20-minute sessions of psychotherapy without a follow-up, which is hardly an adequate exposure to this treatment. In Whorwell et al.'s (1984) study, the patients in the control group had seven 30-minute sessions of supportive psychotherapy. There was a small and significant improvement in this group. Although the three studies differed in the amount of psychotherapy and outcome, one might argue that the authors among themselves established a dose-response curve. It is impressive that a mean of only seven sessions of psychotherapy in Svedlund et al.'s study produced lasting and progressive improvement in IBS patients in contrast to the deterioration seen in the control group.

Berndt and Maercker (1985) also reported a successful outcome of psychotherapy combined with autogenic training in a small study. However, they found the treatment to be successful only in the patients who also had neuroses.

The study by Whorwell et al. (1984) is a striking demonstration of the efficacy of hypnotherapy, which appears to be the most effective treatment in IBS. In patients who had a severe disorder who had not responded to any of the previous treatments, all 15 patients' symptoms after treatment were either "mild or absent" (p. 1232). The authors' understatement merits quotation: "This study suggests that hypnotherapy is useful in the treatment of IBS" (p. 1233). The authors also added that because hypnosis is time consuming and many patients respond to simple measures, it is probably best to reserve hypnosis for refractory cases.

Voirol and Hipolito's study (1987) showed significant changes after a group treatment that combined autogenic training and group psychotherapy. The treatment in this study lasted for about 50 sessions and was thus substantially more time consuming than the other methods.

Neff and Blanchard (1987) found a combination of psychological treatments to be effective. The study was small, but the findings suggest that their method might help patients who do not respond to verbal psychotherapy.

There are several reports from uncontrolled studies. Based on their clinical experience, Whitehead and Schuster (1985) have advocated systematic desensitization in imagery to stressful stimuli. In an uncontrolled study of group therapy of patients with IBS, Wise et al. (1982b) found a substantial reduction of symptoms, and this improvement was largely maintained on follow up.

Recommended Treatments

The choice of treatment depends to a large extent on the nature and severity of IBS, on the patient's personality and psychopathology, on the duration of the disorder, and on the physician's specialty and special skills. It is beyond the scope of this volume to recommend treatments for the primary physician or gastroenterologist of IBS uncomplicated by psychiatric disorders; these have been discussed elsewhere by numerous authors (see Thompson 1986).

Psychiatrists and psychologists encounter mainly patients who have been referred or who are seeking treatment for unrelated emotional disorders. If the patient is already being treated for IBS, the psychiatrist will need to work in conjunction with the patient's physician. In some patients the diagnosis of IBS has been previously made and physical disease has been excluded, but the patient has had no treatment. In milder cases explanation on the nature of IBS and reassurance may be all that is required. If the main symptom is spastic constipation, prescription of one of the bulking agents may constitute adequate treatment. Often the treatment of the coexisting psychiatric disorder (e.g., anxiety or depression) also alleviates the symptoms of IBS. In other cases it is feasible to choose a treatment (e.g., a tricyclic antidepressant) that has beneficial effects on the psychiatric disorder as well as on the IBS. In patients who have panic attacks and IBS, successful treatment of panic may also improve symptoms of the IBS. Loperamide may help if diarrhea and pain are not relieved by other measures.

In view of the possibility of habituation with minor tranquilizers and the risk of tardive dyskinesia with neuroleptics, tranquilizers are best avoided in the treatment of IBS. Antianxiety drugs should be limited to those cases in which severe anxiety is not adequately controlled by other treatments.

In view of the promising effects of psychotherapy in the controlled studies described above, this modality should be tried if the effects of simple measures are inadequate. For the same reason, hypnosis should be tried if psychotherapy is unsuccessful. The combinations of psychological methods as described by Neff and Blanchard (1987) are an alternative treatment. Autogenic training combined with group therapy may be tried, but the treatment in the controlled studies took substantially more time than other psychological treatments.

If these treatments fail, other treatments that have shown promise in uncontrolled series, such as desensitization to events or situations the patient finds stressful, may be tried, particularly if the patient has noticed that these stressful events precede bowel symptoms. In view of the good results of applied relaxation in the treatment of non-ulcer dyspepsia, this treatment may be tried if anxiety appears to induce symptoms of the IBS.

Case History

D.B. was a 38-year-old history professor who had been treated by a competent psychologist for the past 18 months. The treatment consisted predominantly of cognitive psychotherapy. The patient said that he had benefited from treatment; the referral was made because he still suffered from severe anxiety. He did not have spontaneous panic attacks, but frequently anxiety built up to a crescendo, which was extremely distressing and incapacitating. The patient missed time from work frequently; he avoided many social situations, because on days when he felt anxious he could not tolerate being with company.

The patient had diverticulosis with occasional attacks of diverticulitis. He also had IBS with severe abdominal pain and constipation. He took chlordiazepoxide regularly, up to 70 mg daily. The patient remarked that "if the anxiety is unchecked the colon symptoms get worse, which in itself creates more anxiety." The drug did not relieve anxiety, nor the IBS symptoms, adequately. At a later stage, after the patient had improved, he described his previous life as a continous nightmare: "The nightmares at night were dreadful and waking up was no better."

I first tried to treat him with imipramine, but a single dose of 25 mg made him more anxious and the nightmares worse, and a dose of 10 mg had no beneficial effects. Amitripyline, 25 mg at night, controlled his anxiety as well as his bowel symptoms, but made him so tired and sleepy that he could not function; again, smaller doses were ineffective. Fortunately, after several experiments with different doses, 25 mg of doxepin controlled his anxiety as well as the symptoms of the IBS. Attempts at discontinuing the medication or at lowering the dose led to rapid recurrences of symptoms of anxiety as well as of IBS.

On follow-up, which at the time of writing has lasted for 5 years, the patient has only had one episode of diverticulitis. He has had no more symptoms of IBS. He continues to take doxepin each night and rarely takes one capsule (10 mg) of chlordiazepoxide.

D.B. commented on his progress on various occasions: "I lived my whole life in fear. My fear and my colon made my life miserable. I envied other people. I never thought that life could be so good. I am very happy. I am much more sociable than I used to be. I feel the best I have felt my whole life. One little pill is [all there is] between my present state and living in a nightmare."

There are numerous reports of successful treatments of IBS, and results from controlled studies attest to the efficacy of diverse methods. The present case illustrates a psychiatric referral that would not have been made if the patient had not had also a severe psychiatric disorder. It seems unlikely that the drug treatment was predominantly a placebo effect, because some drugs were repeatedly ineffective and others made him feel worse. Patients with IBS benefit often from doses of tricyclic drugs that are far lower than those used in the treatment of psychiatric disorders (Greenbaum et al. 1983), and often several attempts need to be made before the most suitable one is found. In this case, fortunately, the same drug controlled the symptoms of both IBS and his incapacitating anxiety disorder.

Prognosis

A large proportion of patients with IBS will improve with placebo alone, but there is a tendency for recurrences (Waller and Misiewicz 1969). In view of the intermittent course of the disorder, a single evaluation on follow-up will not adequately assess outcome (Whitehead and Schuster 1985). A substantial proportion of patients improve with various treatments. Holmes and Salter (1982), in a 6- to 8-year follow-up, found that 38% of the patients had no further bowel symptoms. Sullivan (1983) found that after 2 years 79% of the patients had improved or were symptom free.

Harvey et al. (1987) examined over 100 patients with IBS, first for a few weeks, and then afterward for at least 5 years. The patients were treated with high-fiber diets, bulking agents, and explanation. Eighty-five percent of the patients were virtually symptom free in the short term, and almost 70% were virtually symptom free 5 years later. The response to treatment was better in men than in women, in those with constipation than in those with diarrhea, and in those with a relatively short history.

Svendsen et al. (1985) reported a substantially worse prognosis in a retrospective study of 112 patients 5 years after the initial diagnosis. Diagnostic errors had occurred in 4.5% of these patients. Half of the patients were either unimproved or worse.

Blanchard et al. (1988) examined in an uncontrolled study predictors of improvement in 45 patients suffering from IBS. The authors used numerous psychological tests, including the MMPI, the BDI, and the Spielberger State-Trait Anxiety Inventory. A multiple regression analysis showed that low trait anxiety scores predicted a 70% chance of successful treatment and no likelihood of complete failure of treatment. It appears that highly anxious patients need longer and more intensive treatment.

Lancaster-Smith et al. (1982) also found an association of psychiatric ill health and poor prognosis. Patients with high scores on the General Health Questionnaire had poorer outcome of most IBS symptoms than did those patients with low scores. Similarly, Chaudhary and Truelove (1962) found on follow-up that a significantly larger proportion of patients with psychosocial stressors or emotional disorders failed to improve compared with other patients. There were more patients among those who improved whose psychosocial stressors had become less burdensome and whose life had changed for the better. Ford (1985) found that interpersonal style of behavior was the best predictor of good outcome after biofeedback-relaxation training.

In an older series, 40% of the IBS patients had abdominal surgery (Keeling and Fielding 1975). This applied particularly to patients with the RDC diagnosis of hysteria (Young et al. 1976). Patients with IBS not only had more abdominal surgery but also had more nonabdominal surgery than did matched control subjects (Fielding 1983). Although there is no evidence of increased mortality in patients with IBS, there is a greater risk of surgical explorations with the risks that these procedures entail.

Various treatments were used in the outcome studies above. The prognosis may be better with current methods of treatment. For example, the outcome of treatment after hypnosis in Whorwell et al.'s (1984) study was good, and patients who had psychotherapy in Svedlund et al.'s (1983) study continued to improve on follow-up.

Summary and Main Conclusions

The conclusions that follow are largely summaries of selected reviewers' opinions quoted in this chapter. Other conclusions are based on research that has been published since these reviews were written.

The symptoms of IBS are mainly diarrhea, constipation, or both; abdominal pain and gaseousness are present to a variable degree. Symptoms that occur more often in IBS than in organic disease are pain relieved by defecation, more frequent stools with pain onset, looser stools with pain onset, abdominal distension, mucus in stool, and feeling of incomplete evacuation after defecation.

IBS patients who seek treatment also have noncolonic gastrointestinal symptoms such as nausea, dyspepsia, and esophageal symptoms. They also tend to have nongastrointestinal symptoms such as bladder symptoms, back pain, and tiredness.

There is incomplete agreement on the prevalence of IBS; in two studies it was estimated as 17% and 21%, respectively. However, the majority of subjects with IBS do not seek treatment. Yet, between 20% and 50% of all gastrointestinal consultations are because of IBS.

In IBS the bowel is more sensitive to experimental stretch and probably also to distension by gas and feces, which causes pain. Experimental distension leads to an increase in bowel motility that is larger in IBS patients than in non-IBS control subjects. Various biochemical abnormalities have been reported in IBS, but their significance is unknown. Lactose malabsorption appears to cause similar symptoms but is an unrelated disorder.

Patients with IBS who are seeking medical treatment have higher distress scores on psychological tests than do patients with gastrointestinal diseases of organic origin and healthy control subjects. IBS patients have substantially more psychiatric disorders than other patients. Intestinal motility increases in patients with IBS, as well as in healthy subjects, after emotional stress. A large proportion of patients with IBS report stressful events such as losses preceding either the onset or the exacerbation of symptoms. Psychosocial stress appears to be one of the factors that induces abnormal motility as well as symptoms.

When subjects in community surveys who have symptoms of IBS but have not sought treatment (particularly when restrictive diagnostic criteria for IBS are used) are compared with control subjects who have no abdominal symptoms, the difference between the two groups on self-rating scales of distress is either small or nonexistent. This finding would suggest that the majority of *noncolonic* symptoms, including symptoms of psychiatric ill health, are associated with seeking medical help rather than being an integral part of the IBS syndrome.

There is some evidence from retrospective studies that the IBS symptoms are, in part, learned. For example, patients with IBS report that in childhood they had more parental attention and more treats when ill than other patients.

Thus, patients who attend for treatment with IBS have a more responsive alimentary tract to various stimuli that include mechanical as well as psychosocial stressors. Some have perhaps acquired conditioned reflexes of abnormal bowel motility acquired through Pavlovian or other forms of conditioning. Some others, because of their emotional distress, appear to be unable to cope with their abdominal symptoms.

The results of various studies suggest that the psychopathology of patients with IBS is not uniform. The degree of physiological abormality, as well as the role and nature of psychological factors and social stressors, differs from one individual to the next.

None of the drugs used in the treatment of IBS have been uniformly effective. Patients who are predominantly constipated may benefit from substances that increase bulk. Patients who have predominantly diarrhea are likely to benefit from small doses of tricyclic antidepressants that are gradually increased; there is at present no evidence that one tricyclic antidepressant is better than another.

Antispasmodic agents that are widely used have a logical appeal, but their efficacy has not been adequately supported in controlled studies, and these agents should not be the drug of first choice. Overall, there is little evidence to date that supports treatment with antianxiety drugs unless they are needed for the treatment of coexisting anxiety. The evidence for other drugs at present is sparse, but a few of the new drugs are promising.

Explanation, reassurance, and support constitute adequate treatment in some patients. Several psychological treatments have been found to be effective in IBS in controlled studies. Fewer than eight sessions of psychotherapy were substantially more effective than routine medical care, and the difference between the groups became larger on follow-up. Hypnosis was strikingly effective in a controlled study in patients with severe IBS who had failed to respond to all previous treatments. Other psychological treatments that were found to be effective in controlled studies are psychotherapy combined with autogenic training, and a stress management program that consisted of a combination of treatments. The controlled studies of relaxation treatment alone have not shown conclusive results, but it seems likely that some patients benefit from this treatment.

A large proportion of patients improve with routine medical treatment, but there is a tendency for recurrences. Some patients remain severely distressed; the proportion of these patients varies across studies.

References

Almy TP: Experimental studies on the irritable colon. Am J Med 10:60–67, 1951

Almy TP, Tulin M: Alterations in colonic function in man under stress, I: experimental production of changes simulating the "irritable colon." Gastroenterology 8:616–626, 1947

Almy TP, Hinkle LE Jr, Berle B, et al: Alterations in colonic function in man under stress, III: experimental production of sigmoid spasm in patients with spastic constipation. Gastroenterology 12:437–449, 1949a

Almy TP, Kern F, Tulin M: Alterations in colonic function in man under stress, II: experimental production of sigmoid spasm in healthy persons. Gastroenterology 12:425–436, 1949b

Arapakis G, Lyketsos CG, Gerolymatos K, et al: Low dominance and high intropunitiveness in ulcerative colitis and irritable bowel syndrome. Psychother Psychosom 46:171–176, 1986

Arvanitakis C, Chen GH, Folscroft J, et al: Lactase deficiency: comparative study of diagnostic methods. Am J Clin Nutr 30:1597–1602, 1977

Barsky AJ: Investigating the psychological aspects of irritable bowel syndrome. Gastroenterology 93:902–904, 1987

Baume P, Cuthbert J: The effect of medazepam in relieving symptoms of functional gastrointestinal distress. Aust N Z J Med 3:457–460, 1973

Bennett P, Wilkinson S: A comparison of psychological and medical treatment of the irritable bowel syndrome. Br J Clin Psychol 24:215–216, 1985

Berndt H, Maercker W: Psychotherapy of irritable colon. Z Gesamte Inn Med 40:107–110, 1985

Blanchard EB, Radnitz CL, Evans DD, et al: Psychological comparisons of irritable bowel syndrome to chronic tension and migraine headache and nonpatient controls. Biofeedback Self Regul 11:221–230, 1986

Blanchard EB, Schwarz SP, Neff DF, et al: Prediction of outcome from the self-regulatory treatment of irritable bowel syndrome. Behav Res Ther 26:187–190, 1988

Bueno L, Fioramonti J, Frexinos J, et al: Colonic myoelectrical activity in diarrhea and constipation. Hepatogastroenterology 27:381–389, 1980

Burns TW: Colonic motility in the irritable bowel syndrome. Arch Intern Med 140:247–251, 1980

Burton R: The Anatomy of Melancholy (1611). London, Oxford University Press, 1883

Cann PA, Read NW, Holdsworth CD, et al: Role of loperamide and placebo in management of irritable bowel syndrome (IBS). Dig Dis Sci 29:239–247, 1984

Chadda VS, Joshi KG, Chadda S: A double-blind crossover study of diphenylhydantoin in irritable bowel syndrome. J Assoc Physicians India 31:425–427, 1983

Chasen R, Tucker H, Palmer D, et al: Colonic motility in irritable bowel syndrome and diverticular disease (abstract). Gastroenterology 82:1031, 1982

Chaudhary NA, Truelove SC: Human colonic motility: a comparative study of normal subjects, patients with ulcerative colitis, and patients with the irritable colon syndrome. Gastroenterology 40:1–36, 1961

Chaudhary NA, Truelove SC: The irritable colon syndrome. Q J Med 31:307–322, 1962

Clouse RE, Eckert TC: Gastrointestinal symptoms of patients with esophageal contraction abnormalities. Dig Dis Sci 31:236–240, 1986

Connell AM, Jones FA, Rowlands AN: Motility of the pelvic colon, part IV: abdominal pain associated with colonic hypermotility after meals. Gut 6:105–112, 1965

Cook IJ, van Eeden A, Collins SM: Patients with irritable bowel syndrome have greater pain tolerance than normal subjects. Gastroenterology 93:727–733, 1987

Creed F, Guthrie E: Psychological factors in the irritable bowel syndrome. Gut 28:1307–1318, 1987

Creed F, Guthrie E: Psychological treatments of the irritable bowel syndrome: a review. Gut 30:1601–1609, 1989

Da Costa JM: Membranous enteritis. Am J Med Sci 62:321–338, 1871

Dawson AM: Origin of pain in the irritable bowel syndrome, in Irritable Bowel Syndrome. Edited by Read NW. New York, Grune & Stratton, 1985, pp 155–162

Dew MJ, Evans BK, Rhodes J: Peppermint oil for the irritable bowel syndrome: a multicentre trial. Br J Clin Pract 38:394–398, 1984

Drossman DA: Psychosocial treatment of the refractory patient with irritable bowel syndrome. J Clin Gastroenterol 9:253–255, 1987

Drossman DA: Psychological factors in gastrointestinal diseases, in Textbook of Gastroenterology. Edited by Yamada T. Philadelphia, PA, JB Lippincott (in press)

Drossman DA, Sandler RS, McKee DC, et al: Bowel patterns among subjects not seeking health care. Gastroenterology 83:529–534, 1982

Drossman DA, McKee DC, Sandler RS, et al: Psychosocial factors in the irritable bowel syndrome. Gastroenterology 95:701–708, 1988

Enck P, Steckler I, Whitehead WE, et al: Lactose intolerance versus irritable bowel syndrome: physiological and psychological comparison (abstract). Gastroenterology 86:1070, 1984

Enck P, Whitehead WE, Schuster MM, et al: Psychosomatic aspects of irritable bowel syndrome: specificity of clinical symptoms, psychopathological features and motor activity of the rectosigmoid. Dtsch Med Wochenschr 113:459–462, 1988

Esler MD, Goulston KJ: Levels of anxiety in colonic disorders. N Engl J Med 288:16–20, 1973

Fava GA, Pavan L: Large bowel disorders, I: illness configuration and life events. Psychother Psychosom 27:93–99, 1976/1977a

Fava GA, Pavan L: Large bowel disorders, II: psychopathology and alexithymia. Psychother Psychosom 27:100–105, 1976/1977b

Feighner J, Robins E, Guze S, et al: Diagnostic criteria for use in psychiatric research. Arch Gen Psychiatry 26:57–63, 1972

Fielding JF: Timolol treatment in the irritable bowel syndrome. Digestion 22:155–158, 1981

Fielding JF: Surgery and the irritable bowel syndrome: the singer as well as the song. Ir Med J 76:33–34, 1983

Fielding JF: Irritable bowel syndrome: physical signs and investigations, in Irritable Bowel Syndrome. Edited by Read NW. New York, Grune & Stratton, 1985, pp 43–52

Ford MJ, Miller PM, Eastwood J, et al: Life events, psychiatric illness, and the irritable bowel syndrome. Gut 28:160–165, 1987

Ford MR: Interpersonal stress and style as predictors of biofeedback/relaxation training outcome: preliminary findings. Biofeedback Self Regul 10:223–239, 1985

Giles SL: Separate and combined effects of biofeedback training and brief individual psychotherapy in the treatment of gastrointestinal disorders. Dissertation Abstracts International 39(5-B):2495, 1978

Greenbaum DS, Ferguson RK, Kater LA, et al: A controlled therapeutic study of the irritable bowel syndrome: effect of diphenylhydantoin. N Engl J Med 288:13–16, 1973

Greenbaum DS, Abitz L, Vanegeren L, et al: Irritable bowel symptom prevalence, rectosigmoid motility, and psychometrics in symptomatic subjects not seeing physicians (abstract). Gastroenterology 84:1174, 1983

Greenbaum DS, Mayle JE, Vanegeren LE, et al: Effects of desipramine on irritable bowel syndrome compared with atropine and placebo. Dig Dis Sci 32:257–266, 1987

Harvey RF, Mauad EC, Brown AM: Prognosis in the irritable bowel syndrome: a 5-year prospective study. Lancet 1:963–965, 1987

Harvey RF, Hinton RA, Gunary RM, et al: Individual and group hypnotherapy in treatment of refractory irritable bowel syndrome. Lancet 1:424–425, 1989

Heefner JD, Wilder RM, Wilson ID: Irritable colon and depression. Psychosomatics 19:540–547, 1978

Hill OW, Blendis L: Physical and psychological evaluation of "non-organic" abdominal pain. Gut 8:221–229, 1967

Hillman LC, Stace NH, Pomare EW: Irritable bowel patients and their long-term response to a high fiber diet. Am J Gastroenterol 79:1–7, 1984

Hislop IG: Psychological significance of the irritable colon syndrome. Gut 12:452–457, 1971

Holdsworth CD: Drug treatment of irritable bowel syndrome, in Irritable Bowel Syndrome. Edited by Read NW. New York, Grune & Stratton, 1985, pp 223–232

Holmes KM, Salter RH: Irritable bowel syndrome: a safe diagnosis? Br Med J 285:1533–1534, 1982

Hovdenak N: Loperamide treatment of the irritable bowel syndrome. Scand J Gastroenterol 22 (suppl 130):81–84, 1987

Howship J: Practical Remarks on the Discrimination and Successful Treatment of Spasmodic Structure in the Colon Considered as an Occasional Cause of Habitual Confinement of the Bowels. London, Burgess and Hill, 1830

Johnsen R, Jacobsen BK, Forde OH: Associations between symptoms of irritable colon and psychological and social conditions and lifestyle. Br Med J 292:1633–1635, 1986

Johnson JD: Regional and ethnic distribution of lactose malabsorption: adaptive and genetic hypothesis, in Lactose Digestion: Clinical and Nutritional Implications. Edited by Paige DM, Bayless TM. Baltimore, MD, Johns Hopkins University Press, 1981, pp 11–22

Keeling PWN, Fielding JF: Irritable bowel syndrome: 1975 review of 50 consecutive cases. Journal of the Irish Colleges of Physicians and Surgeons 4:91–94, 1975

Klein KB: Controlled treatment trials in the irritable bowel syndrome: a critique. Gastroenterology 95:232–241, 1988

Kock NG, Hutten L, Leandoer L: A study of the motility in different parts of the human colon: resting activity, response to feeding and to progstigmine. Scand J Gastroenterol 3:163–169, 1968

Kullman G, Fielding JF: Rectal distensibility in the irritable bowel syndrome. Ir Med J 74:140–142, 1981

Lancaster-Smith MJ, Prout BJ, Pinto T, et al: Influence of drug treatment on the irritable bowel syndrome and its interaction with psychoneurotic morbidity. Acta Psychiatr Scand 66:33–41, 1982

Langeluddecke PM. Psychological aspects of irritable bowel syndrome. Aust N Z J Psychiatry 19:218–226, 1985

Latimer PR: Irritable bowel syndrome: a behavioral model. Behav Res Ther 19:475–483, 1981

Latimer PR: Functional Gastrointestinal Disorders: A Behavioral Approach. New York, Springer, 1983a

Latimer PR: Irritable bowel syndrome. Psychosomatics 24:205–218, 1983b

Latimer PR, Campbell D, Latimer M, et al: Irritable bowel syndrome: a test of the colonic hyperalgesia hypothesis. J Behav Med 2:285–295, 1979

Latimer PR, Sarna S, Campbell D, et al: Colonic motor and myoelectrical activity: a comparative study of normal subjects, psychoneurotic patients, and patients with irritable bowel syndrome. Gastroenterology 80:893–901, 1981

Lavö B, Stenstam M, Nielsen AL: Loperamide in treatment of irritable bowel syndrome: a double-blind placebo controlled study. Scand J Gastroenterol Suppl 130:77–80, 1987

Lennard-Jones JE: Functional gastrointestinal disorders. N Engl J Med 308:431–435, 1983

Liss JL, Alpers D, Woodruff RA Jr: The irritable colon syndrome and psychiatric illness. Diseases of the Nervous System 34:151–157, 1973

Lowman BC, Drossman DA, Cramer EM, et al: Recollection of childhood events in adults with irritable bowel syndrome. J Clin Gastroenterol 9:324–330, 1987

Lucey MR, Clark ML, Lowndes J, et al: Is bran efficacious in irritable bowel syndrome?: a double-blind placebo-controlled crossover study. Gut 28:221–225, 1987

Lydiard RB, Laraia MT, Howell EF, et al: Can panic disorder present as irritable bowel syndrome? J Clin Psychiatry 47:470–473, 1986

Lyrenas E, Abrahamsson H, Dotevall G: Rectosigmoid motility response to beta-adrenoceptor stimulation in patients with the irritable bowel syndrome. Scand J Gastroenterol 20:1163–1168, 1985

Manning AP, Thompson WG, Heaton KW, et al: Towards positive diagnosis of the irritable bowel. Br Med J 2:653–654, 1978

Mathias JR, Ferguson KL, Clench MH: Debilitating "functional" bowel disease controlled by leuprolide acetate, a gonadotropin-releasing hormone (GnRH) analog. Dig Dis Sci 34:761–766, 1989

Myren J, Lövland B, Larssen SE, et al: Psychopharmacologic drugs in the treatment of the irritable bowel syndrome. Ann Gastroenterol Hepatol (Paris) 20:117–123, 1984

Neff DF, Blanchard EB: A multi-component treatment for irritable bowel syndrome. Behavior Therapy 18:70–83, 1987

Nostrand TT, Barnett JL: Management of irritable bowel syndrome. Modern Medicine 57:100–102, 111–113, 1989

Noyes R Jr, Cook B, Garvey M, et al: Reduction of gastrointestinal symptoms following treatment for panic disorder. Psychosomatics 31:75–79, 1990

Page JG, Dirnberger GM: Treatment of the irritable bowel syndrome with Bentyl (dicyclomine hydrochloride). J Clin Gastroenterol 3:153–156, 1981

Palmer RL, Stonehill E, Crisp AH, et al: Psychological characteristics of patients with the irritable bowel syndrome. Postgrad Med J 50:416–419, 1974

Perez-Mateo M, Sillero C, Cuesta A, et al: Diltiazem in the treatment of the irritable bowel syndrome. Int J Clin Pharmacol Res 6:425–427, 1986

Read NW: Irritable Bowel Syndrome. New York, Grune & Stratton, 1985

Rees WEW, Evans BK, Rhodes J: Treating irritable bowel syndrome with peppermint oil. Br Med J 2:835–836, 1979

Richter JE, Barish CF, Castell DO: Abnormal sensory perception in patients with esophageal chest pain. Gastroenterology 91:845–852, 1986

Ritchie JA: Pain from distension of the pelvic colon by inflating a balloon in the irritable colon syndrome. Gut 14:125–132, 1973

Ritchie JA, Truelove SC: Treatment of irritable bowel syndrome with lorazepam, hyoscine butylbromide, and ispaghula husk. Br Med J 1:376–378, 1979

Ritchie JA, Truelove SC: Comparison of various treatments for irritable bowel syndrome. Br Med J 281:1317–1319, 1980

Ruoff M: The irritable colon syndrome, in Emotional Factors in Gastrointestinal Illness. Edited by Lindner AE. Amsterdam, Excerpta Medica, 1973, pp 156–165

Sandler RS, Drossman DA, Nathan HP, et al: Symptom complaints and health care seeking behavior in subjects with bowel dysfunction. Gastroenterology 87:314–318, 1984

Schonecke OW, Schüffel W: Evaluation of combined pharmacological and psychotherapeutic treatment in patients with functional abdominal disorders. Psychother Psychosom 26:86–92, 1975

Snape WJ, Carlson GM, Matarazzo SA, et al: Evidence that abnormal myoelectrical activity produces colonic motor dysfunction in the irritable bowel syndrome. Gastroenterology 72:383–387, 1977

Sullivan SN: Management of the irritable bowel syndrome: a personal view. J Clin Gastroenterol 5:499–502, 1983

Svedlund J, Ottosson J, Sjödin I, et al: Controlled study of psychotherapy in irritable bowel syndrome. Lancet 2:589–592, 1983

Svendsen JH, Munck LK, Andersen JR: Irritable bowel syndrome—prognosis and diagnostic safety: a 5-year follow-up study. Scand J Gastroenterol 20:415–418, 1985

Swarbrick ET, Bat L, Hegarty JE, et al: Site of pain from the irritable bowel. Lancet 2:443–446, 1980

Taylor I: Colonic motility and the irritable colon syndrome, in Irritable Bowel Syndrome. Edited by Read NW. New York, Grune & Stratton, 1985, pp 89–103

Taylor I, Darby C, Hammond P: Comparison of rectosigmoid myoelectrical activity in the irritable colon syndrome during relapses and remissions. Gut 19:923–929, 1978

Taylor L, Duthie HL, Smallwood R, et al: The effect of stimulation on the myoelectrical activity of the rectosigmoid in man. Gut 15:599–604, 1974

Taylor L, Duthie HL, Smallwood R, et al: Large bowel myoelectrical activity in man. Gut 16:808–814, 1975

Thompson DG, Laidlow JM, Wingate DL: Abnormal small-bowel motility demonstrated by radiotelemetry in a patient with irritable colon. Lancet 2:1321–1323, 1979

Thompson WG: The irritable bowel. Gut 25:305–320, 1984

Thompson WG: The irritable bowel: one disease, or several, or none? in Irritable Bowel Syndrome. Edited by Read NW. New York, Grune & Stratton, 1985, pp 3–16

Thompson WG: A strategy for management of the irritable bowel. Gastroenterology 81:95–100, 1986

Thompson WG, Heaton KW: Functional bowel disorders in apparently healthy people. Gastroenterology 79:283–288, 1980

Voirol MW, Hipolito J: Anthropo–analytical relaxation in irritable bowel syndrome: results 40 months later. Schweiz Med Wochenschr 117:1117–1119, 1987

Waller SL, Misiewicz JJ: Prognosis in the irritable-bowel syndrome. Lancet 1:753–756, 1969

Waller SL, Misiewicz JJ: Colonic motility in constipation or diarrhoea. Scand J Gastroenterol 7:93–97, 1972

Wangel AG, Deller DJ: Intestinal motility in man, III: mechanisms of constipation and diarrhea with particular reference to the irritable colon syndrome. Gastroenterology 48:69–84, 1965

Watson WC, Sullivan SN, Corke M, et al: Globus and headache: common symptoms of the irritable bowel syndrome. Can Med Assoc J 118:387–388, 1978

Welch GW, Hillman LC, Pomare EW: Psychoneurotic symptomatology in the irritable bowel syndrome: a study of reporters and non-reporters. Br Med J 291:1382–1384, 1985

Welch GW, Stace NH, Pomare EW: Specificity of psychological profiles of irritable bowel syndrome patients. Aust N Z J Med 14:101–104, 1984

Welgan P, Meshkinpour H, Beeler M: Effect of anger on colon motor and myoelectric activity in irritable bowel syndrome. Gastroenterology 94:1150–1156, 1988

West KL: MMPI correlates of ulcerative colitis. J Clin Psychol 26:214–229, 1970

Whitehead WE: Psychotherapy and biofeedback in the treatment of irritable bowel syndrome, in Irritable Bowel Syndrome. Edited by Read NW. New York, Grune & Stratton, 1985, pp 245–266

Whitehead WE, Schuster MM: Gastrointestinal Disorders: Behavioral and Physiological Basis for Treatment. New York, Academic, 1985

Whitehead WE, Engel BT, Schuster MM: Irritable bowel syndrome: physiological and psychological differences between diarrhea-predominant and constipation-predominant patients. Dig Dis Sci 25:404–412, 1980

Whitehead WE, Winget C, Fedoravicius AS, et al: Learned illness behavior in patients with irritable bowel syndrome and peptic ulcer. Dig Dis Sci 27:202–208, 1982

Whitehead WE, Bosmajian L, Zonderman AB, et al: Symptoms of psychologic distress associated with irritable bowel syndrome. Gastroenterology 95:709–714, 1988

Whorwell PJ: Hypnotherapy in irritable bowel syndrome. Lancet 1:622, 1989

Whorwell PJ, Clouter C, Smith CL: Oesophageal motility in the irritable bowel syndrome. Br Med J 282:1101–1102, 1981

Whorwell PJ, Prior A, Faragher EB: Controlled trial of hypnotherapy in the treatment of severe refractory irritable bowel syndrome. Lancet 2:1232–1233, 1984

Whorwell PJ, McCallum M, Creed FH, et al: Non-colonic features of irritable bowel syndrome. Gut 27:37–40, 1986

Whorwell PJ, Prior A, Colgan SM: Hypnotherapy in severe irritable bowel syndrome: further experience. Gut 28:423–425, 1987

Wise TN, Cooper JN, Ahmed S: The efficacy of group therapy for patients with irritable bowel syndrome. Psychosomatics 23:465–469, 1982a

Wise TN, Cooper JN, Ahmed S: Group therapy for the irritable bowel syndrome: themes and process. Journal of Psychiatric Treatment and Evaluation 4:511–515, 1982b

Young SJ, Alpers DH, Norland CC, et al: Psychiatric illness and the irritable bowel syndrome: practical implications for the primary physician. Gastroenterology 70:162–166, 1976

Yunus MB, Masi AT, Aldag JC: A controlled study of primary fibromyalgia syndrome: clinical features and association with other functional syndromes. J Rheumatol 16 (suppl 19):62–71, 1989

Chapter 7

Urethral Syndrome

The urethral syndrome, which consists of dysuria and urgency, is a common complaint in medical practice. There are various causes for this syndrome.

Symptoms and Signs

Most authors reserve the term *urethral syndrome* for cases of urethral and bladder symptoms in which there is no definite evidence of urinary tract pathology. This definition has been adopted for this chapter.

The symptoms are urinary frequency, urgency, dysuria, and suprapubic discomfort. There may be other associated symptoms, such as hesitancy, incomplete bladder emptying, weak stream, and symptoms unrelated to the urinary tract (e.g., back discomfort) that are less common (Bodner 1988). The syndrome that is discussed here is either chronic or recurrent.

Prevalence

Lower urinary tract infections in women are common, and dysuria is one of the most common symptoms experienced by adult women (Latham and Stamm 1984). The prevalence of the urethral syndrome is not known with certainty because the proportion of patients with this syndrome who have no evidence of persisting infection varies among studies.

Etiology

Irritation in the urethra, particularly in the area of the external urethral (striated) sphincter (Schmidt 1985), is thought to be the cause of the urethral syndrome. Several authors have discussed the etiology of this syndrome (Barbalias and Meares 1984; Bodner 1988; "Can Kasstigation Beat the Truth Out of the Urethral Syndrome?" 1982; O'Dowd 1985; Schmidt 1985; Scotti and Ostergard 1984). Most women with the urethral syndrome have evidence of bacterial infection caused mainly by *Escherichia coli, Staphylococcus saprophyticus, Chlamydia trachomatis* (Weil et al. 1981), *Neisseria gonorrhoeae, Candida albicans* (Latham and Stamm 1984), and, less often, by other organisms. In most studies, however, there is a substantial proportion of patients in whom there is no evidence of current infection, and the estimates vary across studies ("Can Kasstigation Beat the Truth Out?" 1982). For example, Stamm et al. (1980) found evidence of infection in 70% of patients with urethral syndrome, whereas Tait et al. (1985) found such evidence in only 15%. In a 2-year study of 51 women, there was a significant correlation between high counts of fastidious organisms in the urine and the presence of symptoms (Maskell et al. 1983).

Histological changes suggestive of chronic infection involving the urethra are also found in many patients with this syndrome (Permiakov and Titova 1982; Splatt and Weedon 1981). Even if there is no evidence of concurrent infection, there is often histological evidence of previous infection, such as trigonitis, squamous metaplasia, and lymphocytic infiltration of the lamina propria (Tait et al. 1985).

Causes other than infections concerning musculature and sphincter dysfunction have been suggested by several authors. Dynamic studies have shown spasticity of the urethral musculature with discomfort and urge proportional to the elevations of urethral sphincter pressure (Schmidt and Tanagho 1981). The authors advance the view that physiological imbalance in urethral activity may predispose one to urinary tract infection. Other causes that have been suggested are reflex irritation in the external urethral (striated) sphincter, with poor voiding habits as a contributing cause (Schmidt 1985). Kaplan et al. (1980), in an uncontrolled study, found pelvic floor hyperactivity. Barbalias and Meares (1984), in a controlled study, found increased urethral closure pressure, low urinary flow rates, instability of urethral pressure at rest, and incomplete funneling of the bladder neck. The authors claim that autonomically mediated spasm of the smooth muscle sphincter may explain their findings in part. About one quarter of the patients responded favorably to treatment with an alpha-receptor–blocking drug.

While there is substantial evidence for infection playing important roles, there is also evidence of urinary tract infection in women who are asymptomatic. Therefore, in any one case, it is at least initially uncertain whether the urethral syndrome is caused by the concurrent infection.

Psychological Studies

Carson et al. (1979, 1980) administered the Minnesota Multiphasic Personality Inventory (MMPI) to 56 women who complained of frequency of urination, urgency, and dysuria, in whom the results of excretory urography, cystoscopy, and urine cultures did not reveal urinary pathology. The MMPI scores were scored by computer at the Mayo Clinic and compared with the scores of female medical patients. The F scale was significantly higher in the patients with urethral syndrome. The authors commented that those patients with the high F-scale scores tended to exaggerate symptoms and complaints, but the score was "not high enough to invalidate the test" (Carson et al. 1979, p. 312). The scores of the hypochondriasis (Hs), hysteria (Hy), and schizophrenia (Sc) scales were significantly higher in the patients with urethral syndrome than in the other medical patients. The authors concluded that an increase in the Hs and Hy scales with normal D scores is consistent with the findings of other researchers who have described the "classic V conversion" in patients with chronic pain, lower back pain, and other functional complaints. Typical patients with these findings "[use] somatization in order to achieve neurotic ends, and complaints referred to the back, head, abdomen, or bladder reflect periods of tension and stress in some cases (Carson et al. 1979, p. 313). As the authors later pointed out, "[T]his classical-V configuration [on the MMPI] suggests patients who have psychophysiological reactions and who gain from these symptoms by escaping stressful or anxiety provoking situations" (Carson et al. 1980, p. 610). Carson et al. (1979, p. 313) further noted that "the triad of frequency, urgency, and dysuria—like back pain, malaise, and fatigue—is the result not of organic disease, but of a psychophysiologic process that, in these patients [those administered the MMPI], focuses on the lower urinary tract for its functional symptoms."

O'Dowd et al. (1984b) examined general practitioners' prescribing practices for women with urethral symptoms. The main purpose of this part of the study was to determine which patients had antibacterial treatment before the results of the urinary midstream specimen analysis were known. The authors divided their sample retrospectively into 40 women with the urethral syndrome and 46 women with evidence of urinary tract infection (as determined by urinalysis). Patients with the urethral syndrome had less dysuria and more episodes of abdominal pain and anxiety, and more of the patients had been treated with tranquilizers during the previous year. Physicians prescribed antibiotics in 37 cases (out of 46) of urinary tract infections, but only in 9 (out of 40) cases of the urethral syndrome. Thus, the physicians appeared to anticipate correctly the results of the urinalysis in a substantial proportion of patients.

In a later study, O'Dowd et al. (1986) analyzed family practitioners' records to follow the medical history of patients who had participated in the above study 2 years previously. The authors found that patients with the urethral syndrome attended more frequently for treatment unrelated to the urinary tract than did other patients, requested sterilization more often, and had more psychological and psychophysiological symptoms and difficulties in interpersonal relationships than did matched control patients. When these groups of patients were rated with the Nottingham Health Profile, those with urethral syndrome were more likely to have health problems and were more likely to mention that health problems affected their sex lives than were control patients. The authors commented that the patients with urethral syndrome were "a considerable drain on the doctors' time[,] and management needs to be directed toward the anxious patients who make such demands" (p. 30).

Comments

To my knowledge, there are only three studies that have systematically examined psychological features of patients with urethral syndrome. In the study by Carson et al. (1979), the elevated scores on some of the MMPI scales indicate more psychopathology in these patients than in the control patients, but these scores do not imply diagnoses in accord with the names of the scales such as hysteria, hypochondriasis, or schizophrenia. (The value of MMPI in diagnosis is discussed in Chapter 11, p. 232, this volume.) Because the Hs (hypochondriasis) scale consists predominantly of somatic complaints, the findings in Carson et al.'s study suggest that patients with the urethral syndrome who have no evidence of organic disease do have other functional somatic symptoms. These findings also suggest that these patients have more psychopathology than other medical patients.

The conclusion that the typical patient with these findings uses somatization in order to achieve neurotic ends, and that these reactions might be used to escape from painful or stressful situations, was in accord with the theories of somatization at the time. The scores derived from the MMPI alone, however, are inadequate to support such a conclusion. The other conclusion—that "frequency, urgency, and dysuria—like back pain, malaise, and fatigue, is not the result of organic disease, but of a psychophysiologic process that, in these patients, focuses on the lower urinary tract for its functional symptoms"—is also not warranted from these authors' findings. The authors use the term "functional symptoms" to imply that the symptoms serve a function for the patient and to assert that a single psychological mechanism is responsible for the symptoms in all patients. There is ample evidence that urinary symptoms, as well as back pain and fatigue, can be caused by organic disease as well as by psychophysiological processes. The mechanisms of somatization and bodily complaints are discussed further in Part II of this volume.

The studies by O'Dowd et al. (1984b, 1986) suggest that patients with urethral syndrome have more psychopathology than do other patients. In the first study the general practitioners appeared to be able to distinguish patients with current urinary tract infections from those with the urethral syndrome, and the treatment of the two groups differed even before the results of the midstream specimen of urine were known. In the second study the authors found that patients with urethral syndrome manifested more illness behavior and attended more because of apparently functional somatic symptoms, although these patients did not continue to seek treatment of symptoms related to their urinary tract.

The evidence is convincing that a large proportion of women who seek medical treatment because of the urethral syndrome have acute as well as chronic or recurrent infections that cause this syndrome. Women who are anxious or have other psychopathology, and who have a tendency to perceive bodily sensations, either appear to be perceiving their urethral symptoms more or may be more distressed by these symptoms, or both. Because abnormal tension in the bladder and in the striated muscle of the urethra appears to be responsible for the syndrome in some patients, emotional arousal perhaps induces or aggravates the spasm. Anxiety may contribute to selective perception or induce hypochondriacal concerns. In other words, although infection appears to be the most common cause of urethral syndrome, anxiety and concerns about health may exacerbate the symptoms of some patients and may induce these patients to seek medical care more often. In other patients, anxiety and concerns about health appear to be the predominant cause for the syndrome.

Diagnosis

The urethral syndrome is a diagnosis of exclusion of treatable physical disease. The physician's bias often influences the kind and extent of the evaluations. If urine culture and urine cytology show no evidence of an active infection, and if symptoms persist, cystourethroscopy with biopsy is recommended to exclude other pathology (Bodner 1988).

In a few patients the urethral symptoms are clearly preceded by anxiety; in others the discomfort appears to cause anxiety or tension. In many others, it is difficult or impossible to judge the extent to which local irritation, selective attention, and amplification play a part.

The urethral syndrome is not listed in the DSM-III-R (American Psychiatric Association 1987). Because organic factors, particularly evidence of either current or previous infection, are found in a large proportion of patients, it is inappropriate to classify this syndrome as an undifferentiated somatoform disorder unless urinary tract disease has been meticulously excluded. If psychological factors appear to play a substantial role, the appropriate DSM-III-R classification should be *psychological factors affecting physical condition* (316.00), and on Axis III, urethral syndrome. (The code of the ICD-10 draft [World Health Organization 1988] is F45.34.)

Treatment

When a urinary infection appears to be the cause for the urethral syndrome, it should, of course, be energetically treated with appropriate methods. The studies on treatment, however, yield conflicting results. In some studies, treatment with antibiotics was no more effective than placebo (O'Dowd et al. 1984b). In a controlled study by Bergman et al. (1989), 60 patients with the urethral syndrome were randomly divided into three groups: those patients taking placebo, those taking tetracycline, and those undergoing urethral dilation. Uroflowmetry was performed before treatment and 8 weeks after treatment. Complete relief of symptoms was achieved in 20% of the placebo group, 50% of the tetracycline group, and 75% of the group that had treatment with urethral dilation. Objective improvement in uroflowmetry occurred only in the group undergoing serial urethral dilation. In a study by Carson et al. (1980), instrumentation was no more effective than conservative treatment. Some patients may improve with prazosin, or other alpha-receptor–blocking drugs (Barbalias and Meares 1984).

Other treatments that have been suggested are retraining of voiding, skeletal muscle relaxant, and neurostimulation (Schmidt 1985). Other authors have claimed successes with urethroplasty or cryosurgery (Boreham 1984; Splatt 1982).

Psychological or Psychopharmacological Treatments

If the likely physical causes for urethral syndrome have been treated and the syndrome persists, or if psychological factors appear to play a substantial role, psychological treatments or psychotropic drugs should be considered.

Firlit and Cook (1977) found in a study of children with a syndrome similar to the urethral syndrome in adults, that symptoms were relieved by a substantial proportion with administration of diazepam. Kaplan et al. (1980) found in an uncontrolled study of six patients that diazepam provided clinical relief as well as sphincter synergy as demonstrated by urodynamics after treatment. The patients were treated for 2 to 6 months, and when the patients became symptom free, the dose was tapered. To my knowledge, there are no published controlled studies of either psychotropic drugs or psychological treatments.

In Carson et al.'s (1980) study of 160 patients, 15 were referred for psychiatric treatment. The reason for referral, the kind and duration of the treatment, and the length of follow-up are not described. In 13 of the 15 patients (87%), the authors reported "resolution of symptoms." Patients with urethral syndrome are only seldom referred to psychiatrists or psychologists, and if they are, they usually have a conspicuous psychiatric disorder. A few patients with phobias have a fear of incontinence or a feeling of urgency in phobic situations (see case history below).

Clearly, the empirical literature offers little guidance on psychological or psychopharmacological treatments. The data in Carson et al.'s study do not allow an evaluation of the efficacy of psychiatric treatment. Any recommendations on such treatment are tentative. If the urethral syndrome occurs in the course of a psychiatric disorder, the latter should be, of course, treated. A combination of explanation, reassurance, and psychotherapy in accord with the general principles of treating somatization described in Chapter 10 (this volume) appears to be the appropriate approach. For patients who have urethral symptoms only in certain places or situations or fear incontinence in public, the treatment should involve conventional treatment of phobia (e.g., one of the methods of exposure). There are only a few case reports on the effects of psychotropic drugs;

such drugs may be tried if the patient does not respond to psychotherapy and if the symptoms remain distressing.

Case History

A 22-year-old female student, referred by her family practitioner, had complained of an intermittent urethral syndrome. After exclusion of a current infection, her doctor noted that the patient was anxious and referred her for a psychiatric evaluation. The patient had been treated for a generalized anxiety disorder with supportive psychotherapy and diazepam 3 years previously. She said that she still felt anxious at times, but that her anxiety was distressing when she was supposed to attend lectures. She had no difficulty working in the laboratory or going to libraries; on her way to lectures, however, she experienced bladder discomfort and had a strong need to void urine. She tried to arrive at lectures early in order to find a seat near the exit. If she came late and no place was available near the door, she would leave. Some days she avoided going to the lectures altogether because of the discomfort and fear, and went to the library instead. Because of the urgency, she feared that she would become incontinent and that this would be noticed by other students.

I treated this patient in the early 1960s, in those days when there were several studies on desensitization in imagery combined with deep muscular relaxation but little was known about the treatment of phobias in vivo. The role of psychotropic drugs in the treatment of simple phobias was not known. I suggested to the patient that she take one tablet of diazepam, 5 mg, an hour before the lecture to try to help her ignore her bladder symptoms and to do her best to remain in the lecture room. During the next session the patient told me that taking one tablet of diazepam gave her relief from anxiety as well as from bladder symptoms, and that it had become easier for her to ignore the symptoms. She continued to take diazepam intermittently at other times when her anxiety induced urinary symptoms and the fear of becoming incontinent. After 6 weeks, I advised the patient to try to reduce the dose by taking two 2-mg tablets of diazepam and to keep one half of a 2-mg tablet in reserve in case the symptom became troublesome. Within the next 3 months the patient gradually weaned herself partially off diazepam (while still carrying a supply of this drug with her) and eventually did not require medication before lectures, although she continued to take between 2 and 4 mg on other occasions. On a 6-month follow-up visit, the patient was taking virtually no medication and was attending lectures regularly.

In this patient, anxiety either induced or greatly aggravated her bladder symptoms. If I had a similar case again, I would try to treat the patient with exposure without medication. Although there is no evidence that diazepam enhances recovery from phobias, it appears that the rapid onset of antianxiety effects of diazepam made her less distressed and perhaps reduced the number of occasions when she decided not to expose herself to the phobic situation. It probably played no other role in the recovery from her phobia.

Prognosis

O'Dowd et al. (1984a) carried out a controlled study of doxycycline and placebo in 69 women with the urethral syndrome. On follow-up after 12 months, they found that in the majority, the syndrome was short and without recurrence.

In a later paper, however, O'Dowd et al. (1986) reported a follow-up of these patients after another year (i.e., a total of 2 years). Twenty-five women out of 31 had further symptoms, but only 2 had sought medical help for urethral symptoms; there was, however, evidence from their charts and from the Nottingham Health Profile ratings that they had more emotional problems than other women. Maskell et al. (1983), in a 2-year follow-up of 51 women with the urethral syndrome, found that even when symptom free, these women differed from women of control groups who had a significantly higher count of fastidious organisms.

Thus, most episodes of the urethral syndrome are brief. There is a tendency for recurrences, and in some patients who have no urethral symptoms there is evidence of persisting infection.

Summary and Main Conclusions

Urinary symptoms in adult women are among the most common complaints in medical practice. A large proportion of patients with the urethral syndrome have evidence of infection. The proportion of patients in whom no recent infection can be detected varies across studies; many women with urethral symptoms show histological evidence of previous infections, even in the absence of current infection. In some women there is evidence of spasticity of the urethral musculature that may cause or contribute to symptoms of urethral irritation. Most of the episodes of the urethral syndrome are short lived, but there is a tendency for recurrences.

Three studies have shown more psychopathology in women with the urethral syndrome than in other patients. Although infection is most common cause for urethral symptoms, in the chronic urethral syndrome, anxiety and other psychopathology appear to be contributing factors in a substantial proportion of these patients. In a few patients, emotional distress is probably the main cause for the syndrome: they either perceive their urethral symptoms more or are more distressed by them. Because abnormal tension in the bladder and in the striated muscle of the urethra appear to contribute to the syndrome, in some patients emotional arousal perhaps induces or aggravates the spasm.

Apart from eradicating the infecting organism, various somatic treatments, including surgical procedures, have been used in the treatment of the urethral syndrome. There are no adequate studies in the literature to suggest the most appropriate psychological or psychiatric treatment. If organic causes of the syndrome are identified and treated, yet the syndrome persists, or if psychological factors appear to play a substantial role, the patient should be treated in accord with the principles of psychotherapy of somatizing patients. If the urethral symptom occurs predominantly or only in certain places or situations, attempts may be made to treat it with exposure like other phobias.

Diazepam was found to relieve symptoms in uncontrolled studies. In one study, some patients' symptoms improved with prazosin or other alpha-receptor–blocking drugs. Attempts to treat the patient with psychotropic drugs appear to be appropriate if the symptoms are distressing and if other treatments have failed. In one study of 15 patients referred for unspecified psychiatric treatment, 13 were reported to have recovered.

The studies on prognosis suggest that most women who present to physicians with the urethral syndrome have short, self-limiting episodes, but some patients have chronic and distressing symptoms. A large proportion of those who recover will have recurrences of symptoms, although these patients will not seek further medical care. In some patients, symptomless infections persist; conversely, in other women with the urethral syndrome, there is no evidence of persisting infection.

References

American Psychiatric Association: Diagnostic and Statistical Manual of Mental Disorders, 3rd Edition, Revised. Washington, DC, American Psychiatric Association, 1987

Barbalias GA, Meares EM Jr: Female urethral syndrome: clinical and urodynamic perspectives. Urology 23:208–212, 1984

Bergman A, Karram M, Bhatia NN: Urethral syndrome: a comparison of different treatment modalities. J Reprod Med 34:157–160, 1989

Bodner DR: The urethral syndrome. Urol Clin North Am 15:699–704, 1988

Boreham P: Cryosurgery for the urethral syndrome. J R Soc Med 77:111–113, 1984

Can Kasstigation beat the truth out of the urethral syndrome? Lancet 2:694–695, 1982

Carson CC, Osborne D, Segura JW: Psychologic characteristics of patients with female urethral syndrome. J Clin Psychol 35:312–313, 1979

Carson CC, Segura JW, Osborne DM: Evaluation and treatment of the female urethral syndrome. J Urol 124:609–610, 1980

Firlit CF, Cook WA: Voiding pattern abnormalities in children. Urology 10:25–29, 1977

Kaplan WE, Firlit CF, Schoenberg HW: The female urethral syndrome: external sphincter spasm as etiology. J Urol 124:48–49, 1980

Latham RH, Stamm WE: Urethral syndrome in women. Urol Clin North Am 11:95–101, 1984

Maskell R, Pead L, Sanderson RA: Fastidious bacteria and the urethral syndrome: a 2-year clinical and bacteriological study of 51 women. Lancet 2:1277–1280, 1983

O'Dowd TC: The irritable urethral syndrome: discussion. J R Coll Gen Pract 35:140–141, 1985

O'Dowd TC, Ribeiro CD, Munro J, et al: Urethral syndrome: a self-limiting illness. Br Med J 288:1349–1352, 1984a

O'Dowd TC, Smail JE, West RR: Clinical judgment in the diagnosis and management of frequency and dysuria in general practice. Br Med J 288:1347–1349, 1984b

O'Dowd TC, Pill R, Smail JE, et al: Irritable urethral syndrome: follow-up study in general practice. Br Med J 292:30–32, 1986

Permiakov AN, Titova GP: Izmeneniia slizistoi obolochki uretry i mochevogo puzyria pri uretral'nom sindrome. Arkh Patol 44:42–47, 1982

Schmidt RA: The urethral syndrome. Urol Clin North Am 12:349–354, 1985

Schmidt RA, Tanagho EA: Urethral syndrome or urinary tract infection? Urology 18:424–427, 1981

Scotti RJ, Ostergard DR: The urethral syndrome. Clin Obstet Gynecol 27:515–529, 1984

Splatt AJ: The urethral syndrome: experience with the Richardson urethroplasty: a review after 5 years. Br J Urol 54:566, 1982

Splatt AJ, Weedon D: The urethral syndrome: morphological studies. Br J Urol 53:263–265, 1981

Stamm WE, Running K, McKevitt M, et al: Treatment of the acute urethral syndrome. N Engl J Med 304:956–958, 1980

Tait J, Peddie BA, Bailey RR, et al: Urethral syndrome (abacterial cystitis): search for a pathogen. Br J Urol 57:552–556, 1985

Weil A, Gaudenz R, Burgener L, et al: Isolation of *Chlamydia trachomatis* from women with urethral syndrome. Arch Gynecol 230:329–333, 1981

World Health Organization: Draft of the 10th Revision of the International Classification of Diseases. Geneva, World Health Organization, 1988

Chapter 8

Behavior-Induced Physiological Changes: Hyperventilation and Aerophagia

There are various abnormal behaviors beyond an individual's voluntary control that can cause pathological changes, such as habitual clenching of teeth causing dental abrasion or habitual pulling of eyelashes and eyelids that may lead to conjunctivitis. These maladaptive behaviors lie beyond the scope of this volume. Other involuntary behaviors induce physiological changes that may in turn cause somatic symptoms. Two such behaviors are summarized here: hyperventilation and aerophagia.

Hyperventilation

Excessive breathing may occur in several physical diseases. Hyperventilation may occur, however, in the absence of physical disease and may cause distressing somatic symptoms.

Symptoms and Signs

In severe anxiety, hyperventilation is often striking, with the patient gasping for breath. There are usually associated symptoms caused by the alkalosis that accompanies hyperventilation. The patient may not be aware of his or her breathing pattern, or may admit to or complain of a feeling of not getting enough air into the chest. In some patients hyperventilation is inconspicuous.

Prevalence

Estimates on the prevalence of hyperventilation vary widely. Some authors have reported the prevalence of obvious hyperventilation in anxiety states, whereas others believe that inconspicuous hyperventilation causing symptoms is far more common (see above). In one study, 13% of random employees who responded to a questionnaire survey indicated that they had experienced "breathing difficulties, [and] not enough air" during the preceding week. The corresponding figure in neurotic patients was about 40% (Kellner and Sheffield 1973).

Etiology and Associated Disorders

The diseases that induce hyperventilation are listed below in the section on diagnosis. The physiological changes and the resulting symptoms of hyperventilation have been surveyed by several authors (e.g., Pfeffer [1984] and Bass and Gardner [1985]). The fall in pCO_2 and the consequent alkalosis resulting from increased ventilation may cause neuromuscular irritability with paresthesia and numbness, and, in severe cases, carpopedal spasm. The symptoms caused by reduced cerebral oxygenation may include faintness, lightheadedness, and dizziness. Different mechanisms appear to be responsible for the various types of chest pain (see Chapter 11, this volume).

There is evidence that hyperventilation occurs in some patients with anxiety (Bass and Gardner 1985), particularly in those with panic attacks (Salkovskis et al. 1986), and can cause distressing somatic symptoms. When these symptoms occur in conjunction with a panic attack, it is not always possible to discern initially which of the symptoms are caused by which physiological change. Hyperventilation has also been implicated in the induction of panic attacks (Hibbert 1984). The component sequence, however, appears to be hyperventilation occurring as the consequence of panic (Bass and Lelliott, manuscript in preparation, 1989); the somatic symptoms of hyperventilation cause panic if these are perceived as unpleasant and are interpreted in a catastrophic fashion (Salkovskis et al. 1986). Subsequently, anxiety becomes more severe and induces more hyperventilation. Hyperventilation occurs also in other psychiatric disorders (Pfeffer 1978) such as in depressive states (Damas-Mora et al. 1976), in part because of the coexisting anxiety. Individuals who score high on the Neuroticism Scale of the Eysenck Personality Inventory are more distressed by a brief period of hyperventilation than individuals who score low (Clark and Hemsley 1982).

The association of dyspnea and psychiatric symptoms is also found in patients with respiratory diseases. In one study, more patients with chronic bronchitis whose breathlessness was disproportionate to the severity of their respiratory obstruction had psychiatric symptoms, including anxiety, than did other patients (Burns and Howell 1969). In a longitudinal study of patients with chronic respiratory impairment, the severity of dyspnea varied with the level of anxiety (Gift et al. 1986).

Diagnosis

There are several diseases that cause hyperventilation; for example, lesions of the central nervous system cause maladaptive hyperventilation and metabolic acidosis (such as in severe hypoglycemia or salicylate poisoning), which stimulates compensatory excessive breathing. Hyperventilation can occur in several respiratory diseases but is characteristic of interstitial lung disease and pulmonary edema.

Inconspicuous chronic hyperventilation may induce functional somatic symptoms (Brashear 1983; Gardner et al. 1986; Lum 1976). Some patients may have chest pain which is similar to that of cardiac origin, and the disorder is frequently misdiagnosed (Lum 1976). The reduced plasma bicarbonate level and relatively normal arterial pH (compensated respiratory alkalosis) distinguish chronic hyperventilation from acute hyperventilation with the fall in pCO_2 that frequently accompanies arterial puncture (West 1982). The resting pCO_2 level indicates whether the patient chronically hyperventilates, and deliberate hyperventilation by the patient at the request of the physician reproduces the symptoms.

The psychiatric diagnostic classification should include coexisting psychiatric disorders such as panic disorder or generalized anxiety disorder on Axis I, and, because it needs to be treated, the occurrence of hyperventilation should be noted. In the ICD-10 draft (World Health Organization 1988), the appropriate classification is somatoform autonomic dysfunction (F45.33; respiratory—hyperventilation).

Treatment

When somatic symptoms are caused mainly by hyperventilation, or at least when hyperventilation appears to contribute to the causation of somatic symptoms, the patient needs to be trained to breathe appropriately. A few studies report the beneficial effects of such training.

Lum (1976) reported on 640 hyperventilating patients who had been diagnosed mainly as having anxiety states or else had been mistaken for having physical diseases such as cardiac ischemia or recurrent pulmonary emboli. After breathing exercises administered by physiotherapists, 70% were found to be symptom free, and only 5% failed to benefit from treatment.

Clark et al. (1985) and Salkovskis et al. (1986) treated patients who experienced panic attacks by training them to control their breathing. The method consisted of forced overbreathing as a provocation test of symptoms, with instructions to use a paper bag, and completion of a symptom sheet that included the symptoms of hyperventilation followed by a discussion of the induced symptoms. Patients were also given a handout describing the relationship of respiration and anxiety. The explanation of the nature of somatic symptoms that occurred with the panic attacks helped to replace the images of catastrophic events triggering the attacks, such as having heart disease or going insane. With the aid of an audio tape, the patients were trained to inspire 12 times a minute. The patients were directed to practice with the tape daily and to attempt to control panic by the new technique.

In the first study, there was a substantial reduction in the frequency of panic attacks that was maintained on a 2-year follow-up. Although improvement in panic symptoms occurred, avoidance behavior did not change in several patients. The second study included patients with spontaneous as well as situational panic attacks, and the patients were instructed initially not to expose themselves to the phobic situation in order to observe the effects of the respiratory control treatment alone. Again, a large and rapid reduction of panic attacks occurred with this treatment. The patients' resting pCO_2 values (initially significantly lower than those of healthy control subjects) rose to normal levels during treatment.

Bonn et al. (1984) conducted a controlled study with agoraphobic patients in whom a hyperventilation provocation test reproduced their feared symptoms. Seven patients were treated with two sessions of breathing retraining followed by five sessions of exposure to the phobic situation in real life. The authors noted that "breathing retraining consisted of instructing the patient in diaphragmatic respiration. The patient, lying on a couch, was told to place one hand on the abdomen and another on the chest to ensure that the abdomen was pushed out at each inspiration with minimal movement of the thorax . . . at a rate of 8–10 breaths per minute" (p. 666) A control group of five patients were treated with the same total number of sessions but without breathing retraining. The outcome did not differ significantly between patients and control subjects at the end of this treatment. On 6-month follow-up, however, the control group showed deterioration (a learning decrement), whereas those patients given only two sessions of breathing retraining showed further improvement. These differences were significant for all measures: somatic symptoms, panic attacks, phobias, and resting breathing rate.

Prognosis

Although physical symptoms may remain extremely distressing, physical health in most patients who hyperventilate remains unimpaired. Patients with panic attacks, however, have increased mortality rates, and males show an excess of mortality due to circulatory system disease (Coryell et al. 1982). Hyperventilation is a common symptom in panic attacks, and the profound biochemical changes that occur in hyperventilation contribute perhaps to the causes of death.

Aerophagia

The swallowing of an excessive amount of air is termed *aerophagia*. This condition may cause gastrointestinal symptoms.

Symptoms and Signs

Air swallowing may be inconspicuous, and the patient is often unaware of this habit. Aerophagia is one of the causes of non-ulcer dyspepsia (see Chapter 5, this volume); other complaints are a feeling of distension, belching, and excessive flatulence. Aerophagia can also be a cause of unexplained abdominal pain in children (Stone and Morgan 1971). The patient may swallow frequently and may be observed to be gulping air. The habit may cause distressing symptoms, but it is usually benign. Some of the associated syndromes are discussed in the next section.

Prevalence

The prevalence of aerophagia is not known. It is rarely diagnosed, because most physicians do not recognize it as a medical problem (Whitehead and Schuster 1985) except in the severely mentally retarded, in whom it has been variously reported to occur in 2% to 8% of patients (Holburn and Dougher 1986).

Etiology

Air enters the stomach during normal swallowing, so frequent swallowing alone causes distension of the stomach with air (Maddock et al. 1949) such as in chewing gum or tobacco or other causes of hypersalivation. Other causes that have been put forward are drinking carbonated beverages, eating rapidly, or gulping liquids. Because aerophagia apparently occurs often in patients with peptic ulcer and hiatal hernia, it has been suggested that the patient swallows air in an attempt to relieve discomfort (Roth and Bockus 1957). Others have theorized that excessive air swallowing could contribute to peptic ulcer formation by stimulating gastric acid secretion. In addition, aerophagia may trigger bowel peristalsis because of distension by air and thus contribute to the symptoms of irritable bowel syndrome (Calloway et al. 1982).

Psychological Factors

There are no systematic studies exploring the psychological factors in aerophagia, only a few published case reports. There are several case histories of the treatment of aerophagia in the mentally retarded. Antianxiety drugs have been found to be effective, which suggests that anxiety is one of the causes of this habit.

Diagnosis

Physical disease such as peptic ulcer or hiatal hernia may induce aerophagia. In DSM-III-R (American Psychiatric Association 1987), the appropriate classification appears to be *psychological factors affecting physical conditions* on Axis I and aerophagia on Axis III. In the ICD-10 draft (World Health Organization 1988), aerophagia is classified under somatoform autonomic dysfunction (F45.31: psychogenic aerophagy).

Treatments

There is only one small published controlled study of psychological treatment (Calloway et al. 1983). Twelve patients with hiatal hernia and aerophagia participated and had six treatment sessions each. Six patients were treated with training in muscular relaxation aided by galvanic skin response feedback, and six had audiofeedback of swallowing from a throat microphone. Patients were also taught procedures that interfered with excessive habitual swallowing. The rates of swallowing decreased in both groups; however, the decrease was larger in the audiofeedback group. Clinical improvement occurred only in those who succeeded in decreasing the rate of swallowing. On a 4-week follow-up, one half of the improved patients had relapsed.

The results of Calloway et al.'s study were inconclusive because the number of patients was small and the patients had only a few sessions of treatment. The findings suggest that decreasing the rate of swallowing relieves dyspeptic symptoms in some patients with aerophagia. More treatment sessions of audiofeedback combined with training in habit reversal (Azrin and Nunn 1977) might lead to a sustained decrease in the rate of swallowing.

There are a few published case histories and small series of treatment of children or severely retarded institutionalized patients in whom aerophagia is a form of self-injurious behavior (Holburn 1986; Holburn and Dougher 1985; Schroeder et al. 1981). Various operant conditioning and contingency management techniques were reported to decrease or eliminate air swallowing in such patients (Barrett et al. 1987; Gauderer et al. 1981; Holburn and Dougher 1986).

In a placebo-controlled crossover drug trial, medazepam was decidedly more effective than placebo in relieving abdominal symptoms associated with aerophagia (Baume and Cuthbert 1973). This result was replicated in another crossover trial with benzodiazepines; diazepam, as well as lorazepam, was significantly more effective than placebo in relieving aerophagia symptoms (Baume et al. 1975).

Prognosis

Aerophagia may cause persistent symptoms, but in most patients it does not appear to have ill effects. Structural changes have been reported in chronic aerophagia in some patients (Lekkas and Lentino 1978). Death has been reported from excessive distension and perforation of the stomach, but this is exceedingly rare (Hackl 1973; Hutchinson et al. 1980).

Summary and Main Conclusions

There are various behaviors that may induce physiological or pathological changes that, in turn, can cause bodily symptoms. The disorders discussed in this chapter are hyperventilation and aerophagia.

Hyperventilation

In severe anxiety, hyperventilation is often striking, with the patient feeling a lack of air. In other patients it may be inconspicuous, and the patient may be unaware of breathing excessively. About 13% of random subjects who replied to a questionnaire stated that they had breathing difficulties or not enough air during the preceding week; in neurotic patients the prevalence was about 40%.

The fall in pCO_2 and consequent alkalosis may cause symptoms of tetany, and reduced cerebral oxygenation may cause faintness or dizziness. Hyperventilation occurs in severe anxiety and panic attacks. The somatic symptoms of hyperventilation aggravate anxiety if the sensations are interpreted as symptoms of serious disease.

Reduced plasma carbonate level and relatively normal pH distinguish chronic hyperventilation from acute hyperventilation, with a fall in pCO_2 that frequently accompanies arterial puncture. In patients with this syndrome, the true nature of the disorder may not be recognized. Deliberate hyperventilation may reproduce the symptoms.

There is evidence that retraining of breathing combined with explanatory and cognitive therapy reduces the incidence of panic attacks (which suggests that some panic attacks are induced by hyperventilation). Retraining of breathing reduces resting pCO_2 and decreases the number of recurrences of agoraphobia treated with exposure.

Although the physical symptoms can be extremely distressing, the physical health of most patients with hyperventilation remains unimpaired. Because patients with panic disorder have an increased death rate, it is conceivable that the profound biochemical changes induced by hyperventilation are a contributing cause.

Aerophagia

The excessive swallowing of air may cause gastrointestinal symptoms such as dyspepsia, distension, and flatus. Aerophagia occurs more commonly in hiatal hernia and peptic ulceration, so one of the likely causes is an attempt to relieve symptoms. Other causes are frequent swallowing and habits that cause hypersalivation such as chewing tobacco.

Aerophagia is believed to be more common in anxiety. A small controlled study suggests that audiofeedback with a microphone that amplifies swallowing noises combined with habit reversal techniques decreases the rate of swallowing as well as relieving dyspeptic symptoms. In a crossover trial, lorazepam and diazepam were decidedly more effective than placebo in relieving aerophagia symptoms. Apart from causing symptoms, the prognosis is good in most patients. Deaths caused by stomach rupture have been reported, but are extremely rare.

References

American Psychiatric Association: Diagnostic and Statistical Manual of Mental Disorders, 3rd Edition, Revised. Washington, DC, American Psychiatric Association, 1987

Azrin NH, Nunn GR: Habit Control in a Day. New York, Simon & Schuster, 1977

Barrett RP, McGonigle JJ, Ackles PK, et al: Behavioral treatment of chronic aerophagia. American Journal of Mental Deficiency 91:620–625, 1987

Bass C, Gardner WN: Respiratory and psychiatric abnormalities in chronic symptomatic hyperventilation. Br Med J 290:1387–1390, 1985

Baume P, Cuthbert J: The effect of medazepam in relieving symptoms of functional gastrointestinal distress. Aust N Z J Med 3:457–460, 1973

Baume P, Tracey M, Dawson L: Efficacy of two minor tranquilizers in relieving symptoms of functional gastrointestinal distress. Aust N Z J Med 5:503–506, 1975

Bonn JA, Readhead CPA, Timmons BH: Enhanced adaptive behavioral response in agoraphobic patients pretreated with breathing retraining. Lancet 2:665–669, 1984

Brashear RE: Hyperventilation syndrome. Lung 161:257–273, 1983

Burns BH, Howell JBL: Disproportionately severe breathlessness in chronic bronchitis. Q J Med 38:277–294, 1969

Calloway SP, Fonagy P, Pounder RF: Frequency of swallowing in duodenal ulceration and hiatus hernia. Br Med J 285:23–24, 1982

Calloway SP, Fonagy P, Pounder RE, et al: Behavioral techniques in the management of aerophagia in patients with hiatus hernia. J Psychosom Res 27:499–502, 1983

Clark DM, Hemsley DR: Effects of hyperventilation: individual variability and its relation to personality. J Behav Ther Exp Psychiatry 13:41–47, 1982

Clark DM, Salkovskis PM, Chalkley AJ: Respiratory control as a treatment for panic attacks. J Behav Ther Exp Psychiatry 16:23–30, 1985

Coryell W, Noyer R, Clancy J: Excess mortality in panic disorder. Arch Gen Psychiatry 39:701–703, 1982

Damas-Mora J, Grant L, Kenyon P, et al: Respiratory ventilation and carbon dioxide levels in syndromes of depression. Br J Psychiatry 129:457–464, 1976

Gardner WN, Meah MS, Bass C: Controlled study of respiratory responses during prolonged measurement in patients with chronic hyperventilation. Lancet 2:826–830, 1986

Gauderer MWL, Halpin TC, Izant JR: Pathologic childhood aerophagia: a recognizable clinical entity. J Pediatr Surg 16:301–305, 1981

Gift AG, Plaut M, Jacox A: Psychologic and physiologic factors related to dyspnea in subjects with chronic obstructive pulmonary disease. Heart Lung 15:595–601, 1986

Hackl M: Pathologische Aerophagie als Todesursache. Med Klin 68:667–669, 1973

Hibbert GA: Hyperventilation as a cause of panic attacks. Br Med J 288:263–264, 1984

Holburn CS: Aerophagia: an uncommon form of self-injury. American Journal of Mental Deficiency 91:201–203, 1986

Holburn CS, Dougher MJ: Behavioral attempts to eliminate air-swallowing in two profoundly mentally retarded clients. American Journal of Mental Deficiency 89:524–536, 1985

Holburn CS, Dougher MJ: Effects of response satiation procedures in the treatment of aerophagia. American Journal of Mental Deficiency 91:72–77, 1986

Hutchinson GH, Alderson DM, Turnberg LA: Fatal tension pneumoperitoneum due to aerophagy. Postgrad Med J 56:516–518, 1980

Kellner R, Sheffield BF: The one-week prevalence of symptoms in neurotic patients and normals. Am J Psychiatry 130:102–105, 1973

Lekkas CN, Lentino W: Symptom-producing interposition of the colon-clinical syndrome in mentally retarded adults. JAMA 240:747–750, 1978

Lum LC: The syndrome of habitual chronic hyperventilation, in Modern Trends in Psychosomatic Medicine, Vol 3. Edited by Hill O. Boston, MA, Butterworth, 1976, pp 196–230

Maddock WG, Bell JL, Tremaine MJ: Gastro-intestinal gas. Ann Surg 130:512–537, 1949

Pfeffer JM: The aetiology of the hyperventilation syndrome: a review of the literature. Psychother Psychosom 30:47–55, 1978

Pfeffer JM: Hyperventilation and the hyperventilation syndrome. Postgrad Med J 60 (suppl 2):12–15, 1984

Roth JL, Bockus HL: Aerophagia: its etiology, syndromes, and management. Med Clin North Am 41:1673–1696, 1957

Salkovskis PM, Jones DRO, Clark DM: Respiratory control in the treatment of panic attacks: replication and extension with concurrent measurement of behavior and pCO_2. Br J Psychiatry 148:526–532, 1986

Schroeder SR, Schroeder CS, Rojahn J, et al: Self-injurious behavior: an analysis of behavior management techniques, in Handbook of Behavior Modification With the Mentally Retarded. Edited by Matson JL, McCartney JR. New York, Plenum, 1981, pp 61–115

Stone RT, Morgan MD: Aerophagia in children. Am Fam Physician 3:94–95, 1971

West JB: Pulmonary Pathophysiology: The Essentials, 2nd Edition. Baltimore, MD, Williams & Wilkins, 1982

Whitehead WE, Schuster MM: Gastrointestinal Disorders: Behavioral and Physiological Basis for Treatment. New York, Academic Press, 1985

World Health Organization: Draft of the 10th Revision of the International Classification of Diseases. Geneva, World Health Organization, 1988

Chapter 9

Chronic Pain Syndromes

In several of the syndromes described in the previous chapters, the patient's main complaint was pain. These syndromes include fibromyalgia, some of the esophageal motility disorders, non-ulcer dyspepsia, and the irritable bowel syndrome. Pain syndromes caused by contraction of striated muscle are described in Chapter 10. There are, however, numerous other syndromes in which pain is the main complaint. A brief description of some of these syndromes follows.

Chest Pain

> There are few affections which excite more alarm and anxiety in the patient than this. He fancies himself doomed to become a martyr to organic disease of the heart, of the horrors of which he has an exaggerated idea; it is more difficult to divest him of this impression because the nervous state which gives rise to his complaint imparts a fanciful gloom and desponding tone to his imagination.
>
> J. Hope (1832)
> *A Treatise on the Disease of*
> *the Heart and Great Vessels*

Chest pain is a common symptom of organic disease. Chest pain in the absence of physical disease is also a common source of distress and incapacity. Hope's observations are as valid today as they were one-and-a-half centuries ago.

Causes and Diagnosis

There are numerous organic diseases that cause chest pain. A detailed differential diagnosis, which lies beyond the scope of this chapter, is discussed in textbooks of medicine. Among the cardiac causes, the most important is coronary artery insufficiency resulting in myocardial ischemia; others are insufficiency of coronary microcirculation (Cannon et al. 1985), Prinzmetal (variant) angina, and sensitivity of the coronary vessels (i.e., "the tender heart") (Cannon et al.

165

1990; Shapiro et al. 1988). Another cause of chest pain is skeletal disease such as osteoarthritis of the cervical or thoracic spine and tenderness of the chest wall (Epstein et al. 1979). Chest pain is often caused by gastrointestinal disease (Long and Cohen 1980), including peptic ulceration, esophageal reflux, and esophageal motility disorders (see Chapter 4, this volume). Hyperventilation can cause chest pain as well as electrocardiographic changes that resemble those of myocardial ischemia (Evans and Lum 1977; Lary and Goldschlager 1974). In some patients the cause of the pain remains unknown. Because coronary artery disease is a common and serious cause of pain, the other causes are sometimes referred to as *noncardiac chest pain*.

Prevalence

About 500,000 coronary arteriograms are performed annually in the United States; of these, about one fifth show no arterial disease. Among patients with normal arteriograms, about 10% to 30% have esophageal motility disorders. The number of patients with chest pain is substantially larger because those with atypical pain are usually investigated with noninvasive procedures (Kemp et al. 1986). Many patients with chest pain do not consult a physician; for example, a study in Britain found that only about one person in five with angina sought medical treatment for this condition (Rose 1972).

Psychiatric Studies

Noncardiac chest pain is associated with psychiatric morbidity. In several studies, patients with noncardiac chest pain were found to be more depressed, more anxious, and have more phobias than patients with chest pain and coronary artery disease (Bass and Wade 1984; Beitman et al. 1987; Channer et al. 1985; Cormier et al. 1988: Katon et al. 1988; Klimes et al. 1990; Mayou 1989). Many of these patients believe that they have a serious physical disease (Burns and Nichols 1972).

Treatment

There are a few published studies of the treatment of chest pain associated with esophageal motility disorders (see Chapter 4) and a few other case histories of the treatment of patients in whom the source of the pain was known or who also had another diagnosis. For example, there are a few case reports of apparently successful treatment with controlled breathing and relaxation of patients with chest pain caused by hyperventilation (Evans and Lum 1977; Hegel et al. 1989). In an uncontrolled study of the treatment of chest pain with panic disorder, several patients improved with alprazolam (Beitman et al. 1988).

There are several published case histories of psychotherapy or behavior therapy of patients with atypical chest pain (Levenkron et al. 1985) and of an uncontrolled series of patients with cardiophobia (Sulz 1986) (see Chapter 10, this volume).[1]

Patients with noncardiac chest pain are not usually treated or followed up by cardiologists and are not routinely referred elsewhere (Braunwald et al. 1987, p. 865; Lantinga et al. 1988) except for research purposes. They are a sadly neglected and suffering group of people.

Prognosis

The prognosis for survival is good; patients with normal arteriograms have approximately the same life expectancy as do an age-adjusted control group from the community (Bruschke et al. 1973; Kemp et al. 1973; Pamelia et al. 1985; Proudfit et al. 1980). The proportion of patients with persisting chest pain varies with the duration of the follow-up; between 50% and 80% of these patients have persistent symptoms (Lavey and Winkle 1979; Waxler et al. 1971), and between 40% and 60% still believe that they have cardiac disease. About one third to one half are disabled (Bass et al. 1983; Ockene et al. 1980); the average level of anxiety and depression in patients with chronic chest pain remains unchanged on follow-up (Lantinga et al. 1988). The prognosis for disability and morbidity is worse in idiopathic pain than in pain caused by esophageal motility disorders (see Chapter 4, p. 88, this volume).

Chronic Pelvic Pain

Chronic pelvic pain in women can be extremely distressing. In a substantial proportion of patients, no adequate organic pathology is found to account for the pain. The chronic pelvic pain syndrome has also been termed *enigmatic pelvic pain* (Mills 1978).

Symptoms and Signs

Chronic pelvic pain is typically premenopausal. The characteristic symptoms include a dull ache with intermittent sharp exacerbations, described as stabbing or burning in the suprapubic area or in one or both iliac fossae. The pain may also be referred to the inner thighs. The pain is at its worst before a menstrual period, and there is often deep dyspareunia. The pain is often aggravated by

---

[1]

Since this chapter was written, a review article on atypical chest pain was published (Mayou 1989). The author summarizes an unpublished controlled study of atypical chest pain. Thirty-five patients with chest pain for 3 months or longer and no evidence of physical disease were allocated either to immediate cognitive-behavioral treatment or to assessment and advice. Treated patients significantly improved compared with control subjects "in terms of mood, chest pain, and limitation of activities, and gains were maintained on a three months' follow-up." At the end of the treatment the majority of the improved patients now accepted that psychological factors had been a major cause of their symptoms. The study has subsequently been published (Klimes et al. 1990; Pearce et al. 1990).

postural changes and walking. There may be associated symptoms such as leukorrhea or irritability of the bladder (Beard et al. 1988b; "Enigmatic Pelvic Pain" 1978). There are no consistent physical signs except that there may be severe localized tenderness on pelvic examination (Slocumb 1984).

Prevalence

The estimates of prevalence of chronic pelvic pain vary. Between 36% and 76% of diagnostic laparoscopies for pelvic pain reveal normal tissue (Liston et al. 1972; Lundberg et al. 1973).

Etiology

Various physical causes of chronic pelvic pain have been suggested. These include chronic pelvic inflammatory disease (Frangenheim and Kleindienst 1974) and nerve entrapment (Applegate 1972). However, there has been no conclusive evidence to support these views. Several authors have suggested that pelvic varicosities and congestion are the cause (Beard et al. 1988a; Topolanski-Sierra 1958). Beard et al. (1984) found that vascular abnormalities on venography discriminated between the chronic pelvic pain syndrome and pain from other causes. Slocumb (1984) described trigger points and areas of hypersensitivity with referred hyperesthesia of the dermatomal area.

Psychological and Psychiatric Studies

The authors of several uncontrolled studies have suggested that there is substantial psychopathology in women with chronic pelvic pain (Grandi et al. 1988; Renaer 1980). Controlled studies tend to bear this out, but some of the results are conflicting. For example, Beard et al. (1977) found higher neuroticism scores on the Eysenck Personality Inventory (EPI) in patients with chronic pelvic pain than in a control group of patients without pain. Also, there were no significant differences on the Middlesex Hospital Questionnaire in self-rated anxiety, depression, and somatic symptoms, whereas Magni et al. (1986) found significant differences on the somatic scale of the same questionnaire. Pearce (1986) found no differences on the EPI and Profile of Mood States between patients with chronic pelvic pain syndrome and patients with organic pathology, although the patients with chronic pelvic pain syndrome had had more exposure to death and illness, sexual problems, and concerns about illness. Walker et al. (1988) and Slocumb et al. (1989), using a different scale (the Hopkins Symptom Checklist–90), found significantly higher average levels of anxiety, depression, and hostility, and higher averages on several other subscales between patients with pain and patients without pain; Symptom Questionnaire scores yielded similar results. Patients with the chronic pelvic pain syndrome scored higher than healthy control subjects on the General Health Questionnaire (Byrne 1984) and higher than patients with pain and endometriosis on the

Minnesota Multiphasic Personality Inventory (MMPI) scales of hypochondriasis (Hs), depression (D), hysteria (Hy), and anxiety (Renaer 1980).

In a study by Walker et al. (1988), more of the patients with chronic pelvic pain had a history of previous depression (in the majority of cases depression preceded the onset of pain), evidence of current depression, a history of drug abuse, and current sexual difficulties. Substantially more patients with pelvic pain had been sexually abused both as children and as adults than had control subjects. Although there were several indicators of an increased prevalence of psychiatric disturbance in the patients with pain, on an independent evaluation these patients had the same degree of organic pathology as the control group without pain.

Kellner et al. (1988) found that in spite of thorough investigations and explanations of the nature of the disorder, 44% of women with chronic pelvic pain syndrome (a figure substantially higher than in other patients) believed that they had a disease and that their physician had not diagnosed their illness correctly. These women also scored higher on several scales of the Illness Behavior Questionnaire.

There appear to be substantial differences in psychological profiles among women with chronic pelvic pain. Prill (1964) found no psychiatric abnormality in a substantial proportion of patients. In the psychometric studies, many of the patients did not have elevated scores; for example, in one study, over one half of the patients scored within the normal ranges on all scales of the Hopkins Symptom Checklist and the Symptom Questionnaire (Slocumb et al. 1989).

Diagnosis

Numerous diseases of pelvic organs can cause chronic pain, and these are discussed among the differential diagnoses in textbooks of gynecology. Such an extensive list lies beyond the scope of this volume. A classification is of little practical use other than to remind the clinician of the possibilities to be considered (Beard et al. 1986). Because the exact cause of the pain is unknown, the psychiatric diagnosis should not be that of a somatoform pain disorder. If the patient has substantial psychopathology, the appropriate psychiatric classification appears to be *psychological factors affecting physical conditions* of the DSM-III-R (316.00) (American Psychiatric Association 1987) and its code counterpart (F54) of the ICD-10 draft (World Health Organization 1988).

Treatment

Numerous treatments for chronic pelvic pain have been suggested. Most gynecologists believe that after thorough physical investigations, initial treatment consists of reassurance and explanation of the nature of the disorder in keeping with current knowledge (and, inevitably, with the physician's biases). Nondirective counseling, psychotherapy, pain management, and tricyclic antidepressant drugs have been recommended, and successes have been claimed in uncontrolled studies (Quan 1987; Rapkin and Kames 1987).

Because ovarian hormones are believed to be responsible for the dilation of pelvic veins, Beard et al. (1988a) suppressed ovarian activity with medroxyprogesterone acetate (MPA) in an uncontrolled study ($N = 21$). Of the 16 patients who stopped menstruating, all but one had a marked diminution of pain; the remaining five had breakthrough bleeding without diminution of pain intensity.[2]

Slocumb (1984), in an uncontrolled study, found a high success rate with injections of a local anesthetic into trigger points.

Psychotherapy. Beard et al. (1977) reported good results from relaxation training in an uncontrolled study. Beard et al. (1988a) also carried out a controlled study of psychological treatments in chronic pelvic pain syndrome. One group was allocated to "stress analysis," and these patients received a form of cognitive and behavioral stress management and relaxation training. Discussion of pelvic pain and its associated difficulties was discouraged; instead, the focus of treatment was directed toward identifying current worries and concerns apart from the pain. The patients were also asked to keep a daily record of the main concerns they had. The therapists' aim throughout was, first, to identify cognitive strategies used in response to stressors and, next, to discuss alternative responses. The second group had "pain analysis" that involved close monitoring of the patient's pain and associated antecedent and consequent events. The therapy aimed to identify patterns associated with pain episodes, and alternative strategies for avoiding or reducing pain episodes were discussed. These strategies included cognitive, behavioral, and environmental manipulations. Graded exercise programs were instituted for each patient. Spouses were encouraged to prompt and to reinforce "well behaviors." A random control group had the same explanations as the treatment groups about their disorder: that medical or surgical treatments were of no value. Several methods were used to assess treatment outcome, including a blind rating by gynecologists. On all measures of outcome, both treatment groups performed significantly better than the minimal intervention control group at 6-month follow-up, although there was no difference between the conditions at 3-month follow-up. This would suggest that the ability of coping with stress and pain was assimilated and used to advantage during the follow-up period.

Twelve percent of all hysterectomies are done because of pelvic pain, and good results have been claimed for presacral neurectomies (Beard et al. 1986).

2

Since this chapter was written, Farquhar et al. (1989) published a controlled study of MPA alone, MPA plus brief psychotherapy, placebo alone, and placebo plus brief psychotherapy (average about five sessions). MPA was found to be significantly more effective than placebo. There was no evidence of efficacy of brief psychotherapy and placebo on a 9-month follow-up, but there was an interaction effect of psychotherapy and MPA.

There is still a controversy about the indications for surgery. According to one school of thought, the results of surgery are disappointing (Renaer 1981), and surgery is inappropriate in most cases (Beard et al. 1986); according to another view—which is apparently losing support—hysterectomy has a place in the treatment of unexplained pelvic pain and should not be regarded by the gynecologist as a confession of defeat ("Enigmatic Pelvic Pain" 1978).

Prognosis

The prognosis for chronic pelvic pain varies across studies with the duration of follow-up and the kind of treatment used. About 70% of patients either have substantially less pain or are free of pain on follow-up. Some treatments have higher success rates; for example, Slocumb (1984) reported at least some relief from pain in almost 90% of patients. Because all studies have been uncontrolled, the differences in outcome may be largely due to differences in the populations studied and in the nature of the outcome criteria.

Proctalgia Fugax

Proctalgia fugax is a syndrome in which the main feature is intermittent pain in the rectum. The term was coined by Thaysen (1935). There are several published reviews, including those by Douthwaite (1962), Thompson (1981), Whitehead and Schuster (1985), and Peery (1988), in which the literature is referenced. The syndrome has entered the American English language as a vulgar idiom describing a psychophysiological response that reflects disapproval of another person.

Prevalence

In studies using questionnaires and interviews, the prevalence of rectal pain ranged from 13% to 25% in various groups of nonpatients (Panitch and Schofferman 1975; Thompson and Heaton 1980). The prevalence varies with the population studied.

Symptoms and Signs

The pain is severe and cramplike, usually lasting seconds or minutes, and the onset is sudden. Sometimes the attacks are accompanied by flatus or occur after bowel movement, and less frequently after sexual activity. Other symptoms such as syncope or priapism are rare and occur either concurrently or shortly after the attack. Most patients have fewer than six attacks a year, but some have frequent attacks.

Etiology

The cause of proctalgia fugax is not known. It has been attributed to "tension myalgia of the pelvic floor" (Sinaki et al. 1977), to a spasm of the levator ani (Smith 1935), and to a vascular disturbance (Pradel et al. 1967). Harvey (1979) observed with a sigmoidoscope two patients during an attack and found that the pain coincided with contractions of the sigmoid colon. In an uncontrolled study, Pilling et al. (1972) found that 52% of patients with proctalgia fugax had functional abdominal somatic symptoms. Thompson and Heaton (1980), in a study of healthy volunteers, found that patients with a history of proctalgia also had significantly more symptoms suggesting an irritable bowel syndrome than did other subjects. Thompson (1984) compared the prevalence of proctalgia in patients with irritable bowel syndrome, peptic ulcer, and inflammatory bowel disease. About one third had proctalgia, and only two of the irritable bowel symptoms were more common in the proctalgia patients. Thus, it appears that proctalgia is only weakly associated with the irritable bowel syndrome and is probably a somewhat different disorder that occurs more often in patients with gastrointestinal disease than in nonpatients.

Psychological Factors

To my knowledge, there is only one published systematic psychological study of patients with this syndrome. Pilling et al. (1972) administered the MMPI, the Shipley Institute of Living Scale for Measuring Intellectual Impairment, and a checklist of previous illnesses and socioeconomic circumstances to 48 patients with proctalgia fugax at the Mayo Clinic. The authors also examined the patients in an unstructured psychiatric interview. The patients were found to have above-average intelligence. The MMPI scores of the neurotic triad (hypochondriasis, depression, and hysteria) were slightly higher than those of other patients. Based on the various methods of investigation, 73% of the patients were judged to be anxious and tense, 67% perfectionistic, 40% hypochondriacal, and 33% had neurotic symptoms in childhood.

   Comment. Because Pilling et al.'s study was uncontrolled, it is uncertain whether these results pertain specifically to proctalgia or are largely the function of self-selection or selective referral to the clinic (Thompson 1981; Whitehead and Schuster 1985). The only controlled feature of the study was the comparison of MMPI profiles, and these did not differ substantially from those of other patients. The authors concluded that proctalgia fugax was of psychogenic origin; the data, however, are inadequate to support this conclusion.

Treatments and Prognosis

Various treatments for proctalgia fugax have been suggested, but there are no controlled studies to date. Most authors recommend that the patient should be reassured and that if the symptoms are distressing, various methods of relieving the pain may be tried. These methods include pressure on the perineum and simple treatments that relieve symptoms of the irritable bowel syndrome (see

Chapter 6, this volume). Other treatments that have been suggested based on the experiences with a few patients include distraction ("Some Observations on Proctalgia Fugax" 1952), heat (Dodi et al. 1986), and the administration of either clonidine (Swain 1987) or diltiazem (Boquet et al. 1986). The condition is benign, and the attacks tend to wane later in life.

Hysterical Pain (Conversion Pain or Psychogenic Regional Pain)

In the literature, hysterical pain and two other terms—conversion pain and psychogenic regional pain—have been used synonymously. Several features of this disorder are still a matter of controversy.

Symptoms and Signs

There is incomplete agreement on the characteristic features of this disorder. Walters (1961) published the study with the largest series of patients; the description of the symptoms and signs in that study can be summarized as follows: the pain cannot be explained by peripheral nerve stimulation because it does not have an anatomical pattern consistent with nerve distribution and cannot be explained as a consequence of physiological activity such as contraction of striated or smooth muscle. The pain occurs in a variety of psychiatric syndromes.

The pain is associated with one or more of the following physical signs: motor deficit, tenderness, and, in most cases, motor weakness and hyperalgesia. There are rarely vegetative changes over the body surface.

Prevalence

The prevalence of hysterical pain is unknown. The syndrome as defined by the symptoms and signs given above appears to compose only a small proportion of patients with chronic pain.

Etiology

There is disagreement among authors on the nature of regional pain. A few authors regard most cases of regional pain as hysterical. For example, Weintraub (1988) examined 35 consecutive patients with the chronic pain syndrome who were involved in litigation and concluded that 71% displayed elements of hysterical conversion reactions. He based his judgment on signs such as *la belle indifférence* or, conversely, excessive concern about the pain and wearing a cervical collar.

In reply to Weintraub's report, Merskey (1988) expressed the opposite view—that regional pain is rarely hysterical—and argued that there are numerous diseases that cause regional pain and that organic diseases can mimic symptoms and signs of conversion disorder. Several of these go undetected unless special investigations are used, so on routine investigations alone, some of the patients with regional pain may be misdiagnosed as having a conversion disorder. Many of the signs of hysteria can also be found in patients with definite organic lesions (Gould et al. 1986). Moreover, symptoms and signs of conversion disorder are unreliable in the presence of pain; for example, when voluntary power is tested in a limb, some patients show an inconsistent response that may be the consequence of pain or the patient's fear of getting hurt. Also, because the threshold for noxious stimulation is increased in patients with severe pain, the sensory loss interpreted as evidence of a conversion disorder may be the sequel of the patient having endured long-standing and severe pain. There are also varied patterns of sensory disturbance that accompany deep injury, so even organic pain may have a nonanatomical distribution (Woolf and Wall 1986).

In cases in which regional pain occurs in conjunction with definite symptoms and signs of conversion disorder, it seems likely that the two conditions share the same etiology (see Chapter 11, pp. 230–231, this volume). The psychological as well as physiological processes and central nervous system pathways that are involved in conversion pain are unknown. In some of the cases that I have seen, there was no apparent motive and the patient did not appear to gain from the symptoms. The pain usually started at a time of unbearable strain and made an agonizing situation even worse. One of the theories that has been put forward is an activation of a "central pattern generating mechanism" or "reverberating circuit" (Kellner 1986, p. 127), concepts that have been used to explain central pain mechanism (Melzack and Loeser 1978). However, such concepts leave a great deal unexplained.

Diagnosis

After organic pathological causes of regional pain have been meticulously excluded, and if the symptom cannot be explained on grounds of a physiological process (such as muscle contraction), the choice of the anatomical label *regional pain* is unobjectionable. The determination as to whether the pain is hysterical or a conversion disorder is, of course, far more difficult, particularly because the nature of the phenomenon is not understood and there is incomplete agreement of what constitutes conversion pain. The terms *hysterical* or *conversion* should not imply that the pain replaces emotion or that it solves a conflict, because it tends to complicate a situation rather than solve it. The patient seldom gains from acquiring this new and distressing symptom.

Conversion pain appears at a time of severe emotional strain. There may or may not be other conversion phenomena present. Whether conversion (as opposed to other processes of somatization [see Chapter 10]) contributes to the amplification of pain of organic origin is unknown. The term should not include dramatic elaborations of symptoms by a histrionic person.

The diagnostic classification does not pose a problem because the term is *somatoform pain disorder* (307.80) in the DSM-III-R and *persistent pain disorder* (F45.4) in the draft of the ICD-10. Because the phenomenon is of theoretical interest, it should be a topic for further research, and its recognition may have implications for treatment.

There are numerous studies using rating scales, diagnostic schedules, and personality inventories in patients with chronic pain. The results of these studies suggest that such investigations do not help to determine whether regional pain in a particular patient is a conversion phenomenon or not (see Chapter 11, pp. 231–232, this volume).

Shoichet (1978) found that regional pain was relieved under light amobarbital sodium anesthesia, whereas pain caused by organic pathology or pain inflicted by the examiner, such as squeezing the Achilles tendon, was relieved less. This study has not been replicated, so the value of amobarbital sodium as a diagnostic test has not been conclusively established.

Treatment

Walters (1961), who has described the largest series of patients, reported that his patients' disorder was treated "in principle no different from any other psychiatric disorder and [that] the background of their emotional troubles . . . [was] the center of the attack" (p. 14). There are no controlled studies of the treatment of regional pain, and it is unknown whether any of the treatments accelerate recovery. Judging by published case histories, the therapist should try to alleviate existing conflicts and relieve distress.

Prognosis

Little is known about the prognosis of hysterical pain, because in reports on the treatment of chronic pain there is usually no separate description of the outcome of regional pain. Walters (1961) (see above) reported that "three quarters [of the patients] obtained relief from pain." Further studies are needed in order to judge whether prognosis changes with different treatments.

Case Histories

Several authors have described cases of hysterical pain in which the site of the pain was associated with either an idea or with some minor physical trauma. For example, Merskey (1979, p. 116) described a 25-year-old woman who had amblyopia and episodic jabbing pain in her left eye and a continuous dull ache in that area, present for 2 years, which commenced when the buckle of a car safety belt struck her accidentally. The car belonged to a boyfriend whom her parents disliked. At the time when she decided to give up her boyfriend, she was treated with hypnosis and made a complete recovery.

There are other cases in which there is no obvious connection between the site of the pain and a patient's idea or image, but perhaps in which there is a connection that is not revealed during a routine diagnostic interview. The history that follows describes regional pain; it is suggestive of a conversion process, but I did not learn enough about this patient to reach a definite conclusion.

A 35-year-old housewife was referred to me because of severe pain in her ear. She was an immigrant who had arrived in England 18 months previously. Elaborate investigations had failed to discover an organic cause. Her husband, a laborer who earned only a very small income, had left her 6 months previously because of another woman. Two months later she was told that her 3-year-old daughter, her only child, had inoperable sarcoma and was going to die. Four days later, she developed severe pain in her left ear, which she described as unbearable. The pain was constant, and she had not found anything that either relieved or aggravated the pain; there were no other symptoms or signs suggestive of a conversion disorder. She came to see me only twice and failed to keep subsequent appointments. I learned that the pain had persisted for 2 years, and she was examined by several other physicians. Later she moved to another city and I lost touch with her.

Somatoform Pain Disorder (Persistent Pain Disorder)

The predominant feature of this disorder of the DSM-III-R (and the draft of the ICD-10) is persistent pain for which no adequate cause is found. There are numerous patients with chronic pain who cannot be classified among the other syndromes described in this volume. Because there are several published books and numerous articles on chronic pain, the topic will be discussed only briefly.

Symptoms and Signs

Various characteristics of patients with persistent pain have been described. These include a continuing search for an organic diagnosis, exposure to most standard medical treatment and surgical techniques, an implicit appeal to the physician to take responsibility for a cure, behaviors that sustain the sick role, environmental rewards that maintain the sick role, and avoidance of healthy roles. These descriptions are based on patients attending pain clinics or persistently seeking medical care for pain, and they are also found in patients whose pain is clearly caused by a physical disease (Blackwell et al. 1989). The characteristics of people with chronic pain who do not seek treatment may be different from those of the patients who are self-selected or who are selectively referred to pain clinics (Egan and Katon 1987). Moreover, most of these behaviors can be understood as consequences of unmitigated suffering.

Etiology

The etiology of chronic pain is complex; several factors appear to interact, and the exact nature of pain in many patients remains elusive. (For example, Melzack [1973] published a monograph on pain that was aptly titled *The Puzzle of Pain.*)

Various theories, including learning and other reinforcement (Fordyce 1976) and social modeling (Fordyce et al. 1968), have been put forward to explain the nature of persistent pain (Pilowsky 1978). Several theories connect chronic pain with psychopathology, usually with depression. For example, Blumer and Heilbronn (1982) regard the "pain prone syndrome" as being a masked depression. Several authors have argued that although many patients with chronic pain are depressed, there appears to be no single mechanism or psychopathology that accounts adequately for this syndrome (Black 1980; Merskey 1982). It seems unlikely that this syndrome is merely a variant of depression, because of its several different features, including an unremittent course and poorer response to antidepressant treatment. When chronic pain, depression, and anxiety occur together, the psychopathology may be a consequence of the pain rather than an etiological factor. (Another kind of pain that is associated with depression is described below in the section on diagnosis.)

Several studies have shown that patients with chronic pain are distressed regardless of whether the pain is caused by physical disease or whether no obvious organic cause is found. Woodforde and Merskey (1972) found that patients with pain caused by neurological disease had even higher scores on the Middlesex Hospital Questionnaire than patients in whom no physical disease was found to account for the pain, and both groups scored in the range of neurotic patients. Renaer (1980) found no difference in scores on the MMPI and other psychological tests between women who had pelvic pain of unknown origin and those who had pain caused by endometriosis. Rosenthal et al. (1984) found a large degree of psychopathology on the MMPI in women who had pelvic pain regardless of whether the pain was caused by physical disease or of unknown origin. Sternbach and Timmermans (1975) found a decrease in MMPI scores in patients whose lower back pain was relieved by surgery. These findings suggest that anxiety, depression, and neuroticism, as measured by self-rating scales, can be the consequences of severe and persisting pain and are not necessarily etiological factors (Kellner 1986).

There are numerous features associated with chronic pain that are likely to be predisposing and maintaining factors (Merskey and Spear 1967; Sternbach 1968). In any individual case, it is often difficult to determine the extent of the contribution of various factors; for example, it is difficult to judge why two people who have a similar damage to a joint after an accident differ strikingly in the extent of their disability and social impairment resulting from the injury. It seems likely that the mechanisms responsible for somatization in general (which are described in Chapter 10 of this volume) play varying roles in the perception of pain as well as in the response to pain.

Diagnosis

Apart from the exclusion of physical disease as the cause of the pain, major depression should be excluded as the primary cause. In a small minority of patients with chronic pain who are severely depressed, intense, localized, atypical pain occurred after the patients had become depressed; in these patients, apparently the pain is an atypical manifestation of the depression, and the pain tends to remit with effective antidepressant treatment (Bradley 1963).

The somatoform pain disorder of the DSM-III-R (307.80) and the persistent pain disorder of the draft of the ICD-10 (F45.4) share the description of persistent complaints of pain that cannot be explained fully by physiological processes. There are, however, somewhat different emphases on other features in these two classification systems. The ICD-10 draft regards as one of the diagnostic features the "pain occurring in association with emotional conflict or psychosocial problems that are sufficient to allow the conclusion that they are the main causative influences" (p. 126). In many patients with chronic pain in which "social and occupational impairment appears grossly in excess of what would be expected from the physical findings" (which is one of the diagnostic features of the DSM-III-R), there are often no conspicuous emotional stressors that would satisfy the ICD-10 criteria.

Numerous psychological inventories have been used for the evaluation of patients with chronic pain. It is often difficult to establish whether the test results measure personality traits, causative factors, or the consequences of severe pain (Kellner 1986, p. 210). There is no evidence to date that a complex and expensive psychological evaluation enhances the effectiveness of the choice of treatments.

Because the contribution of the various etiological factors is often uncertain, it is also difficult to choose the appropriate psychiatric diagnostic category in these cases. Many of the patients also have other Axis I diagnoses (Blackwell et al. 1984), and these need to be listed. If a physical disease or injury is one of the etiological factors, it needs to be described on Axis III. In view of the complex diagnostic problems, the exclusion criteria of the diagnostic manuals need to be carefully considered when making the diagnosis in patients with chronic pain syndromes.

Treatments and Outcome

There are only a few controlled studies of individual treatment modalities in persistent pain, and there are no adequate controlled studies of the usual combination of treatments practiced at pain centers. There are substantial variations in outcome reported from uncontrolled studies. On the average, over one half of the patients attending pain clinics are reported to have improved on follow-up.

There have been numerous published reviews on research and recommendations for treatment and outcome studies of treated chronic pain (Benjamin 1989; Blackwell et al. 1989; Fordyce et al. 1973; Kocher 1976; Roberts and Reinhardt 1980; Sternbach 1974; Swanson et al. 1979; Turk et al. 1983; Weisenberg 1987). The treatment of chronic pain has become a subspecialty. In view of the magnitude of the field and the many published reviews, another survey of such studies and recommendations for treatment of chronic pain in general lie beyond the scope of this volume.

Summary and Main Conclusions

Noncardiac Chest Pain

There are various causes of noncardiac chest pain. About 100,000 people in the United States evaluated each year because of chest pain have normal coronary arteriograms; many others are investigated for cardiac disease by noninvasive procedures. Psychiatric disorders—particularly panic disorder, depression, and hyperventilation—are substantially higher in patients with normal arteriograms than in patients with coronary artery disease. There are a few small uncontrolled series and a few published case histories of patients with chest pain who also had psychiatric disorders and in whom the treatment was apparently successful. Results of a controlled study of cognitive-behavioral therapy suggest the efficacy of such treatments. Patients with chest pain and normal arteriograms have the same life expectancy as the rest of the population. Although about 50% to 80% of these patients still have symptoms on follow-up, and between one third and one half remain disabled on follow-up, most are not referred for treatment.

Pelvic Pain

Laparoscopies in women with chronic pelvic pain reveal normal tissue in one third to three quarters of these cases. The pain can be extremely distressing and incapacitating. The various causes that have been proposed include chronic pelvic infections, nerve entrapment, and localized areas of hypersensitivity with referred pain. Varicosities and vascular abnormalities are more common in these patients than in other women.

On the average, women with this syndrome show more evidence of psychiatric ill health than do other patients, including those who have pelvic pain caused by organic disease such as endometriosis. A substantial proportion believe that they have an undiagnosed disease. In one study, patients with pelvic pain had experienced substantially more sexual abuse in childhood as well as in adult life; they had a history of depression and drug abuse that preceded the onset of the pain. The patients with this syndrome appear to be psychologically heterogeneous, with about one half scoring in the normal ranges on distress scales.

The cause of pelvic pain remains unknown. Because vascular abnormalities are more common, congestion appears to be an important factor. Since ovarian hormones tend to dilate pelvic veins, this would explain the occurrence of the pain during the reproductive years. In some patients, pain appears to originate with severe sexual trauma in childhood and is accompanied by disturbed adult sexuality; in others, psychological distress appears to be the consequence of severe chronic pain.

Uncontrolled studies suggest benefits from tricyclic antidepressant drugs. Furthermore, in a controlled study, suppression of ovarian activity with medroxyprogesterone acetate (MPA) relieved pain. In a recent controlled study of psychotherapy, cognitive-behavioral therapy combined with relaxation training was found to be superior in outcome to that in a control group in which patients received explanation only. In another study, there was an interaction effect of five sessions of psychotherapy and MPA, but no evidence of efficacy of brief psychotherapy alone on follow-up.

There is disagreement among authors about treatment, and the recommendations on treatment that follow are also subject to personal biases. The initial management consists of a thorough examination with an unqualified assurance about the benign nature of the pain, repeated if necessary. The patients who do not respond should be referred to psychotherapy and pain management, which may include antidepressant drugs, in conjunction with gynecological follow-up.

Injection of trigger points may be tried if the above treatments fail. The value of surgery is controversial and should be regarded as the last resort.

Proctalgia Fugax

Proctalgia fugax is a syndrome in which the main feature is intermittent pain in the rectum. It is usually severe, of sudden onset, cramplike, and brief. The cause is unknown. It is more common in patients with gastrointestinal disease than in other patients. In a study with two patients, the pain coincided with contractions of the sigmoid colon. In an uncontrolled study, clinic patients with proctalgia fugax were judged to have various neurotic traits, a finding that may have been caused by a biased selection of patients. Various treatments have been suggested based on uncontrolled studies. The condition is benign and tends to wane later in life.

Hysterical (or Conversion) Pain

The terms *hysterical pain, conversion pain,* and *regional pain* have been used synonymously, and there is incomplete agreement on the nature of the disorder. The distribution of the pain is inconsistent with that of peripheral nerves and cannot be explained on grounds of physiological activity such as muscle contraction. There are usually also symptoms and signs of a conversion disorder. The presence of conversion symptoms by themselves, however, is not diagnostic, because these symptoms can be the consequences of severe pain from organic causes. The pain usually occurs at a time of severe stress; sometimes there is no apparent motive, and the patient does not appear to gain from pain.

The prevalence of this type of chronic pain is not known; it probably comprises only a small proportion of all chronic pain syndromes. The mechanisms and nervous pathways are not known and are perhaps similar to those of central pain. There are no controlled studies of treatment. In one uncontrolled series of treated patients, three quarters obtained relief from pain.

Somatoform Pain Disorder (Persistent Pain Disorder)

There are many patients with chronic pain who cannot be classified among the pain syndromes described in this volume. Somatoform pain disorder (a category of the DSM-III-R) and persistent pain disorder (a category of the draft of the ICD-10) both share as the main diagnostic feature persistent pain that cannot be explained fully by physiological processes. The emphases on other features differ in the two classification systems. Because there is a large body of literature on the nature and treatments of chronic pain, only the main characteristics and theories are briefly discussed in this chapter.

References

American Psychiatric Association: Statistical and Diagnostic Manual of Mental Disorders, 3rd Edition, Revised. Washington, DC, American Psychiatric Association, 1987

Applegate WV: Abdominal cutaneous nerve entrapment syndrome. Surgery 71:118–124, 1972

Bass C, Wade C: Chest pain with normal coronary arteries: a comparative study of psychiatric and social morbidity. Psychol Med 14:51–61, 1984

Bass C, Wade C, Hand D, et al: Patients with angina with normal and near normal coronary arteries: clinical and psychosocial state 12 months after angiography. Br Med J 287:1505–1508, 1983

Beard RW, Belsey EM, Lieberman BA, et al: Pelvic pain in women. Am J Obstet Gynecol 128:566–570, 1977

Beard RW, Pearce S, Highman JH, et al: Diagnosis of pelvic varicosities in women with chronic pelvic pain. Lancet 2:946–949, 1984

Beard RW, Reginald PW, Pearce S: Pelvic pain in women. Br Med J 293:1160–1162, 1986

Beard RW, Reginald PW, Pearce S: Psychological and somatic factors in women with pain due to pelvic congestion. Adv Exp Med Biol 245:413–421, 1988a

Beard RW, Reginald PW, Wadsworth J: Clinical features of women with chronic lower abdominal pain and pelvic congestion. Br J Obstet Gynaecol 95:153–161, 1988b

Beitman BD, Basha I, Flaker G, et al: Major depression in cardiology chest pain patients without coronary artery disease and with panic disorder. J Affective Disord 13:51–59, 1987

Beitman BD, Basha IM, Trombka LH, et al: Alprazolam in the treatment of cardiology patients with atypical chest pain and panic disorder. J Clin Psychopharmacol 8:127–130, 1988

Benjamin S: Psychological treatment of chronic pain: a selective review. J Psychosom Res 33:121–131, 1989

Black RG: The clinical syndrome of chronic pain, in Pain, Discomfort, and Humanitarian Care, Vol 4. Edited by Ng LKY, Bonica JJ. New York, Elsevier North-Holland, 1980, pp 207–219

Blackwell B, Galbraith JR, Dahl DS: Chronic pain management. Hosp Community Psychiatry 35:999–1008, 1984

Blackwell B, Merskey H, Kellner R: Somatoform pain disorders, in Treatments of Psychiatric Disorders: A Task Force Report of the American Psychiatric Association. Washington, DC, American Psychiatric Association, 1989, pp 2120–2138

Blumer D, Heilbronn M: Chronic pain as a variant of depressive disease: the pain-prone disorder. J Nerv Ment Dis 170:381–406, 1982

Boquet J, Moore N, Lhuintre JP, et al: Diltiazem for proctalgia fugax. Lancet 1:1493, 1986

Bradley JJ: Severe localized pain associated with the depressive syndrome. Br J Psychiatry 109:741–745, 1963

Braunwald E, Isselbacher KJ, Petersdorf RG, et al: Harrison's Principles of Internal Medicine, 11th Edition. New York, McGraw-Hill, 1987

Bruschke AVG, Proudfit WL, Sones FM JR: Clinical course of patients with normal, and slightly or moderately abnormal coronary arteriograms: a follow-up study on 500 patients. Circulation 47:936–945, 1973

Burns BH, Nichols MA: Factors related to the localisation of symptoms to the chest in depression. Br J Psychiatry 121:405–409, 1972

Byrne P: Psychiatric morbidity in a gynaecology clinic: an epidemiological survey. Br J Psychiatry 144:28–34, 1984

Cannon RO III, Leon MB, Watson RM, et al: Chest pain and "normal" coronary arteries: role of small coronary arteries. Am J Cardiol 55:50B–60B, 1985

Cannon RO III, Quyyumi AA, Schenke WH, et al: Abnormal cardiac sensitivity in patients with chest pain. J Am Coll Cardiol 16:1359–1366, 1990

Channer KS, Papouchado M, James MA, et al: Anxiety and depression in patients with chest pain referred for exercise testing. Lancet 2:820–823, 1985

Cormier LE, Katon W, Russo J, et al: Chest pain with negative cardiac diagnostic studies: relationship to psychiatric illness. J Nerv Ment Dis 176:351–358, 1988

Dodi G, Bogoni F, Infantino A, et al: Hot or cold in anal pain? Dis Colon Rectum 29:248–251, 1986

Douthwaite AH: Proctalgia fugax. Br Med J 11(July 21):164–165, 1962

Egan KJ, Katon WJ: Responses to illness and health in chronic pain patients and healthy adults. Psychosom Med 49:470–481, 1987

Enigmatic pelvic pain (editorial). Br Med J 2:1041–1042

Epstein SE, Gerber LH, Borer JS: Chest wall syndrome: a common cause of unexplained cardiac pain. JAMA 241:2793–2797, 1979

Evans DW, Lum LC: Hyperventilation: an important cause of pseudoangina. Lancet 1:155–160, 1977

Farquhar CM, Rogers V, Franks S, et al: A randomized controlled trial of medroxyprogesterone acetate and psychotherapy for the treatment of pelvic congestion. Br J Obstet Gynaecol 96:1153–1162, 1989

Fordyce WE: Behavioral Methods for Chronic Pain and Illness. St. Louis, MO, CV Mosby, 1976

Fordyce WE, Fowler RS Jr, Lehmann JF, et al: Some implications of learning in problems of chronic pain. J Chron Dis 21:179–190, 1968

Fordyce WE, Fowler RS Jr, Lehmann JF, et al: Operant conditioning in the treatment of chronic pain. Arch Phys Med Rehabil 54:399–408, 1973

Frangenheim H, Kleindienst W: Chronic pelvic disease of unknown origin. J Reprod Med 13:23–26, 1974

Gould R, Miller BL, Goldberg MA, et al: The validity of hysterical signs and symptoms. J Nerv Ment Dis 174:593–597, 1986

Grandi S, Fava GA, Trombini G, et al: Depression and anxiety in patients with chronic pelvic pain. Psychiatr Med 6:1–7, 1988

Harvey RF: Colonic motility in proctalgia fugax. Lancet 2:713–714, 1979

Hegel MT, Abel GG, Etscheidt M, et al: Behavioral treatment of angina-like chest pain in patients with hyperventilation syndrome. J Behav Ther Exp Psychiatry 20:31–39, 1989

Katon W, Hall ML, Russo J, et al: Chest pain: relationship of psychiatric illness to coronary arteriographic results. Am J Med 84:1–9, 1988

Kellner R: Somatization and Hypochondriasis. New York, Praeger-Greenwood, 1986

Kellner R, Slocumb JC, Rosenfeld RC, et al: Fears and beliefs in patients with the pelvic pain syndrome. J Psychosom Res 32:303–310, 1988

Kemp HG Jr, Vokonas PS, Cohn PF, et al: The anginal syndrome associated with normal coronary arteriograms. Am J Med 54:735–742, 1973

Kemp HG Jr, Kronmal RA, Vlietstra RE, et al: Seven year survival of patients with normal or near normal coronary arteriograms: a CASS registry study. J Am Coll Cardiol 7:479–483, 1986

Klimes I, Mayou RA, Pearce MJ, et al: Psychological treatment for atypical non-cardiac chest pain: a controlled evaluation. Psychol Med 20:605–611, 1990

Kocher R: The use of psychotropic drugs in treatment of chronic pain. European Neurology 14:458–464, 1976

Lantinga LJ, Sprafkin RP, McCroskery JH, et al: One-year psychosocial follow-up of patients with chest pain and angiographically normal coronary arteries. Am J Cardiol 62:209–213, 1988

Lary D, Goldschlager N: Electrocardiogram changes during hyperventilation resembling myocardial ischemia in patients with normal coronary arteriograms. Am Heart J 87:383–390, 1974

Lavey EB, Winkle RA: Continuing disability of patients with chest pain and normal coronary arteriograms. Journal of Chronic Diseases 32:191–196, 1979

Levenkron JC, Goldstein MG, Adamides O, et al: Chronic chest pain with normal coronary arteries: a behavioural approach to rehabilitation. Journal of Cardiopulmonary Rehabilitation 5:475–479, 1985

Liston WA, Bradford WP, Dowie J, et al: Laparoscopy in a general gynecological unit. Am J Obstet Gynecol 113:672–677, 1972

Long WB, Cohen S: The digestive tract as a cause of chest pain. Am Heart J 100:567–572, 1980

Lundberg WI, Wall JE, Mathers JE: Laparoscopy in evaluation of pelvic pain. Obstet Gynecol 42:872–876, 1973

Magni G, Andreoli C, de Leo D, et al: Psychological profile of women with chronic pelvic pain. Arch Gynecol 237:165–168, 1986

Mayou R: Chest pain in the cardiac clinic. J Psychosom Res 17:353–357, 1973

Mayou R: Invited review: atypical chest pain. J Psychosom Res 33:393–406, 1989

Melzack R: The Puzzle of Pain. New York, Basic Books, 1973

Melzack R, Loeser JD: Phantom body pain in paraplegics: evidence for central "pattern generating mechanism" for pain. Pain 4:195–210, 1978

Merskey H: The Analysis of Hysteria. London, Ballière, Tindall & Cassell, 1979

Merskey H: Comments on "Chronic pain as a variant of depressive disease: the pain-prone disorder." J Nerv Ment Dis 170:409–411, 1982

Merskey H: Regional pain is rarely hysterical. Arch Neurol 45:915–918, 1988

Merskey H, Spear FG: Pain: Psychological and Psychiatric Aspects. London, Ballière, Tindall and Cassell, 1967

Mills WG: The enigma of pelvic pain. J R Soc Med 71:257–260, 1978

Ockene IS, Shay MJ, Alpert JS, et al: Unexplained chest pain in patients with normal coronary arteriograms: a follow-up study of functional status. N Engl J Med 303:1249–1252, 1980

Pamelia FX, Gibson RS, Watson DD, et al: Prognosis with chest pain and normal thallium-201 exercise scintigrams. Am J Cardiol 55:920–926, 1985

Panitch NM, Schofferman JA: Proctalgia fugax revisited (abstract). Gastroenterology 68:1061, 1975

Pearce MJ, Mayou RA, Klimes I: The management of atypical non-cardiac chest pain. Q J Med 76:991–996, 1990

Pearce S: A psychological investigation of chronic pelvic pain in women. Unpublished doctoral dissertation, University of London, London, 1986

Peery WH: Proctalgia fugax: a clinical enigma. South Med J 81:621–623, 1988

Pilling LF, Swenson WM, Hill JR: The psychologic aspects of proctalgia fugax. Dis Colon Rectum 8:372–376, 1972

Pilowsky I: Pain as abnormal illness behavior. Journal of Human Stress 4:22–27, 1978

Pradel E, Hernandez C, Alloy A: Le syndrome dit de "proctalgie fugace." Ann Chir 21:691–699, 1967

Prill HJ: Psychosomatische Gynakologie. Munchen-Berlin, Urban and Schwarzenberg, 1964

Proudfit WL, Bruschke AVG, Sones FM Jr: Clinical course of patients with normal or slightly or moderately abnormal coronary arteriograms: 10-year follow-up of 521 patients. Circulation 62:712–717, 1980

Quan M: Chronic pelvic pain. J Fam Pract 25:283–288, 1987

Rapkin AJ, Kames LK: The pain management approach to chronic pelvic pain. J Reprod Med 32:323–327, 1987

Renaer M: Chronic pelvic pain without obvious pathology in women: personal observations and a review of the problem. Eur J Obstet Gynecol Reprod Biol 6:415–463, 1980

Renaer M: Chronic Pelvic Pain in Women. Heidelberg, Springer-Verlag, 1981

Roberts AH, Reinhardt L: The behavioral management of chronic pain: long-term follow-up with comparison groups. Pain 8:151–162, 1980

Rose G: Epidemiology of ischaemic heart disease. Br J Hosp Med 7:285–288, 1972

Rosenthal RH, Ling FW, Rosenthal TL, et al: Chronic pelvic pain: psychological features and laparoscopic findings. Psychosomatics 25:833–841, 1984

Shapiro LM, Crake T, Poole-Wilson PA: Is altered cardiac sensation responsible for chest pain in patients with normal coronary arteries?: clinical observation during cardiac catheterisation. Br Med J 296:170–171, 1988

Shoichet RP: Sodium amytal in the diagnosis of chronic pain. Can Psychiatr Assoc J 23:219–228, 1978

Sinaki M, Merritt JL, Stillwell GK: Tension myalgia of the pelvic floor. Mayo Clin Proc 52:717–722, 1977

Slocumb JC: Neurological factors in chronic pelvic pain: trigger points and the abdominal pelvic pain syndrome. Am J Obstet Gynecol 149:536–543, 1984

Slocumb JC, Kellner R, Rosenfeld RC, et al: Anxiety and depression in patients with the abdominal pelvic pain syndrome. Gen Hosp Psychiatry 11:48–53, 1989

Smith RNC: Proctalgia fugax (letter). Lancet 2:581, 1935

Some observations on proctalgia fugax. Lancet, January 5, 1952, p 52

Sternbach RA: Pain: A Psychophysiological Analysis. New York, Academic, 1968

Sternbach RA: Pain and depression, in Somatic Manifestations of Depressive Disorders. Edited by Kiev A. New York, Elsevier, 1974, pp 107–119

Sternbach RA, Timmermans G: Personality changes associated with reduction of pain. Pain 1:177–181, 1975

Sulz SK: Verhaltenstherapie der Herzphobie: ein klinischer Erfahrungsbericht uber ein Training kognitiver Angstbewaltigung. Psychiatr Prax 13:10–16, 1986

Swain R: Oral clonidine for proctalgia fugax. Gut 28:1039–1040, 1987

Swanson DW, Maruta T, Swenson WM: Results of behavior modification in the treatment of chronic pain. Psychosom Med 41:55–61, 1979

Thaysen EH: Proctalgia fugax. Lancet 2:243–246, 1935

Thompson WG: Proctalgia fugax. Dig Dis Sci 26:1121–1124, 1981

Thompson WG: Proctalgia fugax in patients with the irritable bowel, peptic ulcer, or inflammatory bowel disease. Am J Gastroenterol 79:450–452, 1984

Thompson WG, Heaton KW: Functional bowel disorders in apparently healthy people. Gastroenterology 79:283–288, 1980

Topolanski-Sierra R: Pelvic phlebography. Am J Obstet Gynecol 76:44–45, 1958

Turk DC, Meichenbaum D, Genest M: Pain and Behavioral Medicine: A Cognitive-Behavioral Perspective. New York, Guilford, 1983

Walker E, Katon W, Harrop-Griffiths J, et al: Relationship of chronic pelvic pain to psychiatric diagnoses and childhood sexual abuse. Am J Psychiatry 145:75–80, 1988

Walters A: Psychogenic regional pain alias hysterical pain. Brain 84:1–18, 1961

Waxler EB, Kimbiris D, Dreifus LS: The fate of women with normal coronary arteriograms and chest pain resembling angina pectoris. Am J Cardiol 28:25–32, 1971

Weintraub MI: Regional pain is usually hysterical. Arch Neurol 45:914–919, 1988

Weisenberg M: Psychological intervention for the control of pain. Behav Res Ther 25:301–312, 1987

Whitehead WE, Schuster MM: Gastrointestinal Disorders: Behavioral and Physiological Basis for Treatment. New York, Academic, 1985

Woodforde JM, Merskey H: Personality traits of patients with chronic pain. J Psychosom Res 16:167–172, 1972

Woolf CJ, Wall PD: Relative effectiveness of C primary afferent fibers of different origins in evoking a prolonged facilitation of the flexor reflex in the rat. J Neurosci 6:1433–1442, 1986

World Health Organization: Draft of the 10th Revision of the International Classification of Diseases. Geneva, World Health Organization, 1988

PART II

MECHANISMS OF BODILY COMPLAINTS

The disorders which are the subjects of the following observations have been treated of by authors, under the names of Flatulent, Spasmodic, Hypochondriac, or Hysteric. Of late, they have also got the name of NERVOUS; which appelation having been commonly given to many symptoms seemingly different, and very obscure in their nature, has often made it to be said, that physicians have bestowed the character of nervous, on all those disorders, whose nature and causes they were ignorant of. To wipe off this approach and, at the same time to throw some light on nervous, hypochondriac, and hysteric complaints, is the design of the following observations.

Robert Whytt (1768)
Observations on Nature,
Causes, and Cure of Those
Disorders Commonly Called
Nervous, Hypochondriac, or
Hysteric

Some of the mechanisms by which symptoms are induced in the absence of disease or damage to tissues are illustrated in the discussion of the etiology of the individual syndromes in the chapters in Part I. Some other mechanisms by which bodily changes are perceived and result in discomfort that, in turn, may lead to complaints brought to the attention of physicians are discussed in Part II. This entails a discussion of theories of somatization as well as empirical studies that address these theories. Part II also addresses the ways the various manifestations of somatization relate to psychiatric classification.

Chapter 10

Somatization

Somatization has become a frequent topic in the theoretical as well as in the research literature, and current textbooks of psychiatry contain separate sections or chapters on somatoform disorders. Somatization causes personal suffering and can have a detrimental effect on a person's interactions with his or her family. It also is a burden on the community and an important matter of public health. It is a common cause of absenteeism, and a large part of physicians' time and effort is spent investigating and treating somatizing patients (Kellner 1990). It has been estimated that between 10% and 20% of the medical budget is spent on patients who somatize or have hypochondriacal concerns (Ford 1983). A recent editorial described somatization as medicine's "unsolved problem" (Lipowski 1987, p. 297).

Various theories have been put forward over the years to explain somatization. One of the aims of this chapter is to summarize the main theories and some of the empirical studies that address the etiological factors in somatization.

Somatizing patients have been described throughout the history of medicine. The term *somatization* was first used by Steckel (1943), who defined it as a bodily disorder that arises as the expression of a deep-seated neurosis, especially of a "disease of the conscious" (p. 580). Steckel tended to coin new terms for existing ones, and he regarded somatization as identical to Freud's concept of conversion. In theoretical writings on somatization, the distinction among conversion disorder, psychosomatic disease, and somatization has not always been clearly made, whereas modern textbooks and diagnostic manuals do attempt to distinguish among these categories. Even in current diagnostic manuals, some of the divisions, although useful, are arbitrary. The boundaries of the construct and the difficulties in demarcating somatization from similar phenomena are discussed later in this chapter in more detail.

In DSM-III-R (American Psychiatric Association 1987) the disorders that have traditionally been labeled as somatization are classified largely in the categories of somatoform disorders, and some belong to the category of *psychological factors affecting physical conditions*. In the ICD-10 draft (World Health Organization 1988) somatization syndromes are classified among the somatoform disorders (F45), the dissociative (conversion) disorders (F44), and neurasthenia

(480), and a few are classified in the category of behavioral syndromes and medical disorders associated with physiological dysfunction (F50).

There is incomplete agreement among authors on the definition of somatization. For example, Katon et al. (1982) define it as an idiom of distress in which patients with psychosocial and emotional problems articulate their distress primarily through physical symptomatology. Kleinman and Kleinman (1986) define somatization as the expression of personal and social distress in an idiom of bodily complaints with medical helpseeking. Ford (1983, 1986) defined it as the use of somatic symptoms for psychological purposes. Bridges and Goldberg (1985) chose operational criteria for somatization that consist of consulting behavior; the patient attributes the somatic manifestations to a physical problem, but his or her condition is a psychiatric illness and responds to psychiatric treatment. Lipowski (1987) defined somatization as the experience and communication of psychological distress in the form of physical symptoms. Kellner (1986), Kirmayer (1986), and several other authors concluded that somatization is neither a discrete clinical entity nor the result of a single pathological process, and that somatization cuts across diagnostic categories.

For the purposes of the present overview I have chosen a broad definition of somatization that is in accord with one of the criteria from DSM-III-R. This definition includes part of the criteria for undifferentiated somatoform disorder and, with slight variations, for the other somatoform disorders. Somatization indicates "one or more physical complaints (e.g., fatigue, loss of appetite, gastrointestinal or urinary complaints)" and either 1) "appropriate evaluation uncovers no organic pathology or pathophysiologic mechanism (e.g., a physical disorder or the effect of injury . . .) to account for the physical complaints," or 2) "when there is related organic pathology, the physical complaints or resulting social or occupational impairment is grossly in excess of what would be expected from the physical findings" (American Psychiatric Association 1987, p. 267).

Prevalence and Duration

About 80% of healthy individuals experience somatic symptoms in any one week (Pennebaker et al. 1977; Reidenberg and Lowenthal 1968). Therefore, when the statistical concept of normality is used, bodily discomfort is the normal experience even in good physical health, and perhaps a fortunate few do not experience some somatic symptoms (see Table 10-1).

The prevalence of somatization has been examined in numerous studies by evaluating attendances to primary-care physicians. In most studies the proportion of patients with somatic complaints for which no adequate physical cause was detected ranged from 10% to 30% (Kessel 1960; Shepherd et al. 1966). In specialty clinics this proportion is usually higher (Kellner 1986, p. 17). The exclusion of substantial physical disease, however, does not necessarily mean that there is no physical cause for the symptoms. A physical cause can be difficult or

Table 10-1. **One week prevalence of somatic symptoms in two countries**

Serial number of items	Symptoms	England		New Mexico	
		Neurotic patients (%)	Employees (%)	Neurotic patients (%)	Employees (%)
1	Headache, head pains	60	32	64	48
2	Dizzy or faint	54	9	60	14
3	Stomach pains	34	22	51	20
4	Sick, nauseated	49	20	62	22
6	Muscle pains, aches, rheumatism	51	42	53	27
7	Parts of body felt weak	63	11	57	23
8	Palpitations, pounding of heart	54	8	44	7
9	Chest pains	32	9	46	14
10	Breathing difficulties, not enough air	40	10	46	13
11	Trembling, shaking	62	2	62	10
12	Tired, lack of energy	78	47	85	40
13	Pressure, tightness in head or body	54	11	58	19
14	Tense	82	22	93	35
17	Poor appetite	44	10	61	5
18	Numb, tingling sensations	34	9	36	12
19	Worry	86	29	93	43
20	Unhappy, depressed	82	24	88	25
21	Poor memory	50	21	63	17
22	Irritable	68	34	80	31
23	People looked down, thought badly of you	43	11	57	18
24	Loss of interest	70	15	78	12
26	Concentration	73	26	69	26
27	Unworthy, failure	60	12	69	16
28	Sleep	65	32	75	33
30	Anxious, frightened	74	15	65	17

Note. Selected affective symptoms are listed for the purpose of comparison. From a questionnaire study of neurotic psychiatric patients ($n = 100$) and random employees ($n = 100$) (Kellner and Sheffield 1973a).

sometimes impossible to distinguish by means of conventional diagnostic methods without investigations that may be of research interest but are not used routinely in clinical medicine. This is the case whether minor symptoms are caused by transient tissue pathology (Mayou 1976) such as gastritis or muscular sprains, by physiological overactivity, or by other mechanisms described below, or whether they are the atypical manifestation of a psychophysiological disorder (Bennett 1987; Whorwell et al. 1986) or minor conversion symptoms (Merskey 1988).

In random subjects, somatic symptoms are more prevalent than emotional ones (Kellner and Sheffield 1973a). It is estimated that over 4% of subjects in a community have multiple chronic functional somatic symptoms (Escobar et al. 1987). Most of the published studies on prevalence were carried out before the DSM-III classification (i.e., before 1980). In a recent study of DSM-III disorders in primary care, 26% of the patients presented with somatization. These findings suggest that somatization is a common presentation of distress even in western cultures (Bridges and Goldberg 1985).

Prevalence studies show that the severity as well as the incidence of somatic symptoms forms a continuum ranging from the common, mild, and transient to the chronic, extremely distressing, and incapacitating (Mayou 1976). The prevalence of somatization apparently varies with the population but depends largely on the diagnostic criteria used for the study.

Little is known about the prevalence of the individual DSM-III-R categories of somatoform disorders. The prevalence of somatization disorder (300.81) in community surveys ranges from 0.03% (Escobar et al. 1987) to 0.7% (Canino et al. 1987), with a median of 0.1% (Myren et al. 1984). In order to diagnose an undifferentiated somatoform disorder (300.70), the duration of symptoms must be 6 months or longer. The duration of most functional somatic symptoms in family practice ranges from a few weeks to a few months, and many other individuals do not seek treatment (Kellner 1963; Thomas 1978); therefore, the most prevalent DSM-III-R somatoform disorders appear to be *adjustment disorder with physical complaints* and *somatoform disorder not otherwise specified*.

Theories and Empirical Studies

Genetic Factors

Genetic factors have played only a minor role in theoretical discussions of somatization. Several studies, particularly in the past two decades, have addressed the role of genetics in somatoform disorders. A study (using the Minnesota Multiphasic Personality Inventory [MMPI]) of identical and fraternal adolescent twins suggests that the contribution of genetics to somatic symptom formation in this age group is small (Gottesman 1962). Twin studies of adult psychiatric patients do not lend themselves to definite conclusions on the extent of the genetic component in somatization (Torgersen 1986). However, results from self-rating scales administered to identical and fraternal twins from the general population suggest a genetic factor for somatic anxiety (Kendler et al. 1987).

A new understanding of the role of genetics and that of early environment in somatization comes from recent adoption studies. Certain somatoform syndromes are associated with psychopathology in the biological parent, whereas other syndromes are associated with psychopathology in the adoptive parent. For example, the biological fathers of female "high frequency somatizers" (whose chief complaint was headache, backache, and abdominal distress on different occasions) had often committed violent crimes, whereas the adoptive fathers of female "diversiform somatizers" (who had a greater diversity of complaints but less frequent disability) were more often alcohol abusers (Cloninger 1986a).

In women, there is a familial aggregation for Briquet's syndrome that is greater than that for somatization disorder (Cloninger et al. 1986). Furthermore, adoption studies also reveal a genetic factor in somatization disorder (Cadoret 1978). Thus, the evidence so far suggests that genetic factors play a substantial role in some syndromes of somatization, whereas other syndromes are determined predominantly by other factors, including environmental stresses.

Masked Depression, Depressive Equivalent, Manifestation of Depression

Numerous writers have emphasized the association of somatization, including somatoform pain disorder, with depression. Research evidence for this association has been consistent regardless of the design of the study. Depressed patients tend to have more somatic symptoms than do nondepressed individuals, and somatizing patients tend to be more depressed than patients with physical disease. Within groups, there is a consistent positive correlation between depressive and somatic symptoms (Cadoret et al. 1980; Katon et al. 1982; Kellner 1986, p. 20; Lloyd 1986). There are, however, substantial differences among individuals, and depression and somatic symptoms do not necessarily improve simultaneously (Katon et al. 1984).

Several authors have described somatization as a masked depression or a depressive equivalent. There is no conclusive evidence that somatization is a true depressive equivalent, meaning that it has the same etiology, course, and response to treatment as depression. Some depressed patients emphasize somatic symptoms for various reasons and may not reveal that they feel depressed. Functional somatic symptoms may occur after losses and stressful life events (Kellner et al. 1983). Some individuals may respond to stresses largely with somatic symptoms rather than with overt emotional ones; but in most of these patients, some affective symptoms are present. Numerous studies show that depression and somatization occur together in various proportions; in patients who complain mainly of somatic symptoms, these symptoms may mask the underlying mood disorder. This may occur more frequently with nonpsychiatric physicians who tend to focus on bodily complaints.

Manifestations of Anxiety

Numerous authors have described somatic symptoms in anxiety. Several have described general anxiety and panic disorder as important, if not the most important, causes of somatization (Kellner 1988).

As with depression, the association of anxiety and somatic symptoms is consistent (Tyrer 1976, p. 91). This finding also applies to studies in which the anxiety or depression scale had no somatic items; thus, the correlations were not spurious (Kellner et al. 1972). Somatic symptoms are invariably more numerous in patients with anxiety disorders than in healthy individuals. Correlation studies show robust positive correlations of anxiety symptoms and somatic symptoms both in patients and in healthy individuals (Kellner 1988).

Patients with panic disorder have numerous somatic symptoms, and frequently these patients present with bodily complaints to general physicians. In a study of panic disorder on a psychiatric consultation service, the most common symptoms were related to the heart (chest pain, tachycardia, and irregular heartbeat); others included gastrointestinal symptoms (especially epigastric distress) and neurological symptoms such as headache, dizziness, vertigo, syncope, and paresthesias. Misdiagnosis had continued often for months or even years (Katon 1984). Some patients may have only paroxysmal attacks of a few somatic symptoms without a conspicuous affective component (Katon et al. 1987; Rosenbaum 1987); other patients with panic disorder have occasional attacks that consist only of the somatic symptoms (Beitman et al. 1987).

The study of the relationship of somatic symptoms on the one hand and anxiety and depression on the other is complicated by the coexistence of anxiety and depression in a large proportion of patients (McNair and Fisher 1978; Von Zerssen 1986). In a correlational study with neurotic patients, somatic symptoms were somewhat more strongly associated with anxiety than with depression (Kellner et al. 1972). Based on psychophysiological research and clinical studies, certain symptoms such as anorexia and tiredness have been regarded as characteristic of depression, whereas symptoms of sympathetic adrenergic arousal such as tachycardia and sweating are characteristic of anxiety. Numerous other functional somatic symptoms (e.g., some gastrointestinal symptoms) are found in both anxious patients and depressed patients. In addition, there may be individual differences in the kind of emotion that leads to various symptoms.

Although there is a consistent positive correlation of emotional and somatic symptoms, there are substantial differences in their ratios among healthy subjects as well as among psychiatric patients. Some patients who are severely anxious or severely depressed report only few or slight somatic symptoms, while a few others who have severe somatic symptoms rate their anxiety or depression as low or virtually absent (Kellner et al. 1972).

Manifestation of Physiological Activity

Many of the symptoms of somatization or functional somatic symptoms are consequences of physiological activity that is often accentuated by stress and emotion. This relationship appears to be one of the reasons for the consistent correlation of emotional and somatic symptoms.

The research on the effects of emotion on physiological functioning is formidable (for reviews, see Black 1970; Grings and Dawson 1978; Lader 1975). By the middle of the 1950s there were already 1,200 publications on the electrical resistance of the skin in response to stress alone (Nimii 1956). Several physiological processes play a role in somatization, and the common ones are summarized below.

Smooth-muscle contraction. Some of the important and most common components of somatization are symptoms caused by smooth-muscle contraction. For example, motility disorders of the esophagus may cause symptoms. Abnormal intestinal motility may cause non-ulcer dyspepsia, and excessive contractions of the sphincter of Oddi may cause right upper-quadrant abdominal pain (Toouli 1984). In addition, generalized colicky abdominal pain may be caused by contractions of the colon in the diarrhea-predominant type of irritable bowel syndrome or by pressure changes in the small intestine (Holdstock et al. 1969). Several of the studies that demonstrate these effects have been listed in the previous chapters.

Striated-muscle contraction. Contraction of voluntary muscle is another common source of physiological activity that gives rise to somatic symptoms. Some of the studies pertaining to these symptoms are summarized below.

There is increased activity of striated muscle during emotion. During experimental stress, neurotic patients have higher electromyographic levels than do nonneurotic individuals (Bartoshuk 1959). Patients with anxiety neurosis show an increase in electromyographic activity that is larger, and a return to baseline levels that is slower, than that of control subjects (Malmo et al. 1950). In a few muscles, a resting difference can be detected between anxious patients and control subjects, and the number of muscles in which such a difference can be detected increases during experimental stress (Goldstein 1964). Resting electromyographic levels are higher in dysthymic (anxious and depressed) patients than in hysterical patients or in control subjects; in one study, during an interview the electromyographic levels were significantly higher in the neurotic patients than in the control subjects (Martin 1956). During psychotherapy, electromyographic activity was found to be greater in forearm muscles during hostility themes and in leg muscles during sexual themes (Shagass and Malmo 1954).

Electromyographic potentials are larger in neck muscles during experimental stress in patients who complain of headaches than in other psychiatric patients (Malmo and Shagass 1949). Muscle tension is increased in parts of the body that are aching or painful compared with other parts of the body (Sainsbury and

Gibson 1954). Electromyographic activity of the temporalis muscle is significantly higher in patients with muscle-contraction headaches than in healthy
control subjects; there are no significant differences, however, in the electromyographic activity of patients who have a headache at the time of measurements and of those who do not (Fujii et al. 1981), and some headache patients
have lower tension than do control subjects. Patients with headaches or neck
pain develop greater electromyographic activity during experimental pain inflicted on the forearm than do other patients (Malmo et al. 1953). Some patients
with lower back discomfort have elevated electromyographic levels in
paravertebral muscles (Dolce and Raczynski 1985), particularly when these patients are emotionally stressed (Flor et al. 1985; Malmo et al. 1950).

Changes in blood flow and endocrine secretion. There are several
well-known syndromes in which the main features are changes in blood flow.
In some of these, there is an associated tissue pathology, such as in transient
ischemic attacks or in many of the cases of coronary artery spasm in variant
(Prinzmetal's) angina. In other cases, there is an instability of blood flow regulation in the absence of tissue damage. The most common of this kind is the
vascular spasm followed by dilation in migraine headaches. Other examples are
cold sensitivity of the Raynaud type, acrocyanosis, and erythromelalgia. One
study has suggested that the pain in nutcracker esophagus is also caused by
impaired blood flow (see Chapter 4, p. 77, this volume).

Studies in psychophysiology show profound endocrine changes in response
to emotions, particularly to fear and anger. These changes involve predominantly the adrenergic and corticosteroid systems. Changes in the former accen-
tuate the effects of sympathetic autonomic arousal, causing peripheral physiological changes. These changes include rise in blood pressure, increased heart
rate and stroke volume, redistribution of blood from the viscera and skin to
striated muscle, and increased respiration rate. It is likely that some somatic
symptoms that appear to be functional on a routine physical examination are
caused by changes in blood flow or other changes that occur during arousal and
are mediated by the endocrine and autonomic nervous system.

Psychophysiological disorders that become aggravated by stress are important causes of somatization. These issues are discussed in further detail below in
the section on diagnosis.

Emotions can also lead to changes in behavior that can cause physiological
changes that, in turn, may lead to somatic symptoms. Some of these behaviors
are described in Chapter 8 (this volume).

The relationship of physiological arousal to symptoms. Adaptation
processes in the central nervous system, such as those producing augmentation
or reduction, influence the degree of physiological changes (Grings and Dawson 1978) as well as the frequency of reported somatic symptoms (Petrie 1967).
There is an association between arousal, the perception of such arousal, and the
experience of somatic sensations (Mandler et al. 1958).

Individuals have a characteristic pattern of physiological responses to stress (Anderson 1981). In some individuals the response remains similar regardless of the kind of stressor used (Lacey and Lacey 1958; Lacey et al. 1953). The idiosyncrasy of physiological responses probably explains in part the differences among individuals in the kind of recurring functional somatic symptoms that are exhibited.

In patients who are morbidly anxious or complain primarily of somatic symptoms (who perhaps have greater physiological changes), the symptoms correlate highly with physiological changes, whereas in healthy subjects (Katkin et al. 1981) and morbidly anxious ones who have predominantly psychological symptoms, bodily feelings correlate poorly with physiological changes (Tyrer 1976, p. 90). In this latter group, either 1) the symptoms are caused by some other mechanisms, or 2) the sensitivity of standard physiological measures is inadequate to detect subtle physiological changes that induce these symptoms.

The evidence across studies is consistent and points to the conclusion that, in some patients, somatization is the consequence of physiological activity that tends to be idiosyncratic, and that physiologic activity tends to become greater and somatization more severe at times of stress. These patients, who may be severely distressed, do not necessarily use bodily metaphors, and some may not "express distress in the only language they have learned" (Kreitman et al. 1965, p. 613). Although they may have various motives for reporting symptoms, they may be accurate in describing bodily sensations that are percepts of physiological activity.

William James (1884) complained in the previous century about attitudes in medical research:

> Many people nowadays seem to think that any conclusion must be very scientific if the arguments in favor of it are derived from the twitching of frogs' legs—especially if the frogs are decapitated—and that on the other hand any doctrine chiefly vouched for by the feeling of human beings—with heads on their shoulders—must be benighted and superstitious.

The present volume has dealt largely with human psychology and physiology, and I have tried to avoid views that are derived entirely from observations on decapitated amphibians. Many of the conclusions on psychosomatics presented here are, however, based on laboratory studies. Chaudhary and Truelove (1961), commenting on their study of the effects of emotionally charged topics on colonic motor activity, wrote that the motor response observed in the laboratory may be "only a pale and incomplete reflection of what actually occurs under conditions of genuine stress" (p. 35). The findings from most laboratory studies are probably only approximations of the physiological changes that occur at times of emotional turmoil that some people endure. Thus, the exact nature and degree of many physiological changes remain usually undetected, and because physiological responses differ widely among individuals (Lacey and Lacey 1958), in some cases, these changes may be extreme.

Learning

Several theories have been put forward to describe somatization as learned abnormal perceptions or as a cognitive style. There is a large body of research that supports the view that learning plays a substantial part in bodily sensations. Various experiences in childhood may act as predisposing factors, while events in adult life can contribute to the precipitation of symptoms as well as to their maintenance (Kellner 1985).

Children's symptoms are often a copy of symptoms occurring in other members of the family (Apley et al. 1978). There are several retrospective studies that suggest that adult somatization and hypochondriacal attention to bodily sensations are associated with parental interest and attention to symptoms in the patient's childhood; however, the extent to which reports are distorted by errors in recall or other factors is not known. Subjects with the irritable bowel syndrome recalled more attention and treats in childhood when ill than did other people, including patients with peptic ulcer (Whitehead et al. 1982). (See Chapter 6, pp. 122–123] for results from other studies that suggest learning in the irritable bowel syndrome.) It has been suggested, based on a prospective study, that generalized distress in adults is, in part, learned illness behavior, but the study did not confirm that maternal attitudes toward a child's illness were crucial factors (Mechanic 1979).

Adoptive studies suggest that certain stresses in early home environment—for example, an alcoholic adoptive (not biological) father—are associated with somatization in adult life (Bohman et al. 1984). Certain kinds of trauma seem to be particularly pernicious. Pelvic pain and abdominal functional symptoms are more common in women who have been sexually abused in childhood (see Chapter 9, pp. 168–169). Abuse in childhood is also associated with anxiety and depression (Kellner and Schneider-Braus 1988). Furthermore, socioeconomic class, education (Kirmayer 1984b; Srole et al. 1962), culture, and subculture influence the rate by which emotional distress is expressed as somatic complaints (Escobar et al. 1987; Kirmayer 1984a; Koss 1990) and may condition certain kinds of physiological arousal (Averill et al. 1969; Lazarus et al. 1966).

There is evidence that selective perception will affect bodily sensations. For example, the kind of instructions to the subject before an experiment will influence whether a bodily sensation is perceived by the patient or not (Pennebaker 1983; Pennebaker and Skelton 1978). Flu symptoms are more likely to be reported if the subjects are reminded that there is a flu epidemic (Pennebaker 1982). Perceptions of diverse physiological changes are positively correlated, and there appears to be a generalized tendency to be aware of, or to attend to, visceral events (Whitehead and Dresher 1980). With training, experimental subjects can learn to improve the perception of sensations from within their body (Adám 1967). It also seems likely that habitual attention to one part of one's body will improve a person's skill in perceiving sensations. The above mechanisms tend to produce an amplification of symptoms (Barsky 1979; Barsky et al. 1988), whereas in other individuals, suppression of bodily percepts is likely to cause minimization or denial of bodily sensation (Mayou 1976; Pilowsky 1969). Thus, the symptoms are caused by percepts, they are not imagined, and numerous processes influence their magnitude. Some other effects of learning are discussed in the next section.

Hypochondriasis

Several authors have advanced the view that somatization is a manifestation of disease phobia. Others view somatization as motivated by a false belief of having a disease, or that hypochondriasis and somatization are merely different manifestations of the same phenomenon. There are, in turn, numerous theories that try to explain the phenomenon of hypochondriasis (Barsky and Klerman 1983; Kellner 1986, p. 10; Kenyon 1965; Starcevic 1989). The DSM-III-R and the ICD-10 draft both distinguish between hypochondriasis and other somatoform disorders.

In published studies there is a consistent association of somatic symptoms on the one hand and fear of disease and conviction of having a disease on the other (Burns and Nichols 1972; Stenbäck and Jalava 1962). About one third of patients with functional somatic symptoms have hypochondriacal concerns (Kellner 1986; Kirmayer and Robbins 1990; Mechanic 1972), whereas severely hypochondriacal patients form a small minority (Mayou 1976). There are various ways in which hypochondriacal concerns and somatic symptoms can interact. Hypochondriacal patients are more likely than other patients to experience somatic symptoms they have heard or read about (Kellner et al. 1987), a phenomenon that is also more common in medical students (Kellner et al. 1986). Hypochondriacal patients are more accurate than other patients in perceiving physiological changes (Tyrer 1976). Also, bodily changes are more likely to be perceived if they constitute a threat (Jones et al. 1981; Mechanic 1972).

Persistent distressing somatic symptoms tend to induce fear of disease or belief of having a disease; for example, peptic ulcer pain can induce the false belief of having another, more serious disease (Stenbäck 1960). False beliefs of having a serious disease can also occur with chest pain (Burns and Nichols 1972) and chronic pelvic pain (see Chapter 9, p. 167). In patients who have chronic pain, other cognitive distortions also occur (Le Febvre 1981). Conversely, patients who fear disease or are convinced they have a disease may let bodily sensations become the focus of their attention; these sensations may be diffuse, as in AIDS phobia, or they may be focused in one area of the body, such as in cardiophobia (Conti et al. 1989). One of the mechanisms in the maintenance of somatic symptoms, as well as in a common hypochondriacal reaction, is the experience of new somatic symptoms at times of anxiety or depression. This is followed by selective perception of bodily sensations, motivated by fear of disease, and results in a subsequent increase in anxiety with more somatic symptoms. These elements appear to be linked in a vicious cycle, and with frequent repetition become overlearned; thus, the chain becomes predictable (Kellner 1985). A similar sequence occurs in many patients during periods of panic (Clark 1986).

Patients who have hypochondriacal concerns seek medical care more frequently than others (Pilowsky et al. 1987). They may need this interaction with physicians for various reasons. There are, however, many somatizing patients, particularly those who have had long-standing or recurring symptoms, who have gained adequate insight. They understand that the symptoms indicate neither a threat to life nor evidence of disease, and yet the symptoms persist (Kellner and Schneider-Braus 1988). In these patients, hypochondriacal fears or beliefs do not appear to be essential in maintaining somatization. The contribution of hypochondriacal concerns to the enhancement of symptoms varies from one individual to another and also varies with the passage of time in the same individual. The attitudes toward symptoms need to be explored in each patient before the extent of the contribution of hypochondriacal fears to the reinforcement and perpetuation of symptoms can be assessed (Barsky and Klerman 1983).

Hypochondriacal patients tend to be more concerned than other individuals about their own appearance (Barsky and Wyshak 1989). Body dysmorphic disorder (dysmorphophobia) often occurs in the absence of hypochondriasis and is one of the motives for seeking medical treatment. Patients with this disorder do not fear disease or believe that they have a disease, but they are convinced that a part of their body is conspicuously deformed or ugly. There have been reports of successful psychological treatment of this disorder (Marks and Mishan 1988) and isolated reports of effective treatment with serotonin reuptake inhibitors (Hollander et al. 1989).

Low Pain Threshold

A lower pain threshold has been found in several groups of people with bodily complaints. Patients with fibromyalgia have a low pain threshold, not only at tender points but at other parts of the muscle as well (see Chapter 1, pp. 10–11). Some of the patients with esophageal chest pain are more sensitive to distension of the esophagus than those patients without pain (Barish et al. 1986; Edwards 1982; Richter et al. 1986). Patients with the "tender heart syndrome" experience pain during catheterization of coronary arteries (Cannon et al. 1985). Conversely, patients with silent myocardial ischemia tend to have a high pain threshold (Droste and Roskamm 1983; Glazier et al. 1986). Patients with the irritable bowel syndrome have a lower pain threshold to distension, and their bowel reacts more when distended, yet they do not have a low pain threshold to cutaneous pain (see Chapter 6, p. 116).

Severely hypochondriacal patients (Merskey and Spear 1967) and patients with disease phobia (Bianchi 1971) have low pain thresholds, and these two diagnostic groups are strongly associated with somatization. In subjects who have an abnormally low threshold for sensations, even slight changes in physiological activity, such as an increase in striated-muscle tension or physiological distension of the viscera, could give rise to distressing percepts.

Hostility

Hostility, particularly repressed hostility, and anger have been described by several authors as crucial factors in somatization. There are several empirical studies that link somatic symptoms to hostility. In one clinical study, depressed women who appeared to hold in their anger were judged to be more prone to somatic symptoms than those who were not angry or who expressed anger (Harris 1951). In another study, more patients in a pain clinic affirmed that they bottle up anger than did patients with chronic pain from other clinics (Pilowsky and Spence 1976). In a study of several populations, somatic symptoms were positively correlated with self-rated anger-hostility scales and negatively correlated with feelings of friendliness. Somatic symptoms, however, tended to be associated more strongly with symptoms of anxiety and depression than with those of hostility (Kellner et al. 1985).

Hostile subjects show greater change in blood pressure and skin conductance than do nonhostile subjects (Hokanson 1961), and hostility has substantial cardiovascular effects in some people (Grings and Dawson 1978). Subjects who supress hostility tend to have higher systolic blood pressure than do other subjects (Williams et al. 1985). Therefore, the physiological concomitants of hostility could be pathways by which anger produces somatic symptoms.

The studies that are available do not support the view that anger and hostility are the main or specific etiological factors in somatization, nor that these factors are the most common ones. There are various possible causes for the association of anger with somatic symptoms. Anger and hostility cause arousal with physiological overactivity and are concomitants of certain kinds of depression (Fava et al. 1982; Overall et al. 1966; Weissman et al. 1971). In one of our recent studies (R. Kellner et al., manuscript in preparation), in a stepwise regression, a question pertaining to inhibited anger predicted self-rated depression but not somatization. Nonpsychotic psychiatric patients have higher self-ratings of anger and hostility than do nonpatient control subjects, so hostility may be the consequence of any chronic distress, including distressing somatic symptoms. While anxiety and depression appear to be more common causes of somatization, anger (and particularly restrained anger) probably plays a major part in a few patients.

Gain and Social Reinforcement

Several authors have expressed views to the effect that somatization is a search for aid, an attention-seeking device, an expression of the wish to assume the sick role, an attempt to manipulate others, or a condition that is maintained and reinforced by gain.

Patients who receive sickness benefits, pensions, or other disability compensation remain disabled longer than those who have no such insurance, even with diseases of similar severity (Better et al. 1979). These findings suggest that disability insurance reduces the incentive to return to the stresses of full-time employment; in some, it acts perhaps as a reinforcer of somatic symptoms, particularly in distressed people with few psychological reserves on which to draw.

In several uncontrolled studies, somatization has been reported in patients involved in compensation proceedings, particularly after accidents (Miller 1961). The anticipation of a financial settlement influences the description of pain caused by physical disease or injury (Leavitt et al. 1982). In a study of neurotic patients, secondary gain appeared to be more common in patients with psychalgia than in other patients (Bishop and Torch 1979). There is inconsistent evidence that litigation increases the reports of severity of pain. There is no evidence to date that it induces, or aggravates, somatization (Leavitt et al. 1982; Pelz and Merskey 1982), that it prolongs the duration of symptoms (Barnat 1985), or that a legal settlement and a favorable verdict lead to recovery in the majority of patients with accident neurosis (Mendelson 1981; Merskey 1984). Gain appears to be a more common etiological factor in conversion disorder than in other somatoform disorders (see Chapter 11).

There are several clinical reports which suggest that in many somatizing and hypochondriacal patients, iatrogenic reinforcement plays a part. For example, patients with functional somatic symptoms reported more ominous and frightening diagnoses from their physicians than patients with similar symptoms who had a physical disease (Burns and Nichols 1972). Uncontrolled studies suggest that many chronic somatizing patients, as well as hypochondriacal patients, had multiple diagnoses from previous physicians and were treated for functional somatic symptoms as though they had had a physical disease. Diagnoses that are understood as threatening apparently can have a suggestive effect when made by a trusted physician.

There are several uncontrolled studies which suggest that other kinds of reinforcements may play a role. For example, in a study of family therapy of patients with chronic pain, the therapist recommended to the family member to withhold reinforcement of pain complaints, which resulted in a subsequent decrease of such complaints and an increase in activity (Hudgens 1979). Loneliness (Katon et al. 1982), reinforcement by family, or interest shown by family members or by a physician probably all contribute to the tendency to attend to bodily sensations or to seek help from physicians, or both. Motivated by gain, a patient may exaggerate the report of the severity of his or her distress, including distress caused by symptoms of physical disease.

Most somatizing patients, however, appear to suffer because of their symptoms rather than to profit from them. Freud's view that hysterical conversions were in part an expression of a wish fulfillment (Freud 1908/1959) has had a pervasive influence on views of somatization in general. There are many convincing published clinical examples of the mechanisms described at the beginning of this section, and it is likely that in some patients such processes do play a crucial role. Reinforcement has such profound effects on behavior that it seems most likely that it also influences somatization. Hypochondriacal fears and beliefs are probably powerful internal reinforcers. It is, however, difficult to design clinical studies that demonstrate the effects of gain; and for most of the views on the role of gain in somatization, there is in fact no conclusive evidence available.

Inhibition, Repression, and Lack of Confiding

Several authors have suggested that denial of, repression of, and lack of confiding about distressing events and emotions are associated with somatization. There is evidence that these mechanisms are linked in various ways to physiological responses, to the report of somatic symptoms, and to illness (Pennebaker 1985, 1989).

A few clinical studies which suggest that repressed anger is associated with somatic symptoms are listed above in the section on hostility. Defensiveness, as measured by the Marlowe-Crowne Scale, is associated with physiological arousal (Weinberger et al. 1979). There is evidence to suggest that repression of threats is associated with increased autonomic arousal. For example, subjects who are repressors as measured by a repression-sensitization scale (Byrne 1964) show greater physiological reactivity than do nonrepressors (Hare 1966; Parsons et al. 1969); this scale, however, may largely measure anxiety or other negative affectivity (Watson and Clark 1984). Suppression of facial expressive responses (which is a concealment of emotion) is generally associated with autonomic arousal, but some of the results have been conflicting (Lanzetta et al. 1976; Notarius and Levenson 1979; Pennebaker 1985). There is also a tendency for the self-rating of the severity of a psychological and of a physical stressor to be negatively correlated with physiological responsiveness in patients as well as in healthy subjects (Anderson 1981).

Some of the findings on repression have been inconsistent. For example, in one study, sensitizers (nonrepressors), as determined by a repression-sensitization scale, reported a greater frequency and severity of illness, and male sensitizers sought medical help more frequently than repressors (Byrne et al. 1968). The reasons for these apparently conflicting findings are unknown; repressors perhaps forget their symptoms and their illnesses more often than sensitizers, and thus may experience symptoms and illness and not report them. Some individuals appear to be highly successful in repressing distressing emotions without ill effects (Pennebaker 1985). A survey of studies suggests that an inhibition of emotion and the lack of confiding may cause physiological arousal, somatic symptoms, and physical disease (Pennebaker 1985, 1989). The findings that are inconclusive or difficult to explain stem usually from studies with self-rating scales of repression; experimental and clinical studies in which the people who confided were compared with those who did not do so have yielded more uniform results.

Confiding about a major traumatic event is associated with fewer symptoms and illness episodes. Among individuals whose spouses died unexpectedly by suicide or automobile accident, the more the survivors had talked with others about the spouse's death, the healthier they reported being (Pennebaker and O'Heeron 1984). Any type of trauma in childhood that was not discussed with others has been correlated with illness in adult life ranging from hypertension and cancer to bouts of influenza and diarrhea (Pennebaker and Susman 1988). Volunteers who were instructed to reveal traumatic events to a tape recorder or were instructed to write repeatedly about these events had significantly fewer visits to physicians than did control subjects on follow-up, particularly among those whose blood pressure had increased during disclosure (which indicates that their disclosure was accompanied by physiological arousal). In another study with a similar design, self-disclosure resulted in improved immune competency. In these studies, the extent of disclosure as assessed by raters, as well as autonomic disturbance during disclosure, positively correlated with improved health indices on follow-up (Pennebaker 1989).

The opportunity for self-disclosure may be one of the ways intimate relationships accomplish their protective effect (Derlega 1984). Inhibition of emotion—and perhaps suppression or repression—and lack of confiding can apparently cause various disturbances including bodily complaints. The studies that show the benefits of confession and confiding appear to have profound implications well beyond the phenomena of somatization.

Communication, Defense, and Conflict Resolution

These theories have been put forward by numerous authors. Steckel (1943), in his original description of somatization, expressed the view that the body was translating into physiological language the mental troubles of the individual. Somatization was seen as a method of communication, often of symbolic significance; that is, an "organ speech of the mind." The disorder was thought to occur in "areas of predilection" that could lead to an organ neurosis (p. 580).

Somatization has also been explained as a defense mechanism—that is, a method of denial, displacement, or rationalization (e.g., the patient blames his failings on his bodily symptoms)—or an attempt at conflict resolution (e.g., the patient becomes preoccupied with bodily sensations instead of dealing with an intolerable conflict).

There are numerous published case histories in which patients who were apparently preoccupied with somatic symptoms were unwilling or incapable of dealing with crucial conflicts. Other case histories suggest that defense mechanisms play an important role (Ford 1983). Conflict resolution was judged to be one of the common features in conversion reactions (Raskin et al. 1966). There can be little doubt that some individuals use bodily metaphors as a method of communication and as an expression of distress (Kirmayer 1984b; Koss 1990; Mechanic 1972). The case reports and clinical experience are convincing, and numerous patients that one sees in clinical practice fit these descriptions. There are also clinical reports of patients who were hypochondriacal and in whom, once they ceased to believe that they had a serious disease, numerous other psychiatric problems were revealed (Kellner 1982); this suggests that either hypochondriacal preoccupations serve as a defense, or that patients attend to their other painful problems after the distressing fears of having a serious disease have receded.

There are only a few empirical studies that have addressed these issues, and the results are inconclusive. For example, in an experiment that included an evaluation of performance, students who scored higher on the MMPI hypochondriasis (Hs) scale apparently used reports of poor health as an excuse for poor performance or as a "self-handicapping strategy" (Smith et al. 1983). Other experiments using different methodologies failed to find evidence that subjects reported symptoms for "ego-preserving reasons" (Pennebaker et al. 1977).

The paucity of studies may be a reflection of 1) the complexity of these concepts and 2) the difficulties of testing them empirically. This does not preclude, of course, the possibility that these mechanisms play a substantial role, at least in some individuals. It appears, however, that some of the consistent concomitants of somatization that have been summarized in previous sections, such as depression, anxiety, and selective perception of physiological activity, are more common etiological factors in somatization than the processes listed here.

Alexithymia

The term *alexithymia* was coined by Sifneos (1973) and means literally "no words for mood." Nemiah and Sifneos (1970a, 1970b) observed that this was a characteristic of patients with psychosomatic disorders. Alexithymic patients have difficulties in expressing emotions in words, and they do not have fantasies expressive of feelings; their thought content is dominated by details of events in their environment (Nemiah 1977). Alexithymic subjects also show a deficit in nonverbal expression of emotion (McDonald and Prkachin 1990). There are several published reviews on this concept (Lesser 1981; Taylor 1984; Taylor and Bagby 1988).

Several empirical studies have examined alexithymia in psychosomatic disorders and somatizing patients. Patients with chronic pain report less cognitive anxiety than nonpatients (DeGood et al. 1985). Alexithymia was found to be more common in hypertensive patients and patients with ulcerative colitis than in other medical patients (Fava and Pavan 1976/1977; Fava et al. 1980; Smith 1983). In other studies, the trait was no more common in patients with psychosomatic diseases than in other patients, and no more common in patients at a psychosomatic clinic than in psychiatric patients (Lesser et al. 1979).

Other studies suggest that patients with commissurotomies have alexithymic characteristics (TenHouten et al. 1986), and these characteristics are also found in patients with other neurological deficits (Weintraub and Mesulam 1983). However, these findings may have no relevance for alexithymic individuals who have no brain damage.

Taylor and Bagby (1988) have reviewed the empirical studies and methods of measurements in alexithymia. They found that the various measures of alexithymia used in empirical studies show little or no relationship to each other. Also, Lesser and Lesser (1983) concluded that many of the views on alexithymia lack empirical support.

Alexithymia is a continuous variable, not a categorical one (Fava and Pavan 1976/1977; Taylor and Bagby 1988). Freyberger (1977) has suggested that apart from being a trait, alexithymia may also occur as a temporary state secondary to bodily distress. In other words, in a medical setting, it may be a reflection of bodily distress, including that caused by physical disease, rather than a predisposing trait. The manifestations depend to a large extent on culture and subculture (Kirmayer 1986, 1987), and, in some studies, it is more common in the lower socioeconomic groups (Smith 1983).

Somatization is associated with certain personality traits such as neuroticism, but little is known about the relationship of alexithymia to these traits. The research on repression and denial may be relevant to the concept of alexithymia because alexithymic patients appear to repress emotions; there are, however, no adequate studies to date that examine the relationship of repression and alexithymia.

Several studies suggest that alexithymia is a valid construct. It is a behavior that probably has various roots. In some patients alexithymia appears to be the manifestation of a state; for example, at times of severe headache, a patient will complain to the physician about his or her physical distress and will refrain from psychic introspection. In other patients it appears to be predominantly a cognitive style, and people with this trait would be more likely to attend to somatic distress rather than psychological events. Alexithymia appears to be one of the several processes that are involved in the ways people interpret and orient to bodily sensations, which, in turn, define the magnitude and meaning of these sensations for the individual (Lesser 1981; Taylor 1984). In some patients, alexithymia is perhaps a manifestation of repression or denial, or it reflects their inability to become aware of their emotions. It awaits further research to determine the boundaries of this trait or cluster of traits and also to examine which are its material components, what are the roles of these components in somatization (as opposed to voicing somatic complaints to physicians), and whether these components predominantly reflect the behavior of somatizers or are etiological factors.

Somatization and Physical Disease

Physical disease and somatization are linked in several ways, as summarized below. The distinction often causes problems in diagnosis and classification, because the two phenomena interact with each other.

1. The first link is an event dreaded by physicians; an undetected physical disease causes symptoms, and these are then misdiagnosed as functional. This can happen in spite of the utmost care, although the opposite error—prolonged, costly, excessive, and, for the patient, worrying investigations—is probably far more common.
2. There is a vague demarcation between physiological changes that cause tolerable sensations and those that cause distressing symptoms. In some disorders, according to Lennard-Jones (1983, p. 431), "there is no dividing line between health and disease, only between those who shrug off their symptoms, seeking little or no medical help, and those whose lives are affected . . . "
3. Some symptoms are labeled functional because of inadequate knowledge and may be caused by an unknown pathological process. For example, in Chapter 9 on chronic pain, some pathological changes are listed that at one time were unexplained and the complaint was regarded as functional. The fibromyalgia syndrome was regarded in the past to be caused by inflammation and later as funtional or psychogenic. (The current views are summarized in Chapter 1.) In other disorders such as the chronic fatigue syndrome, the extent to which the symptoms are caused by organic pathology is often unknown.
4. Even when the etiology is known, there may be uncertainty as to whether the symptom is caused by a physiological or a pathological process. A symptom or a physiological response may be the final common path with various possible causes. A simple example is the shedding of tears; this may be caused by infections, allergies, injuries, tumors, anatomical abnormalities such as a blocked nasolacrimal duct, grief, laughter, other emo-

tions such as gratitude. In psychosomatic disorder, the causation is far more complex, with several etiological factors interacting and summating.

5. Sometimes a psychophysiological process causes tissue pathology, for example, in acute gastric erosions; some types of dyspepsia with and without erosions appear to be on a continuum (see Chapter 5, this volume). Psychosocial stress may decrease immune competence and may increase vulnerability to infection (see Chapter 2). There is a robust association of psychosocial stress and death rates (House et al. 1988). Thus, psychosocial stress may predispose to organic disease as well as induce somatization.

6. Physical disease is one of the predisposing factors for somatization and hypochondriasis (Kreitman et al. 1965). Either the experience of physical disease makes people more aware of bodily sensations, or they become more concerned about the possibility of disease, or both.

7. Physical disease, somatization, and hypochondriacal concerns often coexist (Schwab 1979; Schwab and Kuhn 1986; Stenbäck 1960). The processes of somatization may occur independently of the physical disease, or the patient may focus on the symptoms caused by the disease; particularly if he or she fears the outcome, the symptoms may become a focus of introspection and preoccupation.

8. There is a tendency for patients who are psychologically vulnerable to overreport symptoms of illness. Cluff et al. (1966) reviewed MMPI and California Medical Index (CMI) scores of subjects who were evaluated prior to an influenza epidemic. Subjects with scores suggesting neurotic vulnerability were more likely to report infections than others. Thus, there appeared to be an interaction of physical causes with a psychological predisposition. In the same study, the authors found that significantly more patients with psychological tests indicating depression had a delayed recovery from influenza. This could mean that 1) those patients suffered more distress from bodily sensations, 2) that they amplified symptoms (Barsky 1979), or 3) that their psychological predisposition caused a more virulent infection (Totman et al. 1980).

Because of the availability of specific treatments and the physician's obligation to know as much as possible about the patient's illness, he or she needs to differentiate between symptoms caused by a physiological or psychological process on the one hand and those caused by organ pathology on the other. In many instances, these processes and states coexist, and the physician must weigh the extent of the effect of each.

Clustering of Syndromes and Seeking Care

In patients with psychosomatic disorders, there is a tendency for clustering of syndromes. A person with a psychosomatic syndrome is at risk of acquiring another one; for example, patients with fibromyalgia are more likely than other patients to have also the irritable bowel syndrome and chronic fatigue, and patients with the irritable bowel syndrome are more prone than others to have noncolonic functional syndromes. Because there is also a positive correlation between psychic or cognitive symptoms of anxiety and depression and the number and severity of somatic symptoms, clustering appears to be, in part, a function of the severity of the emotional disturbance. In part, clustering seems to be caused by a person's tendency to react to stress with physiological changes in various systems or somatization, or both. In some patients, the functional symptoms of somatizers can be explained by clustering of psychosomatic syndromes.[1]

In several of the disorders described in previous chapters—for example, in the irritable bowel syndrome—clustering, neurotic symptoms, and abnormal personality traits were predominantly associated with patient status. The term patient status has been used by several authors to describe a self-selected group of people who sought treatment (as opposed to individuals with the same disorder who did not seek medical care). Only a part of symptoms, however, are associated with patient status; functional somatic symptoms are also extremely common in people who do not seek medical care, and there is also a robust correlation of these symptoms with anxiety and depression in people who do not seek treatment.

There are several reasons for some somatizing individuals to repeatedly seek medical care. One reason could be merely the severity of functional symptoms; those individuals with the most severe symptoms seek treatment. When evaluated by a psychiatrist, a substantial proportion of somatizing patients attending clinics are diagnosed as having psychiatric disorders such as depression, anxiety disorders, and personality disorders (Kellner 1985; Lloyd 1986). Because of the vulnerability of these patients, everyday events may be ordeals. They react with stronger emotions to stressful events, which causes more physiological arousal, which, in turn, induces somatic symptoms. Chronic and distressing somatic symptoms are in themselves stressors; they may interfere with work and leisure and may have devastating psychological consequences. In a cross-sectional study, it is difficult or impossible to tease out the extent to which psychological distress (such as depression or irritability) is a cause or a consequence of bodily symptoms, and the extent to which the two reinforce each other. Concern, worry, and depression in turn lend themselves to selective perception of bodily sensations, to amplification (Barsky 1979; Barsky et al. 1988), and to hy-

---

[1]

In a recent study, Kirmayer and Robbins found that the pattern of symptom reporting of somatizers was better characterized by several functional syndromes than by a single somatization disorder (L. Kirmayer, personal communication, 1990).

pochondriacal reactions (see above, pp. 199–200). The anxious, the depressed, and those with personality disorders tend to be less capable of coping with any kind of stress or frustration and thus tend to be dependent on the help of others, including their physicians.

Abnormal Illness Behavior, Personality, and Chronic Somatization

Mechanic (1962) defined *illness behavior* as the way in which a person perceives and evaluates symptoms and the various courses of action he or she may take. Pilowsky (1969) introduced the concept of *abnormal illness behavior* to describe unusual or pathological ways in which a person responds to symptoms or illness. The term subsumes a variety of syndromes and includes both illness-affirming behaviors (such as hypochondriasis, conversion disorder, and factitious disorders) and illness-denying behaviors (such as deliberate denial of illness in order to obtain employment, or denial and noncompliance with treatment of dangerous disease).

Several authors have discussed this concept during the last two decades, including Pilowsky (1986), who redefined abnormal illness behavior with an emphasis on the maladaptive nature of the responses and the persistence of these responses after clarification and discussion with a physician. Blackwell and Gutman (1986) characterized the *chronic illness behavior syndrome,* wherein individuals display to varying degrees the following features: disability disproportionate to detectable disease, search for disease validation, appeal to physician responsibility, attitudes of personal vulnerability and entitlement, avoidance of healthy roles for various reasons, adoption of the sick role because of environmental rewards, and interpersonal behaviors to sustain the sick role.

Mayou (1989, p. 311) has argued that "problems result from . . . a tendency to view illness behavior in a very restrictive manner, covering no more than an unusual rate of consultation and use of medical services." He further argues that the many components of illness behavior require a separate and precise definition and study, and that it would be better to follow the somatoform section of DSM-III-R (as well as the draft of the ICD-10) that defines categories by specific behavioral criteria without referring to illness behavior.

The present volume has been organized in anticipation of and in agreement with Mayou's recommendations. I have tried to examine the various behaviors separately, to use the classification of diagnostic manuals, and to avoid the broad category of abnormal illness behavior. Patients with severe and chronic somatoform disorders do display, however, many of the features enumerated by Pilowsky and Blackwell and Gutman, and the precise diagnostic category is often difficult to assign because more than one diagnosis on Axis I is often appropriate. The personality of somatizing individuals and the chronicity of symptoms are separate constructs, yet they affect each other. The numerous ways in which personality and chronic distress interact, which leads to the presentation of bodily complaints, have been discussed in the previous section.

Some personality traits are associated with a high prevalence of somatic symptoms (Pennebaker 1982); for example, neuroticism (Kellner and Sheffield 1973b) and the trait of novelty seeking (Cloninger 1986b). Clinical studies also suggest that a multitude of personality types exist in somatizing as well as in hypochondriacal patients (Katzenelbogen 1942). Another trait that appears to induce frequent requests for treatment is an unrealistic expectation of freedom from all discomfort and the belief that all ailments and symptoms, no matter how slight, should have the benefit of a physician's advice and care. Furthermore, studies summarized in previous sections have revealed differences among individuals in their physiological responsiveness, their ability to perceive sensation, their tendency to report symptoms, and their tendency to seek medical care. Some of the differences among individuals remain hidden in cross-sectional research; for example, the evaluation of threats and responses to different stressors is idiosyncratic, and some of these differences can be revealed only by subsequent comparisons within each individual (Opton and Lazarus 1967).

The causes for chronicity are also complex, and an attempt to disentangle the contribution of individual etiological factors in chronic patients becomes even more difficult than in disorders of shorter duration, because, usually, several factors combine to produce a chronic outcome. Chronic distress in itself, from any cause, can lead to the characteristic behavior described above as chronic illness behavior (Mechanic 1978).

Traits, affects, attitudes, and behaviors form a characteristic clinical portrait for each individual. The behavior of severe and chronic somatizers, however, is similar in part because these patients share invalidism and suffering; they require treatment and support and often demand it. Somatizing patients are referred to psychiatrists often as a last resort, so many of the observations on the personality of somatizing patients were made by psychiatrists on the uncharacteristic minority rather than on the majority of patients who have functional somatic symptoms (Mayou 1976). Some of the personality traits and mechanisms described in chronic somatizers appear to be the consequences of being ill rather than reflecting the premorbid personality or a predisposition.

Somatization Disorder and Briquet's Syndrome

There is an extensive literature on somatization disorder as well as on Briquet's syndrome, and this has been reviewed by Woodruff et al. (1982). The views on the exact nature of these disorders still differ (Cloninger 1986a; "Briquet's Syndrome or Hysteria?" 1977; Merskey 1979). For example, there is no agreement on whether somatization disorder is the entity that family studies and neuropsychological studies suggest (Flor-Henry et al. 1981), or whether it is the extreme end of the spectrum of functional somatic symptoms with multiple causation. It is, however, beyond the scope of this review to discuss the controversies about this disorder.

Diagnosis and Classification of Somatization

Different processes may be involved in making a diagnosis on the one hand and in labeling or classifying a disorder on the other. The term *diagnosis* means the recognition of the nature of a disease, whereas a *label* is a word or a phrase used with a definition to provide additional information. For example, if a patient has hypochondriacal beliefs for 5 1/2 months, his or her condition is classified in DSM-III-R in the category *somatoform disorder not otherwise specified*, or as an adjustment disorder; whereas if the condition has lasted for 1 month longer, the condition is classified as an *undifferentiated somatoform disorder*. This is one of the examples of when the condition (diagnosis) does not change, but the label or classification does, because of the specific criteria in the diagnostic manual. The description of the differences between diagnosing and labeling in psychiatry lies beyond the scope of the present review and has been discussed elsewhere (Kellner 1986).

Usually the additional steps that are needed to explore psychopathology are more important than the choice of the somatoform label. For example, it is important to evaluate the extent of a coexisting mood disorder (Fabrega et al. 1988) or the kind of hypochondriacal fears or beliefs (Barsky and Klerman 1983), because such knowledge may be helpful in the rational choice of treatments.

At other times, an incorrect psychiatric classification may lead to failure to recognize the exact nature of the disturbance. For example, patients with panic disorders who present predominantly with somatic symptoms may be classified as having one of the somatoform disorders, and such an error may delay appropriate treatment, sometimes for years (Katon 1984).

It may be difficult at times in clinical practice to decide whether to classify a condition among the somatoform disorders (DSM-III-R 300.70) or in the category *psychological factors affecting physical conditions* (316.00). The physiological disturbance may be the same, yet the classification may be different. For example, muscle-contraction headache is classified in the DSM-III-R as code 316.00. If, however, a patient complains of pain elsewhere, the physiological mechanism—in this case, excessive contraction of striated muscle—may be the same in both disorders, yet the patient's condition is likely to be classified among one of the somatoform disorders. Similarly, the irritable bowel syndrome is classified in DSM-III-R as code 316. Persistent abdominal complaints, however, in which the physiology may be the same but not all the characteristic symptoms and signs are present that warrant the diagnosis of irritable bowel syndrome, might be classified under code 300.70. The ICD-10 draft shares some of the same problems. The decision whether to classify this case as *undifferentiated somatoform disorder* (F45.1) or *somatoform autonomic dysfunction* (F45.3) would have to be made.

The DSM-III-R stipulates that in somatization disorder, appropriate evaluation discovers no organic pathology or pathophysiological mechanism. The classification may hinge on the interpretation of what constitutes "appropriate evaluation." In medical practice, as opposed to research, the appropriate evaluation is limited to the exclusion of substantial physical disease, but does not pursue investigations to detect the mechanism responsible for each symptom of a somatizing patient.

The DSM-III-R instruction may be interpreted as follows: if routine clinical evaluation (as opposed to specialized techniques used in research) does not uncover organ pathology or tissue damage, and if the syndrome does not have the characteristic features that merit classification as code 316.00, the syndrome should be classified among the somatoform disorders, even if a physiological disturbance is suspected. It may, however, be justified to add such a suspected disturbance in parentheses.

Exclusion of physical disease in the diagnosis of somatization is, of course, essential. Sometimes physical disease can remain undetected for years unless the disease is first suspected and then specifically looked for (e.g., cholesterolosis) (Jacyna and Bouchier 1987). Physical diseases and injuries (such as in accident neurosis) and somatization often coexist (Merskey 1979); at times the assessment of the relative contribution to symptom formation of physical pathology, functional overlay, and minor conversion symptoms can be exceedingly difficult. For example, patients with disseminated cancer who have a coexisting primary depression have more somatic symptoms than do patients with disseminated cancer and a secondary depression (Robinson et al. 1985). The presence of a serious physical illness may lead to introspection and self-observation and appears to make some patients more prone to somatization than before the onset of their illness. If somatization coexists with physical disease, it is important for the diagnosis to be made, because the former may require treatment as well. The judgment on the extent of somatization may require lengthy observation of the responses to treatments.

Various psychological inventories such as the MMPI have been used in several studies summarized in this volume. It is necessary to interpret these test results with caution. Most of the inventories were validated against psychiatric diagnoses several decades ago, and they reflect the views of psychiatrists' diagnoses at the time (Payne 1958). Thus, a high score on individual scales—for example, the hypochondriasis, hysteria, mania, and schizophrenia scales of the MMPI—does not indicate the same diagnosis by contemporary psychiatrists. Moreover, pain is a stressor, and patients in pain show psychopathology on self-rating scales and personality inventories regardless of whether the pain is caused by physical disease or is idiopathic. Abnormal psychological profiles are often the consequence of pain rather than etiological factors (see Chapter 9). The use of scales and inventories for the measurement of somatization has been discussed elsewhere (see Kellner 1987).

Treatments and Prognosis

The efficacy of treatment in somatizing patients has been underestimated for several reasons. Nonpsychiatric physicians have found that some somatizing patients are resistant to conventional medical treatments, and psychiatrists have often formed opinions about the poor prognosis from chronic, unrepresentative patients. Early studies of psychotherapy suggested that somatizing patients responded less well to conventional insight psychotherapy than did patients with overt emotional symptoms (Rosenberg 1954; Stone et al. 1961), and research in the drug treatment of somatizing patients has been sparse.

Uncontrolled clinical studies show that a large proportion of somatizing patients will have recovered on follow-up with symptomatic treatment alone (Kellner 1989), with minimal treatment, or even without treatment (Thomas 1978). The duration of most somatic complaints ranges from a few weeks to a few months (Kellner 1963). In most patients with recent somatization, explanation and reassurance constitute adequate treatment (Kellner 1986; Sapira 1972). The value of reassurance has also been underestimated by psychiatrists, in part, because of the chronic cases they had to deal with and, in part, because of the prevailing theories on the nature of somatization. Explanation and reassurance have been physicians' important tasks throughout the history of medicine (Kessel 1960; Mayou 1976; Warwick and Salkovskis 1985). Uncontrolled studies of psychotherapy show sustained improvement on follow-up (House 1989; Kellner 1983). Uncontrolled studies also suggest that aerobic exercise is an effective treatment in somatization in general. One controlled has study suggested that aerobic exercise is of benefit in the treatment of fibromyalgia (see Chapter 1).

Controlled studies suggest the following effects of treatment in somatizing patients: psychiatric consultation with the patient's physician leads to substantial reduction in costs of medical treatment in patients with somatization disorder (Smith et al. 1986). In the psychotherapy of patients with some of the somatic syndromes described in previous chapters, the treated group reported substantially more relief than the group treated with routine medical care. For example, patients with muscular pain (see Chapter 1), irritable bowel syndrome (see Chapter 6), and peptic ulcer who also had functional somatic symptoms unrelated to the ulcer (Sjödin et al. 1986) benefited from psychotherapy. Functional somatic symptoms decreased more in the group that had psychotherapy and medical care than they did in the control group that had medical care only. In most controlled studies of treatments in medicine and psychiatry, the difference between the treated group and control group decreases or vanishes on follow-up. However, in two of the studies of psychotherapy of these disorders (Sjödin et al. 1986; Svedlund et al. 1983), the difference between the groups became progressively greater, so psychotherapy apparently reduced the risk of recurrences.

There is consistent evidence that muscle-contraction headache and migraine headache are relieved by relaxation training as well as biofeedback (Blanchard et al. 1980; Jessup et al. 1979; Tarler-Benlolo 1978). Hypnosis is also an effective treatment in migraine headache (Anderson et al. 1975) and in the irritable bowel syndrome (Whorwell et al. 1984), and is likely to be effective in some patients with functional somatic symptoms. The treatment of conversion disorder is discussed in Chapter 11.

The traditional methods of psychotherapy that yielded poor results were insight or analytically oriented ones; if somatic symptoms were addressed at all by the therapist, they were interpreted in accord with the therapist's theoretical orientation, and these theoretical approaches differed widely (Kellner 1986). Patients who complained about bodily sensations at the expense of emotion were judged to lack insight and psychological sophistication, or were regarded as being defensive or denying emotions; alternatively, the symptoms were believed to be the product of reinforcement and subconsciously motivated.

Contemporary psychotherapies of somatic syndromes that show psychotherapy to be an effective mode of treatment tend to adopt differing strategies, yet they have several features in common. The therapist addresses bodily symptoms, attempts to identify stressors that precede the symptoms, helps the patient find strategies to deal with the stressors, and tries to ease the burden and the suffering that severe bodily symptoms entail. Compared with other mental health professionals who participated in previous studies, it also seems likely that therapists who conducted controlled studies with somatizing patients were more interested in somatizers, were more knowledgeable about their psychopathology, did not regard these patients as a burden, may have established a better rapport, and may have been more accepting of them.

The somatizing patient may have regarded the contemporary treatments as more pertinent; the small dropout rate in these studies suggests that this was the case. There may be another reason for the discrepancy between early and later results. The early studies were conducted with psychiatric patients who were somatizers, whereas the later studies were carried out in patients who attended medical clinics. Thus, the former may have had more severe illnesses; many of these individuals were referred to psychiatrists because they had psychiatric disorders in addition to their tendency to somatize. The patients recruited for the studies from medical clinics, however, may have had predominantly a less complicated psychophysiological disorder without coexisting severe neuroses and personality disorders.

There are no controlled studies of psychological treatments of hypochondriasis. Numerous treatment strategies have been advocated (Kellner 1986) that depend on the author's belief about the nature of the disorder. Contemporary therapies tend to address hypochondriacal beliefs and fears directly as opposed to being used to search for the unconscious motives. Several authors have recommended an educational and cognitive approach (Barsky et al. 1988; House 1989; Kellner 1982). If the patient has a persistent false belief that the symptoms are caused by a serious, hitherto undiagnosed disease, various methods of persuasion appear to be essential for interrupting the vicious cycle of fear, somatic symptoms, self-observation, false belief, and more fear (Kellner 1989). In hypochondriacal patients who are disease phobic without the conviction that they suffer from a serious disease, exposure therapy may be adequate and appropriate (Salkovskis and Warwick 1986; Warwick and Marks 1988). In other studies of patients who had hypochondriacal fears as well as other psychopathology, a combination of psychotherapeutic strategies was used (Sulz 1986). Uncontrolled studies suggest that these strategies are helpful in a substantial proportion of patients.

When hypochondriasis is secondary to another disorder such as melancholia or panic disorder, hypochondriacal fears and beliefs remit in a substantial proportion of patients when the primary disorder is effectively treated (Fava et al. 1988; Kellner et al. 1986; Noyes et al. 1986), and no other treatment may be necessary.

Numerous drug trials have shown that antidepressant and antianxiety drugs relieve somatic symptoms in depressed as well as in anxious patients (Kellner 1985). Controlled studies suggest that psychotropic drugs also play an important part in the treatment of psychophysiological disorders such as the irritable bowel syndrome, the fibrositis-myalgia syndrome, aerophagia, and probably in atypical variants of these syndromes that are classified among the somatoform disorders. Overall, there is consistent evidence that both drugs and psychotherapy are effective in reducing the severity of symptoms in somatizing patients, and that psychotherapy reduces the duration of symptoms as well as the tendency for recurrences. Because the mean improvement tends to be greater in the treated groups, the change in some patients in response to treatment is striking, approaching recovery instead of continued suffering.

References

Adám G: Interception and Behaviour: An Experimental Study. Budapest, Akademiai Kiado, 1967

American Psychiatric Association: Statistical and Diagnostic Manual of Mental Disorders, 3rd Edition, Revised. Washington, DC, American Psychiatric Association, 1987

Anderson CD: Expression of affect and physiological response in psychosomatic patients. J Psychosom Res 25:143–149, 1981

Anderson JAD, Barker MA, Dalton R: Migraine and hypnotherapy. Int J Clin Exp Hypn 1:48–58, 1975

Apley J, Keith RM, Meadow R: The Child and His Symptoms: A Comprehensive Approach. Oxford, UK, Blackwell Scientific Publications, 1978

Averill JR, Opton EM Jr, Lazarus RS: Cross-cultural studies of psychophysiological responses during stress and emotion. International Journal of Psychology 4:83–102, 1969

Barish CF, Castell DO, Richter JE: Graded esophageal balloon distention: a new provocative test for noncardiac chest pain. Dig Dis Sci 31:1292–1298, 1986

Barnat MR: Post-traumatic headache patients, adversarial and third-party systems: a pilot study. Headache 25:171–172, 1985

Barsky AJ: Patients who amplify bodily symptoms. Ann Intern Med 91:63–70, 1979

Barsky AJ, Klerman GL: Overview: hypochondriasis, bodily complaints, and somatic styles. Am J Psychiatry 140:273 283, 1983

Barsky AJ, Wyshak G: Hypochondriasis and related health attitudes. Psychosomatics 30:412–420, 1989

Barsky AJ, Goodson JD, Lane RS, et al: The amplification of somatic symptoms. Psychosom Med 50:510–519, 1988

Bartoshuk AK: Electromyographic reactions to strong auditory stimulation as a function of alpha amplitude. Journal of Comparative Physiological Psychology 52:540–545, 1959

Beitman BD, Basha I, Flaker G, et al: Non-fearful panic disorder: panic attacks without fear. Behav Res Ther 25:487–492, 1987

Bennett RM: Fibromyalgia. JAMA 257:2802–2803, 1987

Better SR, Fine PR, Simison D, et al: Disability benefits as disincentives to rehabilitation. Health and Society 57:412–427, 1979

Bianchi GN: Origins of disease phobia. Aust N Z J Psychiatry 5:241–257, 1971

Bishop ER Jr, Torch EM: "Dividing hysteria": a preliminary investigation of conversion disorder and psychalgia. J Nerv Ment Dis 167:348–356, 1979

Black P (ed): Physiological Correlates of Emotions. New York, Academic, 1970

Blackwell B, Gutman M: The management of chronic illness behavior, in Illness Behavior. Edited by McHugh S, Vallis TM. New York, Plenum, 1986, pp 401–408

Blanchard EB, Andrasik F, Ahles TA, et al: Migraine and tension headache: a meta-analytic review. Behavior Therapy 11:613–631, 1980

Bohman M, Cloninger CR, von Knorring AL: An adoption study of somatoform disorders, III: cross-fostering analysis and genetic relationship to alcoholism and criminality. Arch Gen Psychiatry 41:872–878, 1984

Bridges KW, Goldberg DP: Somatic presentation of DSM-III psychiatric disorders in primary care. J Psychosom Res 29:563–569, 1985

Briquet's syndrome or hysteria? Lancet 2:1138–1139, 1977

Burns BH, Nichols MA: Factors related to the localization of symptoms to the chest in depression. Br J Psychiatry 121:405–409, 1972

Byrne D: Repression-sensitization as a dimension of personality, in Progression of Experimental Personality Research. Edited by Maher BA. New York, Academic, 1964, pp 169–220

Byrne D, Steinberg MA, Schwartz MS: Relationship between repression-sensitization and physical illness. J Abnorm Psychol 73:154–155, 1968

Cadoret RJ: Psychopathology in adopted-away offspring of biologic parents with antisocial behavior. Arch Gen Psychiatry 35:176–184, 1978

Cadoret RJ, Widmer RB, Troughton EP: Somatic complaints: harbinger of depression in primary care. J Affective Disord 2:61–70, 1980

Canino GJ, Bird HR, Shrout PE, et al: The prevalence of specific psychiatric disorders in Puerto Rico. Arch Gen Psychiatry 44:727–736, 1987

Cannon RO III, Leon MB, Watson RM, et al: Chest pain and "normal" coronary arteries: role of small coronary arteries. Am J Cardiol 55:50B–60B, 1985

Chaudhary NA, Truelove SC: Human colonic motility: a comparative study of normal subjects, patients with ulcerative colitis, and patients with the irritable colon syndrome. Gastroenterology 40:1–36, 1961

Clark DM: A cognitive approach to panic. Behav Res Ther 24:461–470, 1986

Cloninger CR: Somatoform and Dissociative Disorders. Philadelphia, PA, WB Saunders, 1986a

Cloninger CR: A unified biosocial theory of personality and its role in the development of anxiety states. Psychiatr Dev 4(3):167–226, 1986b

Cloninger CR, Martin RL, Guze SB, et al: A prospective follow-up and family study of somatization in men and women. Am J Psychiatry 143:873–878, 1986

Cluff LE, Canter A, Imboden JB: Asian influenza. Arch Intern Med 117:159–163, 1966

Conti S, Savron G, Bartolucci G, et al: Cardiac neurosis and psychopathology. Psychother Psychosom 52:88–91, 1989

DeGood DE, Buckelew SP, Tait RC: Cognitive-somatic anxiety response patterning in chronic pain patients and nonpatients. J Consult Clin Psychol 53:137–138, 1985

Derlega V: Self-disclosure and intimate relationships, in Communication. Edited by Derlega V. Orlando, FL, Academic, 1984, pp 1–9

Dolce JJ, Raczynski JM: Neuromuscular activity and electromyography in painful backs: psychological and biomechanical models in assessment and treatment. Psychol Bull 97:502–520, 1985

Droste C, Roskamm H: Experimental pain measurement in patients with asymptomatic myocardial ischemia. J Am Coll Cardiol 1:940–945, 1983

Edwards DAW: "Tender oesophagus": a new syndrome (abstract). Gut 23:A919, 1982

Escobar JI, Burnam A, Karno M, et al: Somatization in the community. Arch Gen Psychiatry 44:713–720, 1987

Fabrega H Jr, Mezzich J, Jacob R, et al: Somatoform disorder in a psychiatric setting: systematic comparisons with depression and anxiety disorders. J Nerv Ment Dis 176:431–439, 1988

Fava Ga, Pavan L: Large bowel disorders, II: psychopathology and alexithymia. Psychother Psychosom 27:100–105, 1976/1977

Fava GA, Baldaro B, Osti RMA: Towards a self-rating scale for alexithymia. Psychother Psychosom 34:34–39, 1980

Fava GA, Kellner R, Munari F, et al: Losses, hostility, and depression. J Nerv Ment Dis 170:474–478, 1982

Fava GA, Kellner R, Zielezny MA, et al: Hypochondriacal fears and beliefs in agoraphobia. J Affective Disord 14:239–244, 1988

Flor H, Turk DC, Birbaumer N: Assessment of stress-related psychophysiological reactions in chronic back pain patients. J Consult Clin Psychol 53:354–364, 1985

Flor-Henry P, Fromm-Auch D, Tapper M, et al: A neuropsychological study of the stable syndrome of hysteria. Biol Psychiatry 16:601–626, 1981

Ford CV: The Somatizing Disorders: Illness as a Way of Life. New York, Elsevier, 1983

Ford CV: The somatizing disorders. Psychosomatics 27:327–337, 1986

Freud S: Hysterical phantasies and their relation to bisexuality (1908), in The Standard Edition of the Complete Psychological Works of Sigmund Freud, Vol 9. Translated and Edited by Strachey J. London, Hogarth Press, 1959, pp 155–166

Freyberger H: Supportive psychotherapeutic techniques in primary and secondary alexithymia. Psychother Psychosom 28:337–342, 1977

Fujii S, Kachi T, Sobue I: Chronic headache: its psychosomatic aspect. Japanese Journal of Psychosomatic Medicine 21:411–419, 1981

Glazier JJ, Chierchia S, Brown MJ, et al: Importance of generalized defective perception of painful stimuli as a cause of silent myocardial ischemia in chronic stable angina pectoris. Am J Cardiol 58:667–672, 1986

Goldstein IB: Physiological responses in anxious women patients: a study of autonomic activity and muscle tension. Arch Gen Psychiatry 10:382–388, 1964

Gottesman II: Differential inheritance of the psychoneuroses. Eugenics Quarterly 9:223–267, 1962

Grings WW, Dawson ME: Emotions and Bodily Responses: A Psychophysiological Approach. New York, Academic, 1978

Hare RD: Denial of threat and emotional response to impending painful stimulation. Journal of Consulting Psychiatry 30:359–361, 1966

Harris ID: Mood, anger, and somatic dysfunction. J Nerv Ment Dis 113:152–158, 1951

Hokanson JR: Vascular and psychogalvanic effects of experimentally aroused anger. J Pers 29:30–39, 1961

Holdstock DJ, Misiewicz JJ, Waller SL: Observations on the mechanism of abdominal pain. Gut 10:19–31, 1969

Hollander E, Liebowitz MR, Winchel R, et al: Treatment of body-dysmorphic disorder with serotonin reuptake blockers. Am J Psychiatry 146:768–770, 1989

House A: Hypochondriasis and related disorders. Gen Hosp Psychiatry 11:156–165, 1989

House JS, Landis KR, Umberson D: Social relationships and health. Science 241:540–545, 1988

Hudgens AJ: Family-oriented treatment of chronic pain. Journal of Marital and Family Therapy 5:67–78, 1979

Jacyna MR, Bouchier IAD: Cholesterolosis: a physical cause of "functional" disorder. Br Med J 295:619–620, 1987

James W: What is an emotion? Mind 9:188–205, 1884

Jessup BA, Neufeld RWJ, Merskey H: Biofeedback therapy for headache and other pain: an evaluative review. Pain 7:225–270, 1979

Jones RA, Wiese HJ, Moore RW, et al: On the perceived meaning of symptoms. Med Care 19:710–717, 1981

Katkin ES, Blascovich J, Goldband S: Empirical assessment of visceral self-perception: individual and sex differences in the acquisition of heartbeat discrimination. J Pers Soc Psychol 40:1095–1101, 1981

Katon W: Panic disorder and somatization: review of 55 cases. Am J Med 77:101–106, 1984

Katon W, Kleinman A, Rosen G: Depression and somatization: a review, Part I. Am J Med 72:127–135, 1982

Katon W, Ries RK, Kleinman A: Part II: a prospective DSM-III study of 100 consecutive somatization patients. Compr Psychiatry 25:305–314, 1984

Katon W, Vitaliano PP, Russo J, et al: Panic disorder: spectrum of severity and somatization. J Nerv Ment Dis 175:12–18, 1987

Katzenelbogen S: Hypochondriacal complaints, with special reference to personality and environment. Am J Psychiatry 98:815–822, 1942

Kellner R: Mental ill health in general practice on Deeside. Unpublished M.D. Thesis. Liverpool, UK, University of Liverpool, 1963

Kellner R: Psychotherapeutic strategies in hypochondriasis: a clinical study. Am J Psychother 36:146–157, 1982

Kellner R: The prognosis of treated hypochondriasis: a clinical study. Acta Psychiatr Scand 67:69–79, 1983

Kellner R: Functional somatic symptoms and hypochondriasis: a survey of empirical studies. Arch Gen Psychiatry 42:821–833, 1985

Kellner R: Somatization and Hypochondriasis. New York, Praeger-Greenwood, 1986

Kellner R: Psychological measurements in somatization and abnormal illness behavior, in Research Paradigms in Psychosomatic Medicine, Vol 17. Edited by Fava GA, Wise TN. Basel, S Karger, 1987, pp 101–118

Kellner R: Anxiety, somatic sensations, and bodily complaints, in Handbook of Anxiety, Vol 2: Classification, Etiological Factors, and Associated Disturbances. Edited by Noyes R, Roth M, Burrows GD. New York, Elsevier, 1988, pp 213–237

Kellner R: Undifferentiated somatoform disorder and somatoform disorder not otherwise specified, in Treatments of Psychiatric Disorders: A Task Force Report of the American Psychiatric Association. Washington, DC, American Psychiatric Association, 1989, pp 2147–2152

Kellner R: Somatization: the most costly comorbidity? in Comorbidity of Mood and Anxiety Disorders. Edited by Maser JD, Cloninger CR. Washington, DC, American Psychiatric Press, 1990, pp 239–252

Kellner R, Schneider-Braus K: Distress and attitudes in patients perceived as hypochondriacal by medical staff. Gen Hosp Psychiatry 10:157–162, 1988

Kellner R, Sheffield BF: The one-week prevalence of symptoms in neurotic patients and normals. Am J Psychiatry 130:102–105, 1973a

Kellner R, Sheffield BF: A self-rating scale of distress. Psychol Med 3:88–100, 1973b

Kellner R, Simpson GM, Winslow WW: The relationship of depressive neurosis to anxiety and somatic symptoms. Psychosomatics 13:358–362, 1972

Kellner R, Pathak D, Romanik R, et al: Life events and hypochondriacal concerns. Psychiatr Med 1:133–141, 1983

Kellner R, Slocumb JC, Wiggins RG, et al: Hostility, somatic symptoms, and hypochondriacal fears and beliefs. J Nerv Ment Dis 173:554–561, 1985

Kellner R, Wiggins RG, Pathak D: Hypochondriacal fears and beliefs in medical and law students. Arch Gen Psychiatry 43:487–489, 1986

Kellner R, Abbott P, Winslow WW, et al: Fears, beliefs, and attitudes in DSM-III hypochondriasis. J Nerv Ment Dis 175:20–25, 1987

Kendler KS, Heath AC, Martin NG, et al: Symptoms of anxiety and symptoms of depression. Arch Gen Psychiatry 44:451–457, 1987

Kenyon FE: Hypochondriasis: a survey of some historical, clinical, and social aspects. Br J Med Psychol 38:117–133, 1965

Kessel WIN: Psychiatric morbidity in a London general practice. British Journal of Preventive and Social Medicine 14:16–22, 1960

Kirmayer LJ: Culture, affect, and somatization, Part I. Transcultural Psychiatric Research Review 21:159–188, 1984a

Kirmayer LJ: Culture, affect, and somatization, Part II. Transcultural Psychiatric Research Review 21:237–262, 1984b

Kirmayer L: Somatization and the social construction of illness experience, in Illness Behavior: A Multidisciplinary Model. New York, Plenum, 1986, pp 111–133

Kirmayer LJ: Languages of suffering and healing: alexithymia as a social and cultural process. Transcultural Psychiatric Research Review 24:119–136, 1987

Kirmayer LJ, Robbins JM: Functional somatic syndromes, in Current Concepts of Somatization: Research and Clinical Perspectives. Edited by Kirmayer LJ, Robbins JM. Washington, DC, American Psychiatric Press, 1990, pp 79–106

Kleinman A, Kleinman J: Somatization: the interconnections among culture, depressive experiences, and the meaning of pain, in Culture and Depression. Edited by Kleinman A, Good B. Berkeley, CA, University of California Press, 1986, pp 429–490

Koss J: Somatization and somatic complaint syndromes among Hispanics: overview and ethnopsychological perspectives. Transcultural Psychiatric Research Review 27:5–29, 1990

Kreitman N, Sainsbury P, Pearce K, et al: Hypochondriasis and depression in outpatients at a general hospital. Br J Psychiatry 111:607–615, 1965

Lacey JI, Lacey BC: Verification and extension of the principle of autonomic response-stereotypy. Am J Psychol 71:50–73, 1958

Lacey JI, Bateman DE, Van Lehn R: Autonomic response specificity: an experimental study. Psychosom Med 15:8–21, 1953

Lader M: The Psychophysiology of Mental Illness. London, Routledge & Kegan Paul, 1975

Lanzetta JT, Cartwright-Smith J, Kleck RE: Effects of nonverbal dissimulation on emotional experience and autonomic arousal. J Pers Soc Psychol 33:354–370, 1976

Lazarus RS, Tomita M, Opton E, et al: A cross-cultural study of stress-reaction patterns in Japan. J Pers Soc Psychol 4:622–633, 1966

Leavitt F, Garron DC, McNeill TW, et al: Organic status, psychological disturbance, and pain report characteristics in low-back-pain patients on compensation. Spine 7:398–402, 1982

Le Febvre MF: Cognitive distortion and cognitive errors in depressed psychiatric and low back pain patients. J Consult Clin Psychol 49:517–525, 1981

Lennard-Jones JE: Functional gastrointestinal disorders. N Engl J Med 308:431–435, 1983

Lesser IA: A review of the alexithymia concept. Psychosom Med 43:531–543, 1981

Lesser IM, Lesser BZ: Alexithymia: examining the development of a psychological concept. Am J Psychiatry 140:1305–1308, 1983

Lesser IM, Ford CV, Friedmann CTH: Alexithymia in somatizing patients. Gen Hosp Psychiatry 1:256–261, 1979

Lipowski ZJ: Somatization: medicine's unsolved problem (editorial). Psychosomatics 28:294–297, 1987

Lloyd GG: Psychiatric syndromes with a somatic presentation. J Psychosom Res 30:113–120, 1986

Malmo RB, Shagass C: Physiologic study of symptom mechanisms in psychiatric patients under stress. Psychosom Med 11:25–29, 1949

Malmo RB, Shagass C, Davis JF: A method for the investigation of somatic response mechanisms in psychoneurosis. Science 112:325–328, 1950

Malmo RB, Wallerstein H, Shagass C: Headache proneness and mechanisms of motor conflict in psychiatric patients. J Pers 22:163–187, 1953

Mandler G, Mandler JM, Uviller ET: Autonomic feedback: the perception of autonomic activity. Journal of Abnormal and Social Psychology 56:367–373, 1958

Marks I, Mishan J: Dysmorphophobic avoidance with disturbed bodily perception: a pilot study of exposure therapy. Br J Psychiatry 152:674–678, 1988

Martin I: Levels of muscle activity in psychiatric patients. Acta Psychol (Amst) 12:326–341, 1956

Mayou R: The nature of bodily symptoms. Br J Psychiatry 129:55–60, 1976

Mayou R: Illness behavior and psychiatry. Gen Hosp Psychiatry 11:307–312, 1989

McDonald PW, Prkachin KM: The expression and perception of facial emotion in alexithymia: a pilot study. Psychosom Med 52:199–210, 1990

McNair DM, Fisher S: Separating anxiety from depression, in Psychopharmacology: A Generation of Progress. Edited by Lipton MA, DiMascio A, Killam KF. New York, Raven, 1978, pp 1411–1418

Mechanic D: The concept of illness behavior. J Chronic Dis 15:189–194, 1962

Mechanic D: Social psychologic factors affecting the presentation of bodily complaints. N Engl J Med 286:1132–1139, 1972

Mechanic D: Medical Sociology: A Comprehensive Text, 2nd Edition. New York, Free Press, 1978

Mechanic D: Development of psychological distress among young adults. Arch Gen Psychiatry 36:1233–1239, 1979

Mendelson G: Persistent work disability following settlement of compensation claims. Law Institute Journal 55:342–345, 1981

Merskey H: The Analysis of Hysteria. London, Ballière, Tindall and Cassell, 1979

Merskey H: Psychiatry and the cervical sprain syndrome. Can Med Assoc J 130:1119–1121, 1984

Merskey H: Regional pain is rarely hysterical. Arch Neurol 45:915–918, 1988

Merskey H, Spear FG: Pain: Psychological and Psychiatric Aspects. London, Ballière, Tindall and Cassell, 1967

Miller H: Accident neurosis. Br Med J 1:919–925, 1961

Myren J, Lövland B, Larssen SE, et al: Psychopharmacologic drugs in the treatment of the irritable bowel syndrome. Ann Gastroenterol Hepatol (Paris) 20:117–123, 1984

Nemiah JC: Alexithymia: theoretical considerations. Psychother Psychosom 28:199–206, 1977

Nemiah JC, Sifneos PE: Affect and fantasy in patients with psychosomatic disorders, in Modern Trends in Psychosomatic Medicine, Vol 2. Edited by Hill O. London, Butterworths, 1970a

Nemiah JC, Sifneos PE: Psychosomatic illness: a problem in communication. Psychother Psychosom 18:154–160, 1970b

Nimii Y: Bibliographic survey on galvanic skin response, 2. Philosophia 31:83, 1956

Notarius CI, Levenson RW: Expressive tendencies and physiological response to stress. J Pers Soc Psychol 37:1204–1210, 1979

Noyes R Jr, Reich J, Clancy J, et al: Reduction of hypochondriasis with treatment of panic disorder. Br J Psychiatry 149:631–635, 1986

Opton EM Jr, Lazarus RS: Personality determinants of psychophysiological response to stress: a theoretical analysis and an experiment. J Pers Soc Psychol 6:291–303, 1967

Overall JE, Hollister LE, Pennington V: Nosology of depression and differential response to drugs. JAMA 195:946–948, 1966

Parsons OA, Fulgenzi LB, Edelberg R: Aggressiveness and psychophysiological responsivity in groups of repressors and sensitizers. J Pers Soc Psychol 1:235–244, 1969

Payne RW: Diagnostic and personality testing in clinical psychology. Am J Psychiatry 115:25–29, 1958

Pelz M, Merskey H: A description of the psychological effects of chronic painful lesions. Pain 14:293–301, 1982

Pennebaker JW: The Psychology of Physical Symptoms. New York, Springer-Verlag, 1982

Pennebaker JW: Physical symptoms and sensations: psychological causes and correlates, in Social Psychophysiology: A Sourcebook. Edited by Cacioppo J. New York, Guilford, 1983

Pennebaker JW: Traumatic experience and psychosomatic disease: exploring the roles of behavioural inhibition, obsession, and confiding. Can J Psychol 26:82–95, 1985

Pennebaker JW: Confession, inhibition, and disease. Advances in Experimental Social Psychology 22:211–244, 1989

Pennebaker JW, O'Heeron RC: Confiding in others and illness rate among spouses of suicide and accidental-death victims. J Abnorm Psychol 93:473–476, 1984

Pennebaker JW, Skelton JA: Psychological parameters of physical symptoms. Personality and Social Psychology Bulletin 4:524–530, 1978

Pennebaker JW, Susman JR: Disclosure of traumas and psychosomatic processes. Soc Sci Med 26:327–332, 1988

Pennebaker JW, Burnam MA, Schaeffer MA, et al: Lack of control as a determinant of perceived physical symptoms. J Pers Soc Psychol 35:167–174, 1977

Petrie A: Individuality in Pain and Suffering. Chicago, IL, University of Chicago Press, 1967

Pilowsky I: Abnormal illness behavior. Br J Med Psychol 42:347–351, 1969

Pilowsky I: Abnormal illness behaviour (dysnosognosia). Psychother Psychosom 46:76–84, 1986

Pilowsky I, Spence ND: Pain, anger, and illness behaviour. J Psychosom Res 20:411–416, 1976

Pilowsky I, Smith QP, Katsikitis M: Illness behaviour and general practice utilisation: a prospective study. J Psychosom Res 31:177–183, 1987

Raskin M, Talbott JA, Meyerson AT: Diagnosed conversion reactions: predictive value of psychiatric criteria. JAMA 197:530–534, 1966

Reidenberg MM, Lowenthal DT: Adverse non-drug reactions. N Engl J Med 279:678–679, 1968

Richter JE, Barish CF, Castell DO: Abnormal sensory perception in patients with esophageal chest pain. Gastroenterology 91:845–852, 1986

Robinson J, Bashier M, Dansak D: Depression and anxiety: evidence for different causes. J Psychosom Res 29:133–138, 1985

Rosenbaum JF: Limited-symptom panic attack. Psychosomatics 28:407–424, 1987

Rosenberg S: The relationship of certain personality factors to prognosis in psychotherapy. J Clin Psychology 10:341–345, 1954

Sainsbury P, Gibson JG: Symptoms of anxiety and tension and the accompanying physiological changes in the muscular system. J Neurol Neurosurg Psychiatry 17:216–224, 1954

Salkovskis PM, Warwick HMC: Morbid preoccupations, health anxiety, and reassurance: a cognitive-behavioural approach to hypochondriasis. Behav Res Ther 24:597–602, 1986

Sapira JD: Reassurance therapy. Ann Intern Med 77:603–604, 1972

Schwab JJ: Psychosomatic disturbances, in Psychiatry in General Medical Practice. Edited by Usdin G, Lewis JM. New York, McGraw-Hill, 1979, pp 369–393

Schwab JJ, Kuhn CC: The treatment of physically ill patients' psychiatric illness, in Psychiatry and Health. Edited by Masserman JH. New York, Human Sciences Press, 1986, pp 133–142

Shagass C, Malmo RB: Psychodynamic themes and localized muscular tension during psychotherapy. Psychosom Med 16:295–313, 1954

Shepherd M, Cooper B, Brown AC, et al: Psychiatric Illness in General Practice. London, Oxford University Press, 1966

Sifneos PE: The prevalence of "alexithymic" characteristics in psychosomatic patients. Psychother Psychosom 22:255–262, 1973

Sjödin I, Svedlund J, Ottosson J-O, et al: Controlled study of psychotherapy in chronic peptic ulcer disease. Psychosomatics 27:187–196, 200, 1986

Smith GR Jr: Alexithymia in medical patients referred to a consultation/liaison service. Am J Psychiatry 140:99–101, 1983

Smith GR Jr, Monson RA, Ray DC: Psychiatric consultation in somatization disorder. N Engl J Med 314:1407–1413, 1986

Smith TW, Snyder CR, Perkins SC: The self-serving function of hypochondriacal complaints: physical symptoms as self-handicapping strategies. J Pers Soc Psychol 44:787–797, 1983

Srole L, Langner TS, Michael ST, et al: Mental Health in the Metropolis: The Midtown Manhattan Study. New York, McGraw-Hill, 1962

Starcevic V: Pathological fear of death, panic attacks, and hypochondriasis. Am J Psychoanal 49:347–361, 1989

Steckel W: The Interpretation of Dreams. New York, Liveright, 1943

Stenbäck A: Hypochondria in duodenal ulcer. Adv Psychsom Med 1:307–312, 1960

Stenbäck A, Jalava V: Hypochondria and depression. Acta Psychiatr Scand Suppl 37:240–246, 1962

Stone AR, Frank JD, Nash EH, et al: An intensive five-year follow-up study of treated psychiatric outpatients. J Nerv Ment Dis 133:410–422, 1961

Sulz SK: Verhaltenstherapie der Herzphobie: ein klinischer Erfahrungsbericht uber ein Training kognitiver Angstbewaltigung. Psychiatr Prax 13:10–16, 1986

Svelund J, Sjödin I, Ottosson J-O, et al: Controlled study of psychotherapy in irritable bowel syndrome. Lancet 2:589–592, 1983

Tarler-Benlolo L: The role of relaxation in biofeedback training: a critical review of the literature. Psychol Bull 85:727–755, 1978

Taylor GJ: Alexithymia: concept, measurement, and implications for treatment. Am J Psychiatry 141:725–732, 1984

Taylor GJ, Bagby RM: Measurement of alexithymia: recommendations for clinical practice and future research. Psychiatr Clin North Am 11:351–366, 1988

TenHouten WD, Hoppe KD, Bogen JE, et al: Alexithymia: an experimental study of cerebral commissurotomy patients and normal control subjects. Am J Psychiatry 143:312–316, 1986

Thomas KB: The consultation and the therapeutic illusion. Br Med J 1:1327–1328, 1978

Toouli J: Sphincter of Oddi motility. Br J Surg 71:251–256, 1984

Torgersen S: Genetics of somatoform disorders. Arch Gen Psychiatry 43:502–505, 1986

Totman R, Kiff J, Reed SE, et al: Predicting experimental colds in volunteers from different measures of recent life stress. J Psychosom Res 24:155–163, 1980

Tyrer P: The Role of Bodily Feelings in Anxiety. London, Oxford University Press, 1976

Von Zerssen D: Clinical self-rating scales (CSRS) of the Munich Psychiatric Information System, in Assessment of Depression. Edited by Sartorius N, Ban TA. New York, Springer-Verlag, 1986, pp 270–276

Warwick HMC, Marks IM: Behavioural treatment of illness phobia and hypochondriasis: a pilot study of 17 cases. Br J Psychiatry 152:239–241, 1988

Warwick HMC, Salkovskis P: Reassurance. Br Med J 290:1028, 1985

Watson D, Clark LA: Negative affectivity: the disposition to experience aversive emotional states. Psychol Bull 96:465–490, 1984

Weinberger DA, Schwartz GE, Davidson RJ: Low-anxious, high-anxious, and repressive coping styles: psychometric patterns and behavioral and physiological responses to stress. J Abnorm Psychol 88:369–380, 1979

Weintraub S, Mesulam MM: Developmental learning disabilities of the right hemisphere: emotional, interpersonal, and cognitive components. Arch Neurol 40:463–468, 1983

Weissman M, Klerman GL, Paykel ES: Clinical evaluation of hostility in depression. Am J Psychiatry 128:41–46, 1971

Whitehead WE, Dresher VM: Perception of gastric contractions and self-control of gastric motility. Psychophysiology 17:552–558, 1980

Whitehead WE, Winget C, Fedoravicius AS, et al: Learned illness behavior in patients with irritable bowel syndrome and peptic ulcer. Dig Dis Sci 27:202–208, 1982

Whorwell PJ, Prior A, Faragher EB: Controlled trial of hypnotherapy in the treatment of severe refractory irritable bowel syndrome. Lancet 2:1232–1233, 1984

Whorwell PJ, McCallum M, Creed FH, et al: Noncolonic features of irritable syndrome. Gut 27:37–40, 1986

Williams JRB, Barefoot JC, Shekelle RB: Health consequences of hostility, in Anger and Hostility in Cardiovascular and Behavioral Disorders. Edited by Chesney MA, Rosenman RH. Washington, DC, Hemisphere Publishing Corporation, 1985, pp 173–185

Woodruff RA, Goodwin DW, Guze SB: Hysteria (Briquet's syndrome), in Hysteria. Edited by Roy A. New York, John Wiley, 1982, pp 117–131

World Health Organization: Draft of the 10th Revision of the International Classification of Diseases. Geneva, World Health Organization, 1988

Chapter 11

Hysteria

> ... it becomes evident that much of what has been called
> hysteria at various periods would now no longer be so
> described, and much of what is now recognized as symptomatic
> of hysteria was earlier attributed to other diseases.
>
> Daniel Hack Tuke (1892)
> *Illustrations of the Influence*
> *of the Mind Upon the Body in*
> *Health and Disease*

Among the causes of bodily complaints are hysterical or conversion symptoms. The term *hysteria* has been used by several of the authors of the studies quoted in the previous chapters.

The concept of the nature of hysteria—its origin, symptoms, and management—has undergone many radical changes (Veith 1965). In the epigraph to this chapter, Tuke described accurately the history of the term, and the same judgment applies to the term's fate in the present century. Until the last few decades, most authors failed to distinguish between conversion symptoms and other functional somatic symptoms.

Even in recent studies, authors—including those quoted in this volume—have described different syndromes when using this term, and these disagreements have historical causes. For the same reason, personality inventories that purport to measure hysteria do not necessarily measure the same construct. In order to understand the role of hysteria in psychophysiological syndromes as used by authors whose studies are summarized in this volume, it is essential to define the various meanings of the term.

A person suffering from hysteria or someone described as a hysterical person in the older medical and psychiatric literature had the predominant traits of affective immaturity and affective instability, displaying excessive emotionality and attention-seeking behavior (Slater and Roth 1969, p. 110). Such a person was classified in the ICD-9 (World Health Organization 1979) and the DSM-II (American Psychiatric Association 1968) as having a *hysterical personality dis-*

order, in DSM-III (American Psychiatric Association 1980) this term was re-named the *histrionic personality disorder*. Hysteria in the ICD-9 included sev-eral syndromes such as conversion reaction, dissociative reaction, Ganser syn-drome, compensation neurosis, and multiple personality. Briquet (1859) described a syndrome with multiple somatic complaints that he termed *hysteria*; this meaning of the term was accepted by numerous American authors (includ-ing authors quoted in this volume) until the DSM-III modified this syndrome somewhat and renamed it *somatization disorder*. The draft of the ICD-10 (World Health Organization 1988) has adopted the term *somatization disorder* for this syndrome. The DSM-III divided hysterical neurosis into separate disor-ders that include conversion disorder and dissociative disorder. In the draft of the ICD-10 the new term is *dissociative (conversion) disorder*.

Various theories have been put forward throughout the ages trying to ex-plain hysterical phenomena (Ey 1982). The discussion of research in this chap-ter will be limited to conversion disorder of DSM-III-R. Most of the other syn-dromes that have been classified as hysteria are not directly relevant to the topics of this volume.

Prevalence

There have been substantial differences in estimates of prevalence of hysteria apparently because of differences in diagnostic criteria used by various authors. For example, a history of unexplained neurological symptoms was obtained in 33% of postpartum women (Farley et al. 1968). The point prevalence is not known.

Symptoms and Signs

The summary that follows is derived from DSM-III-R, and I shall use this as the basis for the discussion. The main feature of conversion disorder is "an alter-ation or loss of physical functioning that suggests physical disorder [i.e., organic pathology], but that instead is apparently an expression of a psychological con-flict or need" (American Psychiatric Association 1987, p. 257). When the conver-sion symptoms are limited to pain or are merely the symptoms of somatization disorder, conversion disorder is not diagnosed.

The most obvious conversion symptoms are those that suggest neurological disease, such as paralysis, aphonia, seizures, coordination disturbance, blind-ness, tunnel vision, anesthesia, and parasthesia. In a general hospital, the most common manifestations of conversion disorder are spasms, weakness, parasthesia, and seizures. More rarely, conversion symptoms may involve the autonomic or endocrine system. Vomiting as a conversion symptom represents revulsion and disgust. Pseudocyesis can represent both a wish for and a fear of pregnancy. The definition of conversion disorder is unique in the DSM-III-R classification in that it implies specific psychological mechanisms to account for the disturbance. The person achieves primary gain by keeping an internal conflict or need out of awareness and achieves secondary gain by avoiding a particular activity that is noxious to him or her and by getting support from the environment that otherwise might not be forthcoming.

Usually the symptoms appear suddenly in a setting of extreme psychological stress. Histrionic personality traits are common but not invariably present. *La belle indifférence,* an attitude toward the symptoms that suggests a lack of concern incongruous with the severe nature of the impairment, is sometimes present (American Psychiatric Association 1987).

There are numerous variants on the manifestation and setting of conversion reactions that have been summarized by Merskey (1989, p. 2153). Conversion symptoms can be part of another psychiatric disorder such as schizophrenia or a depressive illness. The symptoms are more likely to develop in individuals with severe personality disorders. Damage to the brain or intoxication with, for example, an anticonvulsant drug will predispose patients to experience conversion symptoms. Conversion symptoms tend to occur as part of a somatization disorder with multiple other symptoms, and conversion symptoms, as well as symptoms of other somatoform disorders, can occur as part of an epidemic. Conversions can occur in otherwise healthy individuals under unbearable stress.

Etiology

Research on the etiology of hysteria has been reviewed by several authors, including Merskey (1979), Roy (1982), and Ford and Folks (1985). It lies beyond the scope of this chapter to present more than a few conclusions about contemporary research and the ways the findings relate to the topics of this volume.

Shields (1962) found a low concordance of hysterical symptoms in identical twins reared apart. The twin studies suggest that the genetic contributions to hysteria are small (Slater and Roth 1969, p. 104).

The classical description of conversion symptoms occurring in persons with histrionic personalities who manifest *la belle indifférence* appears to be contradictory because these two phenomena represent opposite extremes. The prevalence of *la belle indifférence* in patients with conversion disorder has been inconsistent (Barnert 1971; Raskin et al. 1966). Various personalities have been found in studies of series of patients with conversion disorders, including passive-aggressive, emotionally unstable, inadequate, and schizoid personalities. In some studies, histrionic personalities constitute only a small minority (Chodoff and Lyons 1958; Stephens and Kamp 1962). Some studies have found an association of conversion symptoms and depression (Ziegler et al. 1960).

There is evidence from psychophysiological research that consistent differences exist between patients with conversion phenomena and other neurotic patients. For example, on computerized electroencephalographic frequency analysis, there are some differences between patients with conversion disorder and those with other somatoform disorders (Drake et al. 1988). The studies on the psychophysiology of conversions have been reviewed by Lader (1975, 1982). In experiments, healthy individuals and neurotic patients habituate (meaning that correlates of stress such as the galvanic skin response [GSR] gradually decrease when exposed to repeated stressful stimuli). In one study, patients with conversion disorder, on the average, did not habituate, and some became progressively more aroused (Lader and Sartorius 1968). In the same study, spontaneous-fluctuation GSR, which is a measure of sympathetic nervous system activity supplying sweat glands, showed significantly more fluctuation than even in anxious psychiatric patients. The patients with conversion symptoms rated themselves as more anxious than patients with anxiety states, whereas a psychiatrist rated the patients with conversion reactions as significantly less anxious.

Sedation threshold (the amount of a sedative injected at a standard rate that causes an inflection on the electroencephalogram [EEG]) is associated with anxiety. Patients with conversion symptoms have a high sedation threshold, which is further evidence to suggest that these patients have high levels of arousal (Shagas and Naiman 1956).

On neuropsychological testing, patients with conversion disorder show increased field dependency, impaired vigilance-attention, heightened suggestibility, and impairment of recent memory (Bendefeldt et al. 1976). These findings are consistent with the theory that a corticifugal inhibition of afferent stimuli occurs in conversion (Ludwig 1972; Whitlock 1967); however, they also could be the effects of excessive arousal.

Studies with evoked cerebral somatosensory potentials in conversion anesthesia have yielded inconsistent results (Alajouanine et al. 1958; Halliday 1968; Hernandez-Peon et al. 1963). The findings apparently depend on several factors such as the intensity of the stimulus and whether it is applied over the skin or over a major nerve (Levy and Behrman 1970; Levy and Mushin 1973). Overall, the studies suggest that, at least in some patients, there is an inhibition of impulse conduction on the affected side. These results apparently apply only to somatosensory stimulation; normal evoked responses are found in persons with hysterical amblyopia (Behrman 1969), and normal auditory evoked responses are found in persons with hysterical deafness (Cody and Bickford 1965). In patients in whom conversion anesthesia occurs in conjunction with pain after an accident, there is a failure of habituation to somatosensory evoked potentials after repeated stimulation; in some patients the responses increase with repetition (Moldofsky and England 1975).

There are substantial psychophysiological differences between patients with chronic conversion disorders and patients with acute, short-lived conversion symptoms (Meares and Horvath 1972). The degree of physiological responsiveness may be one of the factors that determines whether conversion symptoms become chronic.

Psychological and Psychiatric Studies

The published descriptions of patients' attitudes and beliefs suggest that patients with conversion disorder believe the disorder was caused by physical disease for which they require medical treatment. Raskin et al. (1966) judged that in 93% of patients with conversion, psychological stress preceded the onset of symptoms. There are numerous reports of conversions in soldiers who were exposed to prolonged terrors of combat (Hurst 1940).

Primary gain predominantly as a means of solving a conflict has been reported to be common in conversion reactions; in one study, secondary gain was judged to be present in patients with conversion reactions as well as in patients who were later found to have an organic disease (Raskin et al. 1966).

There are numerous reports of mass hysteria or epidemic hysteria in which people in proximity develop similar somatic symptoms for which no adequate cause is found. Colligan et al. (1982) have surveyed these studies. Many of the patients have various somatic symptoms that do not have the features of conversion reactions. Fear, self-scrutiny, and selective perception appear to be the main psychological processes; the etiological mechanisms to explain symptoms are more akin to acute somatization than they are to conversion phenomena. In most cases there is no evidence of the victims gaining from their symptoms.

Psychological tests have not been helpful in either identifying patients with conversion disorder or helping psychiatrists to understand psychopathology. Some early studies with the Maudsley Personality Inventory yielded conflicting results on differences between hysterical and other neurotic patients (Ingham and Robinson 1964; Sigal et al. 1958). Dysthymic patients (i.e., anxious and depressed patients) tended to be more introverted than hysterical, psychopathic, and healthy patients. Healthy subjects were as extroverted as hysterical patients. Hysterical patients tended to score lower on the neuroticism scale than either dysthymic or psychopathic patients.

Later studies that yielded similar results were reviewed by Eysenck (1982). Ingham and Robinson (1964) found that patients with hysterical personalities (histrionic personality disorder [301.50]) and those with conversion hysteria (conversion disorder [300.11]) had different scores on the Maudsley Personality Inventory (MPI); the latter patients were found to be more introverted.

There are numerous studies in which the Minnesota Multiphasic Personality Inventory (MMPI) was administered to psychiatric patients. These studies were inconclusive and are discussed in the next section.

Thus, there is evidence for 1) a predisposition to conversion disorders and 2) unbearable stress and gain to contribute to the onset of conversion disorders, at least in some patients. Most episodes of conversions are preceded by emotional upheaval, and often another psychiatric disorder coexists. Conversion disorder can occur in a physiologically predisposed individual who is unable to habituate to everyday stressful events, or in patients with severe personality disorder who lack the psychological stamina to cope with even common threats and frustrations, or it may occur in a healthy individual who breaks down when the stress becomes exceedingly severe.

Diagnosis

The most important differential diagnosis is, of course, physical disease. This distinction can be exceedingly difficult because physical disease, particularly brain damage or intoxication, can contribute to conversion symptoms (Slater 1965). Conversion symptoms can occur in all psychiatric disorders (Guze et al. 1971).

Although vomiting is classified in DSM-III-R as a conversion disorder, patients who are vomiting may be suffering from a psychophysiological disorder (somatoform autonomic dysfunction in the draft of the ICD-10). In pseudocyesis, which is also classified as a conversion disorder, there are endocrine changes (Drife 1985), and, thus, the physiological changes in this disorder differ substantially from a conversion disorder that mimics neurological disease. Some psychological mechanisms may be similar to conversion phenomena, because craving for pregnancy is a usual and conspicuous feature and the symptoms and signs reflect an idea and a wish. Physiologically, however, the disorder is unlike other conversion reactions. Thus there are diverse syndromes included in the DSM-III-R category of conversion disorder (300.11).

Psychological tests have not been helpful in the understanding or diagnosis of hysteria or conversion disorder. There may be various causes for this. The selection of the various populations of hysterical patients had not been standardized, and patients with different syndromes appear to have been included. The MMPI hysteria (Hy) scale is of little value; it is correlated with ratings of somatic concerns, but there is no evidence of diagnostic validity in cases of conversion disorders (Zelin 1971). In a factor-analytic study, there was no evidence of a factor that corresponded to conversion disorders (Jackson and Messick 1962).

In DSM-III-R, conversion symptoms are not classified as conversion disorder if the symptom is part of a somatization disorder. Such a distinction is justified for research purposes or for the purposes of classification, but there is no reason to believe that these symptoms are different from other conversion symptoms.

Uses of the Term Hysteria

The various uses of the term *hysteria* may lead to conflicting conclusions. For example, in two studies on the irritable bowel syndrome (Liss et al. 1973; Young et al. 1976) (see Chapter 6, p. 120, this volume), a high proportion of patients had the diagnosis of hysteria. However, the authors defined the term "hysteria" for Briquet's syndrome (which had become with slight modification the somatization disorder of DSM-III). Consequently, it is essential to examine the definition and criteria used in various studies before drawing conclusions.

In the study by Wilson et al. (1988), the authors concluded that the globus sensation was hysterical because of the test results of the Eysenck Personality Inventory (EPI) (see Chapter 3, this volume). These findings are inadequate to reach such a conclusion. The precursor of the EPI, the MPI, was administered as part of a validation study to a group of hysteric patients selected by the diagnostic criteria prevalent at that time. Moreover, subsequent studies have shown that patients with histrionic personalities and those with conversion disorders (both labeled at one time "hysterics") have different EPI extroversion scores. A psychological test score reflects the score of the group that was used for initial validation (Payne 1958). Therefore, if the terminology has changed, or if the selection of the original group is no longer regarded as valid, the test score cannot be used to make a diagnosis.

Treatments

Numerous treatments have been advocated and practiced in conversion disorders. These include long-term psychotherapy, hypnosis, attempts at abreaction under hypnosis, narcoanalysis, suggestion under narcosis, establishing mobility of a paralyzed limb under light narcosis, and various behavioral methods that entail reinforcement, suggestion-contingency management, and encouragement to use the affected part (Caplan and Nadelson 1980; Dickes 1974; Hafeiz 1980; Merskey 1989; Munford and Liberman 1982; Sim 1982).

In treating acute conversion reactions, reassurance, psychological support, encouragement, and easing of stresses constitute adequate treatment to achieve remission in most cases, at least for achieving remission of the acute episode. In epidemic hysteria, many of the patients recover while the bacteriological studies are still in progress; there is evidence, however, that affected individuals have more evidence of neurotic ill health on follow-up than those who were not affected (McEvedy and Beard 1973; Rawnsley and Loudon 1964). Isolating fellow victims from each other during the acute episode is believed to be helpful in accelerating recovery (Lyons and Potter 1970; Sirois 1982).

There are no controlled studies of the treatment of conversion disorder. In uncontrolled studies of ocular conversion disorders, suggestion and training were found to be successful in some patients (Smith et al. 1983). In uncontrolled studies of chronic conversion paralyses, the most impressive results reported so far come from energetic physical rehabilitation (Cardenas et al. 1986; Delargy et al. 1986; Withrington and Parry 1985). This method appears to be adequate in a large proportion of patients even without other psychological or behavioral treatments. In another recent study of four patients with chronic conversion paralysis, a striking improvement occurred after electromyographic biofeedback (Fishbain et al. 1988).

Prognosis

There are substantial differences in outcome of conversion disorders across studies that are probably caused by differences in the populations studied (Ljungberg 1957; Slater 1965; Ziegler and Paul 1954). Most conversion symptoms apparently remit (Farley et al. 1968; Folks et al. 1984). For patients in whom a conversion disorder has persisted for some time, the prognosis for recovery is poor (Louis et al. 1985). Moreover, on follow-up, there is an increased risk of emergence of physical disease than of other psychiatric disorders, and there is an increased mortality (Slater 1965). The few uncontrolled studies suggest that contemporary methods of rehabilitation may substantially improve the outcome.

Summary and Main Conclusions

A review of the psychophysiological studies suggests that the mechanisms of conversion differ from those of the other somatoform disorders. Patients with chronic conversion disorder show high arousal and habituate more slowly than other psychiatric patients. Some fail to habituate and become more aroused as the experiment progresses. Somatosensory evoked potentials suggest a lowering of peripheral sensitivity and a central mechanism of inhibition of afferent pathways. Conversion symptoms can occur in any psychiatric disorder. In one study, a substantial proportion of patients with a conversion disorder had other psychiatric disorders or physical diseases on long-term follow-up. Prognosis in chronic conversion paralysis used to be poor; uncontrolled studies suggest that energetic rehabilitation can be effective even in cases of long-standing conversion paralyses.

References

Alajouanine T, Scherrer J, Barbizet J, et al: Potentiels évoqués corticaux chez des sujets atteints des troubles somesthésiques. Revue Neurologique 98:757–761, 1958

American Psychiatric Association: Diagnostic and Statistical Manual of Mental Disorders, 2nd Edition, Revised. Washington, DC, American Psychiatric Association, 1968

American Psychiatric Association: Diagnostic and Statistical Manual of Mental Disorders, 3rd Edition. Washington, DC, American Psychiatric Association, 1980

American Psychiatric Association: Diagnostic and Statistical Manual of Mental Disorders, 3rd Edition, Revised. Washington, DC, American Psychiatric Association, 1987

Barnert C: Conversion reactions and psychophysiologic disorders: a comparative study. Psychiatry Med 2:205–220, 1971

Behrman J: The visual evoked response in hysterical amblyopia. Br J Ophthalmol 53:839–845, 1969

Bendefeldt F, Miller LL, Ludwig AM: Cognitive performance in conversion hysteria. Arch Gen Psychiatry 33:1250–1254, 1976

Briquet P: Traité Clinique et Thérapeutique de l'Hystérie. Paris, JB Baillière, 1859

Caplan LR, Nadelson T: The Oklahoma complex: a common form of conversion hysteria. Arch Intern Med 140:185–186, 1980

Cardenas DD, Larson J, Egan KJ: Hysterical paralysis in the upper extremity of chronic pain patients. Arch Phys Med Rehabil 67:190–193, 1986

Chodoff P, Lyons H: Hysteria, the hysterical personality and "hysterical" conversion. Am J Psychiatry 114:734–740 1958

Cody DTR, Bickford RG: Cortical audiometry: an objective method of evaluating auditory acuity in man. Mayo Clin Proc 40:273–287, 1965

Colligan M, Pennebaker JW, Murphy LR (eds): Mass Psychogenic Illness: A Social-Psychological Analysis. Hillsdale, NJ, Erlbaum, 1982

Delargy MA, Peatfield RC, Burt AA: Successful rehabilitation in conversion paralysis. Br Med J 292:1730–1731, 1986

Dickes RA: Brief therapy of conversion reactions: an in-hospital technique. Am J Psychiatry 131:584–586, 1974

Drake ME Jr, Padamadan H, Pakalnis A: EEG frequency analysis in conversion and somatoform disorder. Clin Electroencephalogr 19:123–128, 1988

Drife JO: Phantom pregnancy. Br Med J 291:687–688, 1985

Ey H: History and analysis of the concept, in Hysteria. Edited by Roy A. New York, John Wiley, 1982, pp 3–19

Eysenck HJ: A psychological theory of hysteria, in Hysteria. Edited by Roy A. New York, John Wiley, 1982, pp 57–80

Farley J, Woodruff RA Jr, Guze SB: The prevalence of hysteria and conversion symptoms. Br J Psychiatry 114:1121–1125, 1968

Fishbain DA, Goldberg M, Khalil TM, et al: The utility of electromyographic biofeedback in the treatment of conversion paralysis. Am J Psychiatry 145:1572–1575, 1988

Folks DG, Ford CV, Regan WM: Conversion symptoms in a general hospital. Psychosomatics 25:285–295, 1984

Ford CV, Folks DG: Conversion disorders: an overview. Psychosomatics 26:371–383, 1985

Guze SB, Woodruff RA, Clayton PJ: A study of conversion symptoms in psychiatric outpatients. Am J Psychiatry 128:135–138, 1971

Hafeiz HB: Hysterical conversion: a prognostic study. Br J Psychiatry 136:548–551, 1980

Halliday AM: Computing techniques in neurological diagnosis. Br Med Bull 24:253–259, 1968

Hernandez-Peon R, Chavez-Ibarra G, Aguilar-Figueroa E: Somatic evoked potentials in one case of hysterical anaesthesia. Electroencephalogr Clin Neurophysiol 15:889–892, 1963

Hurst AF: Medical Diseases of War. London, Edward Arnold, 1940

Ingham JG, Robinson JO: Personality in the diagnosis of hysteria. Br J Psychology 55:276–284, 1964

Jackson DN, Messick S: Response styles on the MMPI: comparison of clinical and normal samples. Journal of Abnormal and Social Psychology 65:285–299, 1962

Lader M: The Psychophysiology of Mental Illness. London, Routledge & Kegan Paul, 1975

Lader M: The psychophysiology of hysteria, in Hysteria. Edited by Roy A. New York, John Wiley, 1982, pp 81–87

Lader M, Sartorius N: Anxiety in patients with hysterical conversion symptoms. J Neurol Neurosurg Psychiatry 31:490–495, 1968

Levy R, Behrman J: Cortical evoked responses in hysterical hemianaesthesia. Electroencephalogr Clin Neurophysiol 29:400–402, 1970

Levy R, Mushin J: The somatosensory evoked response in patients with hysterical anaesthesia. J Psychosom Res 17:81–84, 1973

Liss JL, Alpers D, Woodruff RA Jr: The irritable colon syndrome and psychiatric illness. Diseases of the Nervous System 34:151–157, 1973

Ljungberg L: Hysteria: A Clinical, Prognostic, and Genetic Study. Copenhagen, Ejnar Munksgaard, 1957

Louis DS, Lamp MK, Greene TL: The upper extremity and psychiatric illness. J Hand Surg [Am] 10:687–693, 1985

Ludwig AM: Hysteria: a neurobiological theory. Arch Gen Psychiatry 27:771–777, 1972

Lyons HA, Potter PE: Communicated hysteria: an episode in a secondary school. Journal of the Irish Medical Association 63:377–379, 1970

McEvedy CP, Beard AW: A controlled follow-up of cases involved in an epidemic of benign myalgic encephalomyelitis. Br J Psychiatry 122:141–150, 1973

Meares R, Horvath T: "Acute" and "chronic" hysteria. Br J Psychiatry 121:653–657, 1972

Merskey H: The Analysis of Hysteria. London, Baillière, Tindall and Cassell, 1979

Merskey H: Conversion disorders, in Treatments of Psychiatric Disorders: A Task Force Report of the American Psychiatric Association, Vol 3. Washington, DC, American Psychiatric Association, 1989, pp 2152–2159

Moldofsky H, England RS: Facilitation of somatosensory average–evoked potentials in hysterical anesthesia and pain. Arch Gen Psychiatry 32:193–197, 1975

Munford PR, Liberman RP: Behavior therapy of hysterical disorders, in Hysteria. Edited by Roy A. New York, John Wiley, 1982, pp 287–303

Payne RW: Diagnostic and personality testing in clinical psychology. Am J Psychiatry 115:25–29, 1958

Raskin M, Talbott JA, Meyerson AT: Diagnosed conversion reactions: predictive value of psychiatric criteria. JAMA 197:530–534, 1966

Rawnsley K, Loudon JB: Epidemiology of mental disorder in a closed community. Br J Psychiatry 110:830–839, 1964

Roy A: Hysteria. New York, John Wiley, 1982

Shagas C, Naiman J: The sedation threshold as an objective index of manifest anxiety in psychoneurosis. J Psychosom Res 1:49–57, 1956

Shields J: Monozygotic Twins Brought Up Apart and Brought Up Together. London, Oxford University Press, 1962

Sigal JJ, Star KH, Franks CM: Hysterics and dysthymics and criterion groups in the study of introversion-extraversion. J Abnorm Psychol 57:143–148, 1958

Sim M: The management of hysteria, in Hysteria. Edited by Roy A. New York, John Wiley, 1982, pp 261–276

Sirois F: Epidemic hysteria, in Hysteria. Edited by Roy A. New York, John Wiley, 1982, pp 101–115

Slater E: The diagnosis of hysteria. Br Med J 1:1395–1399, 1965

Slater E, Roth M: Clinical Psychiatry, 3rd Edition. Baltimore, MD, Williams & Wilkins, 1969

Smith CH, Beck RW, Mills RP: Functional disease in neuro-ophthalmology. Neurol Clin 1:955–971, 1983

Stephens JH, Kamp M: On some aspects of hysteria: a clinical study. J Nerv Ment Dis 134:305–315, 1962

Veith I: Hysteria: The History of a Disease. Chicago, IL, University of Chicago Press, 1965

Whitlock FA: The aetiology of hysteria. Acta Psychiatr Scand 43:144–162, 1967

Wilson JA, Deary IJ, Maran AGD: Is globus hystericus? Br J Psychiatry 153:335–339, 1988

Withrington RH, Parry CBW: Rehabilitation of conversion paralysis. J Bone Joint Surg 67B:635–637, 1985

World Health Organization: International Classification of Diseases, 9th Revision. Geneva, World Health Organization, 1979

World Health Organization: Draft of the 10th Revision of the International Classification of Diseases. Geneva, World Health Organization, 1988

Young SJ, Alpers DH, Norland CC, et al: Psychiatric illness and the irritable bowel syndrome. Gastroenterology 70:162–166, 1976

Zelin ML: Validity of the MMPI scales for measuring twenty psychiatric dimensions. J Consult Clin Psychol 37:286–290, 1971

Ziegler FJ, Imboden JB, Meyer E: Contemporary conversion reactions: a clinical study. Am J Psychiatry 116:901–910, 1960

Ziegler GK, Paul N: On the natural history of hysteria in women. Diseases of the Nervous System 15:301–306, 1954

Chapter 12

Deception

Some patients present bodily complaints in an attempt to deceive the physician. Textbooks and diagnostic manuals distinguish two main categories: *malingering* and *factitious disorder*. These acts are deliberate and differ from the other mechanisms described in this volume. They have been described extensively by other authors and will be reviewed here only briefly.

Malingering

The DSM-III-R (American Psychiatric Association 1987) includes the following description of malingering (ICD-10 draft V65.20–Z76.5):

> The essential feature of Malingering is intentional production of false or grossly exaggerated physical or psychological symptoms, motivated by external incentives such as avoiding military conscription or duty, avoiding work, obtaining financial compensation, evading criminal prosecution, or obtaining drugs, or securing better living conditions. . . .
> Malingering should be suspected if any combination of the following is noted: (1) medicolegal context of presentation, . . .; (2) marked discrepancy between the person's claimed stress or disability and the objective findings; (3) lack of cooperation during the diagnostic evaluation and in complying with the prescribed treatment regimen; and (4) the presence of Antisocial Personality Disorder. (p. 360)

Even if malingering is suspected, it is usually difficult to prove. Various methods have been used to detect deception. These include special interviews, the administration of personality inventories, specialized tests that aim to discriminate between actual and exaggerated deficits, and interviews with the patient under the influence of sedative drugs such as amobarbital sodium. Polygraph testing in combination with specific methods to detect deception has been used in forensic work.

The personality inventory that has been used most often has been the Minnesota Multiphasic Personality Inventory (MMPI) (Hathaway and McKinley 1970). The F scale has been regarded as an index of malingering (Dahlstrom et al. 1972). The F minus K (F–K) dissimulation index has been reported to improve the detection rate (Gough 1950). In most validation studies in which the

239

MMPI or other personality inventories were administered, however, the authors used volunteers who were instructed to fake their responses, a method that has not been validated against criterion groups of malingerers and other patients (Greene 1988; Stermac 1988).

More recent methods consist of the use of structured clinical interviews. Rogers (1986) used the Structured Interview of Reported Symptoms (SIRS) to compare the responses of psychiatric patients with those of forensic patients who were believed to have a motive to deceive the interviewer. Forensic patients tended to show unusual responses, including unusual pairing of symptoms, unusual severity of symptoms, and discrepancies between reported and observed symptoms. Rogers (1988), in reviewing the clinical techniques that have been used in the evaluation of malingering, concluded that such an assessment is "with a few exceptions, more an art of clinical judgment than an empirically based process" (p. 293).

The evaluation of malingering poses numerous problems. Malingering is often an exaggeration of existing symptoms and disabilities rather than an invention of symptoms. Sometimes a patient, while trying to persuade the physician, manages to persuade himself or herself that the symptoms are disabling or severe. In some patients who exaggerate symptoms and who have a motive to feign illness, some of the processes of somatization may contribute to the amplification of sensations.

Probably the most reliable method of detecting malingering is to observe the difference between the patient's behavior in the clinic compared with places where he or she believes himself or herself to be unobserved. For this method to be dependable, it requires careful, independent cross-validated judgments resembling detective work rather than clinical psychiatric or psychological assessments.

It is doubtful whether a person who has no psychiatric disorder and who cheats can be persuaded to desist. To my knowledge, no effective treatments have been reported.

Factitious Disorder With Physical Symptoms

In this disorder (DSM-III-R 301.51; ICD-10 draft F68.1), it is also the intention of the patient to mislead the physician into believing that the physically healthy patient suffers from a disease. The patient's goal, however, is not a reward that can be easily understood—an external incentive such as a financial settlement or disability pension—rather the patient apparently derives satisfaction from being regarded as ill. The person presents with feigned bodily symptoms and usually also with a misleading history. Some patients will fake physical signs or laboratory results, for example, by placing a drop of blood in the urine. Other patients will make themselves ill by injecting pus or some other contaminant into various parts of the body.

The studies on various kinds of factitious disorders have been surveyed by Ford (1983). The best known variant, but the least common, is the Münchausen syndrome, a chronic disorder in which the person manages to get admitted to a hospital on numerous occasions (Asher 1951; Mayou and Hawton 1986). Von Maur et al. (1973) reported a case involving an individual who achieved over 420 documented hospital admissions, which qualifies as the current world record. The less conspicuous factitious disorder variants are probably common; for example, fever of unknown origin was judged to be factitious in 2.2% and 9.6% of the patients in two studies (Aduan et al. 1979; Petersdorf and Bennett 1957; Rumans and Vosti 1978). Factitious disorder is more common under the age of 40. In some studies, females, nurses, paramedical personnel, and patients with borderline personalities were overrepresented (Bayliss 1984). The characteristics of these patients derived from a survey of the literature have been described by Ford (1983).

The various theories that have aimed to explain factitious disorder have been surveyed by Eisendrath (1989b). One theory is that patients with factitious disorder have dependency needs and the expectation to be frustrated, originating from deprivation early in life. Hospitalization early in life when the child's unsatisfied needs were met by doctors and nurses may have been a reinforcing event; conversely, early hospitalization was a major trauma, and admission with a factitious disorder may represent an attempt at mastery. Feigning illness may represent a need to be taken care of in a socially sanctioned way. It has also been theorized that it may be a masochistic attempt to atone for guilt by punishment, by subjecting oneself to invasive diagnostic procedures and surgical operations, and by deliberately letting the deception be discovered, leading to mistreatment by parental figures. Some patients seek narcotics by faking painful diseases; some perhaps get satisfaction from fooling the powerful symbols that doctors and nurses represent. Some others may be hypochondriacal; they may believe that they suffer from a hitherto undiagnosed disease, and they fake signs of disease in order to induce further tests and investigations.

To my knowledge, there are no studies that have aimed at testing the validity of these theories. While numerous views on the patients' motives have been published, I have found only one brief report by Eisendrath (1989b) who asked the patients for the reasons of their behavior. The author has kindly allowed me to summarize a recent prepublication draft in which he also describes other patients' confessions and self-explorations occurring in the course of psychotherapy.

A 30-year-old registered nurse who had been sexually abused by her father when she was 12 years old admitted that she had injected herself with urine because she felt guilty because her boyfriend was being too nice to her in giving her a diamond engagement ring. In another case, a young professional woman revealed that she had caused severe cellulitis (nearly leading to leg amputation) after her boyfriend left her. She terminated psychotherapy after 6 months even though she was still unable to explain fully the reasons for her conduct. In yet another case, a young nurse confessed in psychotherapy that she had injected herself with insulin in order to avoid becoming pregnant when pressured by her husband and friends.

From the little that is known, it appears that there are various motives for factitious illness. Apart from the reasons listed above, there may be some others, and they appear to differ from one person to another. For some people, the drama of admission to a hospital relieves the desperate loneliness and emptiness of their lives. Once they have succeeded in convincing the hospital staff of their illness, they perhaps develop the peculiar mixture of tension and attraction followed by relief, similar to that of kleptomaniacs or fire setters, that makes them seek the same adventure repeatedly.

Recognition of illness as factitious seldom occurs in the early stages of the disorder. Factitious disorder is usually suspected only after the laboratory results are either in themselves bizarre or the findings are incompatible with the clinical picture. In addition to the exclusion of physical disease, the other somatoform disorders and psychophysiological syndromes need to be excluded. Early diagnosis is important in order to avoid unnecessary investigations and treatments, including exploratory surgery (Nadelson 1979).

It is unknown which is the most effective treatment. Psychotherapy appears to be the treatment of first choice if the patient is willing. Various treatments have been advocated (Bursten 1965; Ford 1973; Jefferson and Ochitill 1982; Nadelson 1979), and these have been reviewed by Eisendrath (1989a) and Kooiman (1987). Van Putten and Alban (1977) reported substantial improvement with lithium treatment in a patient who had a factitious disorder as well as a conversion disorder. The therapist should try to explore the patient's motives and aim at changing them. If the patient is not fully aware of the motives, yet feels compelled to repeat the self-damaging acts, treatments similar to those of other disorders of impulse control (Kellner 1982, pp. 329–418) or methods of habit reversal (Azrin and Nunn 1977) may be adopted. Other coexisting psychiatric disorders may require the appropriate treatments.

Summary and Main Conclusions

The main conclusions of this chapter are summarized together with other mechanisms of bodily complaints in Chapter 13 of this volume.

References

Aduan RP, Fauci AS, Dale DC, et al: Factitious fever and self-induced infection: a report of 32 cases and review of the literature. Ann Intern Med 90:230–242, 1979

American Psychiatric Association: Diagnostic and Statistical Manual of Mental Disorders, 3rd Edition, Revised. Washington, DC, American Psychiatric Association, 1987

Asher R: Münchausen's syndrome. Lancet 1:339–341, 1951

Azrin NH, Nunn GR: Habit Control in a Day. New York, Simon & Schuster, 1977

Bayliss RIS: The deceivers. Br Med J 288:583–584, 1984

Bursten B: On Münchausen's syndrome. Arch Gen Psychiatry 13:261–268, 1965

Dahlstrom WG, Welsh GS, Dahlstrom LE: An MMPI Handbook, Vol I: Clinical Interpretation, Revised Edition. Minneapolis, MN, University of Minnesota Press, 1972

Eisendrath SJ: Factitious disorder with physical symptoms, in Treatments of Psychiatric Disorders: A Task Force Report of the American Psychiatric Association, Vol 3. Washington, DC, American Psychiatric Association, 1989a, pp 2159–2164

Eisendrath SJ: Factitious physical disorders: treatment without confrontation. Psychosomatics 30:383–387, 1989b

Ford CV: The Münchausen syndrome: a report of four new cases and a review of psychodynamic considerations. Psychiatry in Medicine 4:31–44, 1973

Ford CV: The Somatizing Disorders: Illness as a Way of Life. New York, Elsevier, 1983

Gough HG: The F minus K dissimulation index for the MMPI. Journal of Consulting Psychology 14:408–413, 1950

Greene RL: Assessment of malingering and defensiveness by objective personality inventories, in Clinical Assessment of Malingering and Deception. Edited by Rogers R. New York, Guilford, 1988, pp 123–158

Hathaway SR, McKinley JC: Minnesota Multiphasic Personality Inventory, Revised. Minneapolis, MN, University of Minnesota, 1970

Jefferson JW, Ochitill H: Factitious disorders, in Treatment of Mental Disorders. Edited by Greist JH, Jefferson JW, Spitzer RL. New York, Oxford University Press, 1982, pp 387–397

Kellner R: Disorders of impulse control (not elsewhere classified), in Treatment of Mental Disorders. Edited by Greist JH, Jefferson JW, Spitzer RL. New York, Oxford University Press, 1982, pp 398–418

Kooiman CG: Neglected phenomena in factitious illness: a case study and review of literature. Compr Psychiatry 28:499–507, 1987

Mayou R, Hawton K: Psychiatric disorder in the general hospital. Br J Psychiatry 149:172–190, 1986

Nadelson T: The Münchausen spectrum: borderline character features. Gen Hosp Psychiatry 1:11–17, 1979

Petersdorf RG, Bennett IL Jr: Factitious fever. Ann Intern Med 46:1039–1062, 1957

Rogers R: Structured Interview of Reported Symptoms (SIRS). Unpublished scale, Clarke Institute of Psychiatry, Toronto, 1986

Rogers R: Current status of clinical methods, in Clinical Assessment of Malingering and Deception. Edited by Rogers R. New York, Guilford, 1988, pp 293–308

Rumans LW, Vosti KL: Factitious and fraudulent fever. Am J Med 65:745–755, 1978

Stermac L: Projective testing and dissimulation, in Clinical Assessment of Malingering and Deception. Edited by Rogers R. New York, Guilford, 1988, pp 159–168

Van Putten T, Alban J: Lithium carbonate in personality disorders: a case of hysteria. J Nerv Ment Dis 164:218–222, 1977

Von Maur K, Wasson KR, DeFord JW, et al: Münchausen's syndrome: a thirty-year history of peregrination par excellence (editorial). South Med J 66:629–632, 1973

Chapter 13

Mechanisms of Bodily Complaints: Main Conclusions

Part II of this volume contains an overview of the various processes that lead to bodily complaints. It includes a list of the theories of somatization, a survey of the empirical studies that pertain to these theories, and a discussion of the evidence.

There is incomplete agreement among authors on the definition of the term *somatization*. One of the recent usages—which has been adopted for this volume—is the presentation of somatic symptoms in the absence of physical disease or tissue damage. This definition subsumes the diagnostic categories of the somatoform disorders.

Etiology

Functional somatic symptoms are common. About 80% of healthy individuals experience somatic symptoms in any one week. Over 4% of subjects in the community have multiple chronic functional somatic symptoms.

Adoption studies suggest that there is a genetic predisposition for some of the somatic syndromes, whereas stress in childhood, such as sexual abuse or living with an alcoholic father, is asociated with others. Other predisposing factors include culturally acquired attitudes and behaviors, lack of education, and lower socioeconomic class. There is some evidence to suggest that learning of attitudes toward illness, and probably learning of some physiological responses, may occur early in life.

There is a consistent association of functional somatic symptoms and anxiety as well as depression. The correlations with hostility are lower. There are large differences among individuals in the ratios of somatic symptoms to emotional ones.

Many of the functional somatic symptoms are consequences of physiological activity that is changed, usually increased, by stress and emotions. This appears to be one of the reasons for the consistent association of emotional and somatic symptoms.

Several of the syndromes described in this volume, particularly if they are atypical or their manifestation is incomplete, are often judged to be features of somatization. The physiological changes that may cause symptoms include 1) smooth-muscle contractions, such as in motility disorders of the esophagus or the diarrhea-predominant type of the irritable bowel syndrome; 2) striated-muscle contraction, such as in tension headaches, or localized pain in other parts of the body; and 3) hyperventilation that causes the symptoms of alkalosis. Symptoms can be caused by numerous physiological changes that occur during sympathetic-adrenergic arousal. Unexplained symptoms are sometimes accounted for by physiological changes that can be detected only by special investigations such as electromyographic recording or esophageal manometry. Individuals have characteristic patterns of physiological responses to stress; this idiosyncrasy explains in part the the tendency for some functional symptoms to recur. Only some of the functional somatic symptoms can be explained by excessive peripheral physiological activity or selective perception of usual activity. This means that either current methods are inadequately sensitive or other mechanisms summarized in Part II of this volume cause symptoms.

In persons who seek treatment, there is a tendency for syndromes to cluster; for example, chronic fatigue, fibromyalgia, and the irritable bowel syndrome occur together in some individuals more often than could be expected by chance. This phenomenon appears to be associated with the severity of emotional disturbance, the tendency to react to such a disturbance with somatization, and concomitants such as excessive physiological responsiveness. In some patients the functional symptoms of somatizers can be explained by clustering of psychosomatic syndromes.

There is a complex relationship of somatization to physical disease. For example, in the chronic fatigue syndrome, fibromyalgia, and the urethral syndrome, there is no clear demarcation between psychophysiological processes and tissue pathology. In many cases, the extent to which one or more of the mechanisms of somatization and tissue pathology are responsible for the symptoms is difficult to assess. Diagnosed physical disease and somatization often coexist. Patients who are psychologically vulnerable also tend to report more symptoms of their physical disease. Physical disease is one of the predisposing factors of somatization as well as of hypochondriasis. A person who has experienced physical disease likely becomes more aware of bodily sensations, or has more fears of physical illness, or both. Psychosocial stress may decrease immune competency and predispose one to infection, and is associated with increased mortality. Thus, psychosocial stressors may predispose one to physical disease as well as induce somatization.

There is a consistent association of somatic symptoms on the one hand and fear of disease or a false belief of having a disease on the other. About one third of patients with functional somatic symptoms have at least transient hypochondriacal concerns. There is experimental and clinical evidence that selective attention enhances a person's awareness of sensations. Attention to a part of one's body, motivated by fear of disease, may cause a person to selectively perceive even normal physiological activity. Hypochondriacal patients are more accurate than others in perceiving physiological changes; conversely, persistent, distressing somatic symptoms, even if caused by physical disease, are likely to induce a false belief of having yet another disease.

In several of the syndromes described in this volume, patients had, on the average, a low pain threshold. For example, patients with fibromyalgia had a lower generalized pressure pain threshold than other patients, and not only at tender points. Others were unduly sensitive to distension of a viscus, for example, patients with the irritable bowel syndrome. Hypochondriacal patients tended to have a lower pain threshold than did others. These findings suggest that in some patients, persistent bodily complaints are a reflection of an abnormally low sensation threshold.

The results on the effects of gain and other reinforcement vary across studies. Patients who receive sickness benefits remain disabled longer than those without such insurance. Secondary gain was judged in one study to be more frequent in patients with idiopathic pain than in other patients. The results of studies of the effects of litigation on the reporting of and persistence of symptoms have been inconsistent. There is some evidence to suggest that iatrogenic reinforcement may occur; hypochondriacal beliefs are apparently induced or maintained when a person is told an unwarranted diagnosis of having a disease.

The inhibition of emotions tends to enhance physiological arousal. Inhibition and lack of confiding are associated with ill health, more frequent attendances for medical care, and probably with somatization, whereas confiding appears to improve health.

There is an association of alexithymia and somatization. Alexithymia appears to be, in part, the effect of a cognitive style that is patterned by the culture. Alternatively, alexithymia may be a person's characteristic response to bodily distress in a medical setting. The findings on the relationship of alexithymia to psychosomatic disease, however, have been conflicting. There is inadequate evidence at present to conclude that alexithymia is an etiological factor in psychosomatic disease or somatization.

Conversion symptoms, like other functional somatic symptoms, may be a part of another psychiatric disorder or may be the predominant symptoms. The psychophysiology of conversion disorder differs from that of other somatoform disorders. Patients with chronic conversion disorder show high levels of arousal and tend to habituate more slowly, or not at all, to stressful stimuli. The results of physiological studies in conversion anesthesia vary with the method, but the findings suggest that there is an inhibition of impulse conduction on the affected side, at least in some patients.

Some patients complain of bodily symptoms or exaggerate disabilities in an attempt to deceive physicians. In malingering, there is an external incentive. Patients with factitious disorder with physical symptoms may give a misleading history, fake laboratory tests, or inflict a physical disease upon themselves. There are only a few case histories that describe the patients' confessed motives; these motives appear to vary substantially from one person to another.

There are several other theories on the nature of functional somatic symptoms. Some patients apparently seek support from physicians, while others use symptoms as bodily metaphors to express distress, and, in others, the illness resolves a conflict or satisfies another need. In empirical studies, it is difficult to separate these motives and behaviors from other features that may contribute to the experience of somatic sensations or the presentation of bodily complaints.

There are some unresolved problems in the classification of somatoform disorders in both the DSM-III-R and the draft of the ICD-10. Often, however, the additional steps that are needed to explore psychopathology are more important than the choice of the diagnostic label. For example, it is important to evaluate the extent and nature of a coexisting mood disorder and the kind of hypochondriacal fears or beliefs, because such knowledge may help in the rational choice of treatment.

Interaction of Etiological Factors

The studies on somatization show that the etiology of somatization is not only multifactorial but also exceedingly complex. No single theory such as a defense mechanism, a conflict resolution, a method of symbolic communication, or reinforcement by gain can explain the various phenomena of somatization. Somatization ranges from minor common symptoms that are a part of normal experience to the most severe and disabling ones that occur in a minority. The psychopathology and its manifestations differ substantially from one individual to another.

The interaction of emotion with bodily symptoms is complex. Anxiety and depression frequently cause somatic symptoms; conversely, severe somatic symptoms may induce concerns, may deprive a person of pleasure, and, like other suffering, may aggravate depression. At times of anxiety or depression, a person evaluates his or her somatic symptoms as having more ominous portent than at other times. Most of the bodily symptoms do not take the place of emotions; they are not conversions, but instead coexist with, result from, and may reinforce emotions. A common mechanism in somatization, as well as in hypochondriasis, appears to be a mood disorder inducing somatic symptoms, followed by selective perception of bodily symptoms, motivated by fear of disease or other concerns. This results in a subsequent increase in anxiety with more somatic symptoms, forming links in a vicious circle.

The physiological changes and the resulting somatic symptoms may be the final common pathway with a variety of causes. For example, the shedding of tears may be caused by numerous diseases, by injuries, by anatomical abnormalities, and by a few emotions such as grief or gratitude. Most psychophysiological processes are more complex than this simple response; predisposing, precipitating, and maintaining factors summate and interact in complex chains.

Etiological factors that appear to be dominant in one patient may play only a minor or fleeting role in another. One person may have distressing somatic symptoms because of physiological disturbances with genetic factors predisposing, whereas another may have somatic symptoms only when he or she is anxious or depressed. Another may attend to somatic symptoms only when she fears that she has a disease, whereas another may habitually attend to bodily sensations because of early learning. Yet another may complain of bodily symptoms because he fears losing his disability payments and returning to his stressful workplace. In most patients, multiple etiological factors appear to play a part, and the relative contribution of each may change with the passage of time. It sometimes takes lengthy and unprejudiced exploration of psychopathology before the approximate contribution of various etiological elements can be gleaned.

Treatments

Clinical studies suggest that there is no treatment method or strategy that is equally suitable for all somatizing patients. Most functional somatic symptoms for which patients seek treatment last for a few weeks or months, and a large proportion remit with explanation and reassurance alone. Controlled studies described in this volume show that psychotherapy, as well as psychotropic drugs, is effective in the treatment of patients with bodily complaints. A few studies suggest that aerobic exercise is an effective treatment in somatization, but there are no prospective controlled studies to date.

There are also no controlled studies of hypochondriasis and conversion disorder. Uncontrolled studies of hypochondriasis suggest that explanation, persuasion, and exposure are effective in a substantial proportion of patients. In chronic conversion paralyses, the best results have been reported with energetic physical rehabilitation.

Many of the patients with bodily complaints who have no physical disease benefit from treatment. In a few, treatment means the difference between suffering and disability on the one hand and recovery on the other.

Index